T0243108

Cambridge History of Medicine
EDITORS: CHARLES WEBSTER AND CHARLES ROSENBERG

Quality and Quantity

Charles Webster, ed.   *Health, medicine, and mortality in the sixteenth century*

Ian Maclean   *The Renaissance notion of woman*

Michael MacDonald   *Mystical Bedlam*

Robert E. Kohler   *From medical chemistry to biochemistry*

Walter Pagel   *Joan Baptista Van Helmont*

Nancy Tomes   *A generous confidence*

Roger Cooter   *The cultural meaning of popular science*

Anne Digby   *Madness, morality, and medicine*

Guenter B. Risse   *Hospital life in Enlightenment Scotland*

Roy Porter, ed.   *Patients and practitioners*

Ann G. Carmichael   *Plague and the poor in Renaissance Florence*

S. E. D. Shortt   *Victorian lunacy*

Hilary Marland   *Medicine and society in Wakefield and Huddersfield, 1780–1870*

Susan M. Reverby   *Ordered to care*

Russell C. Maulitz   *Morbid appearances*

Matthew Ramsey   *Professional and popular medicine in France, 1770–1830*

John Keown   *Abortion, doctors, and the law*

Donald Denoon   *Public health in Papua New Guinea*

Paul Weindling   *Health, race, and German politics between National Unification and Nazism, 1870–1945*

Quality and Quantity

THE QUEST FOR BIOLOGICAL REGENERATION
IN TWENTIETH-CENTURY FRANCE

William H. Schneider

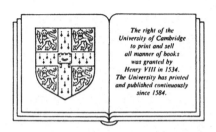

The right of the
University of Cambridge
to print and sell
all manner of books
was granted by
Henry VIII in 1534.
The University has printed
and published continuously
since 1584.

CAMBRIDGE UNIVERSITY PRESS

CAMBRIDGE

NEW YORK   PORT CHESTER   MELBOURNE   SYDNEY

PUBLISHED BY THE PRESS SYNDICATE OF THE UNIVERSITY OF CAMBRIDGE
The Pitt Building, Trumpington Street, Cambridge, United Kingdom

CAMBRIDGE UNIVERSITY PRESS
The Edinburgh Building, Cambridge CB2 2RU, UK
40 West 20th Street, New York NY 10011–4211, USA
477 Williamstown Road, Port Melbourne, VIC 3207, Australia
Ruiz de Alarcón 13, 28014 Madrid, Spain
Dock House, The Waterfront, Cape Town 8001, South Africa

http://www.cambridge.org

First published 1990
First paperback edition 2002

A catalogue record for this book is available from the British Library

Library of Congress Cataloguing in Publication data
Schneider, William H. (William Howard), 1945–
Quality and quantity: the quest for biological regeneration in
twentieth-century France / William H. Schneider.
        p.   cm. – (Cambridge history of medicine)
Includes bibliographical references.
ISBN 0 521 37498 7
1. Eugenics – France – History – 20th century.   2. Eugenics – Moral
and ethical aspects.   I. Title.   II. Series.
HQ755.5.F8S36   1990
304.5–dc20   90-1767   CIP

ISBN 0 521 37498 7 hardback
ISBN 0 521 52461 X paperback

To Ann Laurie

Contents

Preface

The inspiration for this book came from a graduate seminar on comparative eugenics movements in the early 1970s at the University of Pennsylvania. I was working on a dissertation about French views of Africans during the period of colonial expansion, and I decided to study whether eugenics in France was connected to racist attitudes at the end of the nineteenth century. This was not to be the case, alas, and I returned to complete the dissertation, publish it as a book, and take up my first teaching assignment.

When I returned to my investigation of eugenics, I uncovered a vast interconnection of movements that quickly took me in several new directions. Although race was not at the root of these movements – demography and health were – it was always present, and later became an important component. Of greater overall significance was the fact that the various movements for the biological regeneration of France in the twentieth century typified society's relation to science in the modern world that crossed national boundaries and continues to the present day. Because of the interest in eugenics and the social relations of science, and the importance of the comparative perspective, I have written this book to set forth the French experience in its broadest context. Rather than its being the last word on the subject, it will I hope prompt others to add, correct, and above all complete the study of the topic.

Work on this project has lasted for so long that it would be impossible to thank all of those who have helped. I would be remiss, however, if I were not to acknowledge the generous support over the years of grants from the American Philosophical Society, the National Endowment for the Humanities, the National Science Foundation, the Rockefeller Archives Center, the University of

North Carolina at Wilmington, and the School of Liberal Arts of Indiana University at Indianapolis. I would also like to thank Robert Nye and Mark Adams, who were present at the creation, as well as Gar Allen, Toby Gelfand, Everett Mendelson, and Paul Weindling, who have read the work and offered helpful comments. I am grateful for Ronald Cohen's especially conscientious editing work, and for the assistance of Barbara Christmas, Cathy Johnson, Mary Gelzleichter, and Mary Frisby in preparing the manuscript and index. In France, I owe special thanks to Jean-François Picard, who has helped make numerous research trips very productive. I am also deeply grateful to Denis Richet, Gabriel Richet, and Roger Couvelaire – descendants of some of the principals in the story, who were kind enough to allow me access to unpublished materials in family records.

Finally, I wish to thank my wife and children for "supporting" me (in the French and English senses of the word) during the research and writing of this book. Because the work coincided with the founding of a family, I was provided with many personal examples of the broader themes I uncovered. For my family's unwitting service as case studies, I am both grateful and apologetic.

William H. Schneider

1

Introduction

In December 1941, Eugen Fischer, a leading anthropologist of the Nazi Reich, visited the occupied city of Paris. As founder of the Kaiser Wilhelm Institute for Anthropology, Human Heredity, and Eugenics, Fischer delivered a lecture entitled "Problems of race and racial legislation in Germany" at the Maison de la chimie, a noted center of collaborationist propaganda.[1] Fischer was not the first who had come to spread the word to the French about the National Socialist revolution in applied human biology. Earlier in the year, Otmar von Verscheurer, the Frankfurt geneticist whose pupils included the notorious Nazi doctor Josef Mengele, spoke on human heredity and Nazi marriage laws, and others during the year lectured on "Public health in the reich" and "Biology and the organization of the state."[2]

Fischer admitted at the beginning of his talk that he had chosen his topic because "racial problems and German racial legislation are often the subjects of the greatest incomprehension by foreigners."[3] His aim was not only to explain the laws but also to persuade the French to join the Germans in their campaign to preserve the "hereditary health" of the population. He did this in part by flattery, telling his audience of the superiority of "the race called 'Nordic,' to which a great proportion of the French population also belongs." Fischer also played on racial fears, warning that

French laws and institutions permit black blood to infiltrate the organism of the French people . . . [producing] a regression of the intellectual and cultural capacity of France that will have absolutely unavoidable consequences if the mixing continues to spread on a vast scale.

He did not fail to mention another common enemy, the Jews, declaring that their "moral tendencies and all the activities of Jewish Bolsheviks reveal a mentality so monstrous that one can only speak of inferiority and beings of a different species than ours."[4]

Although the talk contained the usual Nazi race propaganda the French had heard before, Fischer's conclusions addressed a specific problem that the French themselves had recognized for decades – their low birthrate. The German racial legislation, said Fischer, did not focus solely on the undesirables. It would do little good to eliminate them, he declared, "if the people no longer had the will to survive." Hence, the people had to do their part by "the pro-creation of large numbers of healthy children in all families." Fischer did not, however, support the blind natalist policy that had been attempted in previous decades in countries such as France, because the result would be the "reproduction of inferior individuals, of those at the lowest social level." Fischer's conclusion, therefore, stressed that "it is not only the number of births that plays a de-cisive role but the quality and the health of the race, without which a people cannot perpetuate itself."[5]

Fischer and the other Germans spoke as if they were bringing the first words of eugenics and biological regeneration to the French, whom they had long considered decadent because of their low birthrate and high incidence of disease and alcohol. Fischer was correct in his assumption that for eugenics to work in France, it had to address the natalists' concerns; but he ignored the fact that for thirty years there had been an organized movement that ad-vocated the necessity of improving both the quantity *and* the qual-ity of the population: the French Eugenics Society. In fact, attend-ing the Fischer lecture was Henri Briand of the Ecole d'anthropologie who reported on the talk for the society in the *Revue anthropologique*.[6] It was to be the last official act of the soci-ety, because the war had disrupted its organization, and the new Vichy and occupation regimes had absorbed many of the interests it represented. So, rather than heralding the beginning of eugenics in France, the Fischer talk signaled the capstone of an era of French eugenic thought and activity that had its own indigenous roots and development.

This incident is very telling about perceptions of France and the history of eugenics that persist to this day. For example, if one mentions the word "eugenics" to a Frenchman, he will shake his head either in ignorance or with a knowing disdain. "Yes," he will agree, if he knows the word at all, "those Germans and Anglo-Saxons certainly did some nasty things in the name of eugenics. Fortunately in France we did not succumb to such folly." This view has been reinforced in recent years by scholars and those in the scientific community who had taken a keen interest in the history of eugenics. Their conclusions generally support this popular attitude.[7] By and large, so the story goes, it was the English who invented eugenics, but the Americans and Germans who were most enthusiastic in giving it practical application, which in the case of the Nazis was carried to the ultimate and horrible extreme of the death camps.

France, in fact, enjoys a reputation for having been strongly anti-eugenic in its history. Observers within the country and outside have boasted or complained (depending on whether they opposed or favored eugenics) that the strong egalitarian tradition of the Third Republic, coupled with the tradition of Gallic opposition to things Anglo-Saxon, provided a strong opposition to the English-inspired and German-perfected science of improving the human race. Writing in 1933 for the English *Eugenics review,* C. B. S. Hodson, secretary of the English Eugenics Society, noted that "France has the reputation of showing little concern for questions of human biology and has an antagonistic outlook on eugenics."[8]

Yet the record of French views on the subject (both scholarly and popular) shows almost no evidence of opposition to eugenics. There were occasional complaints about the Americans or Germans going to extremes. And some French proponents of eugenics complained of resistance to their ideas. Otherwise, the single organized attack came from the Catholic church, and then only after the papal encyclical of 1930 forced French Catholics to abandon a decade-long attempt to define a Christian eugenics. The reknowned French Ligue des droits de l'homme, established to protect individual rights during the Dreyfus affair, supported proposals by eugenicists in the name of protecting "the rights of unborn generations." And although this may have been for non-eugenic reasons, the league certainly never attacked eugenics. Even the French Communist party aligned itself with several eugenic causes by the end of the 1930s.

On one level the characterization of eugenics as being Anglo-Saxon is understandable. The United States and Germany were, by all accounts, the countries where the most extensive eugenic legislation was passed and applied.[9] Although England, as will be seen, is improperly considered to be the sole fount and inspiration for all eugenics movements, the Englishman Francis Galton does deserve credit (or blame) for first setting forth the new ideas and coining the term that has come to be applied to the movements and practices everywhere.[10] But closer analysis simply of the question of the naming of the new science suggests problems with this common view of the history of eugenics. Ideas comparable to Galton's were developed simultaneously and independently both in Germany and France, as reflected in their indigenous names, which persisted well into the twentieth century: in Germany, "race hygiene," and in France, "puericulture."[11]

A major purpose of this book is to show that what the English and Americans called eugenics was only one manifestation of a far more pervasive trend at the time, and that there is a serious risk of distorting the record by defining eugenics narrowly, based on peculiar English or American circumstances. This broader view considers eugenics as a widespread phenomenon found at the turn of the nineteenth century in most industrial societies. Its roots lay in the social class differentiation and conflict that was endemic to those societies, as well as in the economic cycles, growth of government, and increasingly scientific view of the world. Eugenics was a reaction to the perception that society was in a state of decline and degeneration.[12] Its novelty was in the self-proclaimed scientific means it proposed to resolve this decline, but this reaction was common to a long list of countries in the world of 1900. This book examines in detail how eugenics in France provided a broad cover for a variety of movements that aimed at the biological regeneration of the population, such as natalism, neo-Malthusianism, social hygiene, and racist immigration restrictions. Hence, it provides a thorough examination of eugenics beyond the Anglo–Saxon context, and lends further evidence to the increasing number of studies on other countries from Russia to Brazil and Norway to Japan.[13]

The larger view of eugenics as a biologically based movement for social reform also permits a better appreciation of the many social and cultural cross-currents in each of the countries where eugenics developed. The book demonstrates that if scholars take this broader perspective, they can better discern the common features that defined eugenics. In addition, they can see eugenics as much more of a worldwide phenomenon than is currently thought. The early and regular international meetings of eugenicists have long been a clue to this fact, which has yet to be thoroughly examined.[14]

One can immediately see both the need and value of this broader perspective on the history of eugenics by considering the question of its origins. The most common explanation for the beginning of eugenics is that once humans were seen as part of the evolutionary process, proposals were made to try to control it. According to this view, Darwin's theory of evolution was the inspiration for his cousin Francis Galton to propose a new science of eugenics. Galton's goals, as stated in an 1883 definition of eugenics, essentially fit this explanation. He called eugenics

the science of improving stock, which is by no means confined to questions of judicious mating, but which, especially in the case of man, takes cognisance of all influences that tend in however remote a degree to give the more suitable races or strains of blood a better chance of prevailing speedily over the less suitable than they otherwise would have.[15]

As with the naming of eugenics, this oft-repeated account of its origins requires modification if it is to apply to the broader development of the movement. For example, there was a delay of over twenty years between Galton's definition of eugenics and the creation of the first eugenics organizations after the turn of the century in England (1907), Germany (1905), and the United States (1910). It has been argued that the reason for the delay was the need for a better theoretical understanding of how hereditary traits were passed on to subsequent generations; and the rediscovery of Mendel's work in 1900 offered just such an understanding.[16] His laws, based on the assumption that discrete inherited traits were *not* modified by the environment, represented an improvement on Galton's and Darwin's idea of "blending" or averaging of inherited qualities from each parent, opening up eugenics research to the vast empirical experience of plant and animal breeders who had developed many rule-of-thumb ideas similar to Mendel's.

This explanation of the delay is correct in its assumption that there were important theoretical and practical problems in the initial attempt to follow Galton's dictum, but it goes too far in claiming they were all resolved by Mendel's discoveries. Eugenicists, whether Mendelian or not, continually had trouble producing the results they promised from their theories. It is therefore difficult to claim that problems in hereditary theory alone were responsible for the delay. More important, the French experience shows that a Mendelian hereditary theory was not a necessary condition for the development of eugenic thought. Mendelism did not come to France until the 1930s, yet from the beginning of the century Lamarckian hereditary theory, which maintained that acquired characteristics *could* be inherited, was the basis of a eugenics movement with similar goals and some of the same programs as those in Anglo-Saxon countries. Thus, although the spread of Mendel's ideas may have been an important part of the beginning of eugenics in England and the United States, Mendelism was by no means a prerequisite.[17]

There are other equally plausible reasons why eugenics organizations were not immediately established in the 1880s that look at broader social and intellectual developments at the time. Support for this view comes from the fact that the delays transcended significant local differences from country to country. Nowhere in Europe or the United States was a eugenics organization created before 1900; and thereafter, such organizations were established both in places where Mendelism was accepted and where it was rejected. In fact, one feature of eugenics movements showing the most consistency was the timing of the establishment of formal eugenics societies. Only a few years lapsed between the founding of the German Race Hygiene Society in 1905 and the French Eugenics Society in 1912. And in between, more than a dozen such organizations came into existence across Europe, the United States, and eventually Japan. It might be argued that the simultaneity was simply the result of imitation and the spread of English ideas to other countries. But although it is true that in France the immediate impetus for the creation of the French Eugenics Society was the First International Eugenics Congress held in London in 1912, as I will show, the deeper inspiration came from developments in French science and society that began at the same time as in England and the United States. A closer examination of the delay in establishing a eugenics organization in France shows that it came not just from theoretical problems in explaining hereditary causes, but for more mundane reasons such as the personalities of individuals and the difficulty in drawing together the people working in the diverse fields that comprised eugenics.

It is very curious that until recently the French have virtually ignored the history and impact of eugenic thought in their own country. Despite the understandable desire to allow the Anglo-Saxons and Germans to have the dubious distinction of excelling in eugenics, lack of interest in France is all the more striking because French scholars have been among the pioneers during the last twenty years in recognizing the relationship between biological and medical thought on the one hand, and society and politics on the other. The work of Michel Foucault in particular has inspired a whole generation of researchers to see the ever-increasing social and political power of the state during the nineteenth and twentieth centuries as having extended to physical control over individuals, with a justification in biomedical terms.[18]

Foucault's work offers an even broader perspective on the history of eugenics, because it views Darwin's theory as just another tool with which the state and society could order human biological resources. Already by the end of the eighteenth century, according to Foucault, humans were seen as a species whose reproduction was to be measured and assessed to determine the "bio-power" of the state. Another aspect of this development was the state's need to "discipline" the population physically for military, economic, and political purposes. Sexuality, which had previously been a private matter, now became a tool of the state and society. Procreative behavior was thus considered to be a legitimate area of state concern, to be protected from pathogenic influences, and to be increased, limited, or regenerated according to the needs of the state.[19]

The eugenic thought that tied together the movements for the biological regeneration of France and elsewhere beginning at the end of the nineteenth century can clearly be seen as manifestations of Foucault's bio-power. Eugenicists may not have been overtly motivated by power and control as ends in themselves, but their goals involved the state more broadly and deeply in matters previously left to the individual, going beyond a concern for individual or collective health to the quality of future generations. Studies of this phenomenon in France have usually focused on particular biologically based reform movements, such as those against alcohol and prostitution or in favor of birth control. Despite the fact that Foucault considered eugenics along with female hysteria, childhood masturbation, and sexual perversion as central examples (or "strategies") of the exercise of bio-power, his countrymen have yet to produce a full history of eugenics in France.[20] This book examines the specific reform movements in the context of broader eugenic thought, thus taking a position midway between Foucault's sweeping overview and the more limited case-study perspectives. At the same time, the book will show the relevance of the biosocial writings of the French school to the extensive research on Anglo-Saxon eugenics.

The thesis of this book is that eugenics in France provided a theoretical framework linking together several different movements for the biological reform of society in the late nineteenth and early twentieth centuries. Eugenicists were able to do this because of their promise to improve the hereditary quality of the population. Moreover, because of the widespread belief in France in the Lamarckian theory of the inheritability of acquired characteristics, many would-be reformers saw great advantages in a theory maintaining that any physical improvements in the population would be passed to subsequent generations. If eugenicists in other countries were critical of French neo-Lamarckism, they hid it well. For, as will be seen, the French were always prominent at international conferences, including some at which they served as hosts.

A greater difficulty for eugenics in France was the problem of declining birthrate that Eugen Fischer mentioned in his 1941 talk. The fear of depopulation made it difficult for French eugenicists to propose negative measures to eliminate undesirable elements in the population. Natalist organizations, among others, opposed any action that might restrict procreation. Yet French eugenicists were able to maintain a coalition with these groups for a surprisingly long time by stressing positive eugenics and the need to improve both the quality *and* quantity of the population. This position was in direct contrast to the neo-Malthusian eugenicists of the English Malthusian League who in the early twentieth century adopted as their slogan, *Non quantitas sed qualitas*.[21] The strikingly different French position was possible in part because of neo-Lamarckian hereditary theory, which assumed that if one could improve the undesirable conditions of one generation, it would make the next generation better. Toward the end of the 1920s, however, French eugenicists found it impossible to continue the alliance with the natalists, and the result was a greater emphasis on negative eugenic measures in the 1930s and 1940s, much like their Anglo-Saxon and German counterparts.

This book is not meant to be the last word on French eugenics. On the contrary, it is a first attempt to set forth the major components of French eugenics, both for comparison with other countries and to show the interaction of the various movements that comprised it. Some of these, such as the neo-Malthusian and anti-venereal disease movements, have already been examined in detail, whereas others, such as the history of statistics or French anthropology, are just beginning to be studied.[22] For virtually all of these the twentieth century has received the least attention.

The first two chapters give an overview of French perceptions of decline and proposals for regeneration that were typical of turn-of-the-century Europe. In many ways the decline was seen as more pronounced in France than elsewhere, not only because of French political instability and economic stagnation in the nineteenth century, but also because of the fear of demographic decline stemming from recognition of the slowing French birthrate. Among the proposals for reversing the situation were ideas for biological regeneration out of which the French eugenics movement sprang. The most important of these were the natalist, birth control, and social hygiene movements, the latter of which aimed at eliminating the so-called social plagues of alcoholism, tuberculosis, and venereal disease.

Chapter 3 examines the immediate precursors of the French Eugenics Society – that is, proposals stemming from the eugenic thought of the late nineteenth century that failed to produce an organized eugenics movement. This includes an examination of why it took over thirty years before an organization was created that embodied these eugenic ideas. And because there was also a delay in other countries, the answers for France help to shed light on the experience elsewhere. Chapter 4 examines the people and existing organizations that came together to form the French Eugenics Society in 1912. It analyzes the background of the principal leaders, the goals and institutional framework of the organization, and compares the society with organizations in other countries before the First World War. The impact of the war on French

eugenics is covered in Chapter 5, which also looks at related natalist and social hygiene programs during the 1920s. When eugenicists lost control of the social hygiene movement, they began a
campaign for a premarital medical examination law, which is the
subject of Chapter 6. That was not only a turning point as a move
toward negative eugenics, but also a tactic that tested the influence
of eugenics in the country.

Chapter 7 presents an overview of eugenics during the 1930s, a
period of change in France as in other countries.[23] It produced, for
example, the first organized opposition to eugenics by natalists
and the Catholic church, and at the same time brought new support, at least for some eugenic ideas, from the French left. The
most dramatic development, however, was an increasing call for
harsher, negative measures – birth control, sterilization, and immigration restriction. These were only partly the reaction to the
new circumstances of the Depression, because they also coincided
with a change in the way the French Eugenics Society was organized. The result was that by the end of the decade a significant
body of writing and ideas existed in France to support such measures, with a seemingly scientific justification offered by eugenics.
Chapters 8 and 9 provide a more detailed consideration of the
questions of race and immigration that grew in importance during
the 1930s and have continued up to the present.

Chapter 10 looks at the Vichy period from the standpoint of the
changes Vichy brought to eugenics as part of its new call for the
biological regeneration of France. The regime provided opportunities to carry out some of the older racist and social hygiene proposals, and in addition established the Foundation of Alexis Carrel, which set forth some new ones. Many of these developments
survived the end of the Second World War, despite the abrupt
change in the French government in 1944. Hence, the book concludes in Chapter 11 with some observations on the continuity of
eugenics up to the present.

2

Degeneration and regeneration

Proponents always presented eugenics as a progressive movement, a viewpoint that carried over into the work of early historians of eugenics. In light of the Nazi Holocaust, however, most
scholarship of the past two decades has stressed the conservative,
right-wing nature of eugenics, and occasional efforts to redress the
balance have been loudly shouted down.[1] The history of eugenics
in France reveals the existence of both progressive and conservative elements, but eugenics can be better understood from the start
as being fundamentally conservative in nature.

Eugenics in France grew out of several movements for biological regeneration at the end of the nineteenth century such as neo-
Malthusianism and social hygiene, which at first glance appear to
be progressive. But the beginnings of these movements cannot be
fully understood separately from the perceptions of degeneration
that they sought to correct. From this perspective, French eugenics was reactionary – that is, it attempted to restore a previous
status quo or reverse negative trends. It was, therefore, less inspired by utopian visions of a shining city on a hill than by a fear
of regression and decline. What Garland Allen has said of the
American eugenics movement and Progressivism, can also be said
of developments in France:

> It was in large part a reactionary, return to the "good old days" philos-
> ophy which looked backward rather than forward. Its only consistent
> "progressive" (forward looking) aspect was a belief that social ills could
> be cured by some form of community or governmental intervention in
> otherwise laissez-faire processes of the world.[2]

To understand this point of view, one must therefore begin the
story of French eugenics with an analysis of the perceptions

of degeneration that were widespread in the United States and France as well as the rest of Europe at the end of the nineteenth century.

The concern with decline was perhaps an inevitable consequence of overexpectations growing out of the belief in progress that had existed since mid-century. During that time, England in particular and Europe in general had just led the world through an industrial revolution that had increased economic production to unprecedented levels, making the benefits of progress available to more people than ever before. Despite growing socialist rhetoric, the threat of revolution in the streets that had been common in the period up to 1848 was for most countries a thing of the past.[3] In the realm of international relations, after 1871 and into the twentieth century there was no war between major European powers, despite signs of growing national rivalry. Scientific discoveries promised to reveal the innermost secrets of the physical universe and life itself, thanks to the work of publicly recognized geniuses such as Darwin, Maxwell, and Mendeleev. The venerable historian Carlton Hayes, whose best-known epithet for the period was "a generation of materialism," also called it the "climax of the Enlightenment" because of its belief that progress had been rendered automatic.

What then was there to be pessimistic about, and was not this progress so evident as to overshadow the fears of even the most concerned observers? The list of perceptions of decline ranged from reflexive fears prompted by short-term, minor wars and political scandals to theories of broad historical trends such as Spengler's idea of the rise and fall of civilizations. In Britain, growing economic competition from the new German empire and the United States heralded the end of the era when Britain could claim to be "the workshop of the world." In addition, continuing British emigration and the slowing of the birthrate were seen as signs of degeneration and decline that the problems of the Boer War seemed to confirm after the turn of the century.[4] In the United States, the rising number of immigrants from southern and eastern Europe was pointed to by some as a threat to the Anglo-Saxon population, while studies showing a rise in the number of criminals, alcoholics, and the insane were used as additional proof of the overall degeneration of the population.[5] Germany, poised in the heart of Europe between a revanchist France and a rising "Slavic peril" to the east, was always sensitive to any indication of a decline in the birthrate, to the increased incidence of disease, or to threats to the social order that might be exploited by hostile foreign powers.[6] Despite variations from place to place, these perceptions were so widespread toward the end of the nineteenth century that they cannot be attributed simply to peculiar local circumstances. In England, Germany, and the United States as well as in France, alarms were sounded and complaints made about the decay and degeneration of society.[7] As I will show, eugenics movements arose in all these countries, promising solutions to these problems.

In France, perceptions of decline were also in evidence by the end of the 1800s. For example, one frequently cited indicator that seemed to be more prominent in France than elsewhere was its record of political rule – it had been the least stable of major European countries in the nineteenth century. By 1871 the list of regimes that had been in power in the preceding century included two empires, three republics, and two different royal houses. Moreover, the prospects for an end to the instability looked dim after the 1871 uprising of the Paris Commune.[8] Monarchists argued that the civil strife that followed the defeat at the hands of the Prussians only demonstrated a greater need for the stability and order of the old regime, and the ideas and actions of the Communards suggested that the nature of the new regimes, rather than moderating, was becoming increasingly radical. The Third Republic that succeeded the Commune was, in the opinion of all, only a temporary arrangement of convenience, worked out under the guns of the Germans. Even after the institutions of the new government became more permanent in the 1880s, the republic was under constant attack both by aristocratic elements whose positions of power and authority were being usurped and by conservative intellectuals who protested the leveling effect of democracy. This was only in part the result of the mediocrity and demagoguery these groups saw at work in the Third Republic. More fundamental was their opposition to the *égalité* of the French Revolution, a theme that was embellished by such groups as Action Française,[9] and later picked up by eugenicists faced with the problem of justifying the elimination of undesirable elements of the population. The strengths as well as the limits of these critics of the Third Republic were demonstrated by the Dreyfus affair – which the government survived, but only after an extraordinary struggle.

There were also concerns in France about the economic condition of the country at the end of the nineteenth century, indicating that fear of decline went beyond political critics of the republic. Economists who looked at international matters saw Britain as having surpassed France economically in the first part of the nineteenth century thanks to its industrial revolution. With the economic growth of Germany and the United States after mid-century, these economists warned that France was in danger of becoming a fourth-rate economic power.[10] Their warnings were reinforced by the Depression of 1873 and subsequent aftershocks, most notably the crash of the Union Générale in 1882, which indicated that the decline might not just be relative, as absolute figures for unemployment rose and those for trade dropped.

The economic rivalry with Germany was only one of several reasons for concern by Frenchmen looking across the Rhine. The growth of Prussian military and diplomatic strength in the 1860s produced a tension between Bismarck and Napoleon III that reached a climax in the war of 1870–71. The resounding victory of the Germans, which settled the question of continental supremacy, also touched off a wave of soul-searching in France about the cause of the debacle. More will be said later about the far-reaching consequences of this examination, which left few aspects of French life untouched – from army organization to industrial production, and from the quality of scientific education to the demographic pattern of birth and death rates.[11] Suffice it to say now that Germany's rise was seen by most French as having been at France's expense.

One final indication of the decline in France at the end of the nineteenth century came from a group of intellectuals who expressed their ideas in literary form through a movement called the Decadents.[12] Their immediate roots were in nineteenth-century Romanticism and such mid-century writers as Flaubert and the Goncourts; hence their inspiration was not the economic, military, or political events of the 1870s. Their perspective was much broader, involving a comparison of bourgeois nineteenth-century society with other times at least as far back as the Age of Louis XIV, but more typically the Renaissance or ancient Greece, which were considered the high points of the human spirit. As if to flaunt their view, Paul Bourget and other leaders of the Decadents used the name not to describe French society but themselves. Their ironic use of language indicated a preference for their own irrational and "uncivilized" decadence over the complacent, self-satisfied middle class world around them. They were anti-modern, however, seeking a more natural expression of humanity than the scientific positivism that had reigned since mid-century. Hence, they were not a direct influence on eugenicists and others seeking scientific reform of society. They were more directly the inspiration for such philosophers as Nietzsche and Bergson who made anti-rationalism the cornerstone of their work. Nonetheless, they were symptomatic of the times, and added to the mood of *fin-de-siècle* malaise.[13]

BIOLOGICAL DECLINE

The eugenic view of decline at the end of the nineteenth century was different from that of the Decadents because of its scientific perspective.[14] Its roots were biomedical, and as many recent studies have shown, they can be traced back to well before Darwin. By far the earliest and most important of these views in France was demographic, for in an age of industry and statistics, progress and power were seen increasingly in numerical terms.[15] As the French and other countries began compiling vital statistics during the nineteenth century, the overall size of the population became another indicator of national well-being that was watched very closely. Ironically, at the beginning of the century the rapid rise of population was a source of alarm, inspiring most notably Malthus's famous essay on population. The rapid growth of cities added to the perception of population increase; and as late as 1851 the Academie Française offered a 3,000 franc prize for the best work on the following subject: "Happy the country where public and private wisdom unite to prevent the population from growing too rapidly."[16]

After 1850, statistics began to show that the French birthrate was dropping. Rather than considering the decline as a reason to rejoice, some saw it as an augur of impending "depopulation." The years 1854 and 1855 were the first in which the total number of deaths in France exceeded the number of births; and although this quirk (due to a cholera epidemic and the Crimean War) immediately corrected itself, it was duly noted by critics of Napoleon III's empire who were eager to find any signs that his regime would meet the fate of previous imperial regimes. These concerns about the decline in the birthrate were greatly heightened after the Franco-Prussian War, because the smaller size and slower growth of the French population were seen not only as general symptoms of decline but also as direct impediments to future military recruitment.

The nineteenth century also saw the medical profession develop a new language to describe the quality of individual life.[17] It is a common notion that physicians rose in social esteem and importance in France during the nineteenth century, even taking the place of the religious confessor for many important and troubling problems that people faced. In Balzac's words, "Today the peasant prefers to listen to the doctor who gives him a better prescription to save his body than to the priest who sermonizes him about the salvation of souls." Although some have questioned the universal applicability of this observation, it is generally agreed that there was growing concern with health rather than with mere subsistence, thanks to the rise in the standard of living during the century.[18] As medical ideas spread to the general populace, biological language was used increasingly to describe not only diseases such as smallpox, cholera, and tuberculosis, but how people felt – that is, their fears, obsessions, anxieties, and boredom.[19] New terms such as neurasthenia, hysteria, and even degeneration itself were coined to describe the manifestations of decline in individuals. Quantifiable signs of this decline were seen in rejection rates as high as 60–75 percent for prospective military conscripts in some regions of France.[20]

By the late 1860s, these criticisms had become so widespread that Paul Broca, founder of the Paris Anthropological Society, presented a report to the French Academy of Medicine entitled "On the so-called degeneration of the French population." Broca sought in particular to refute the charge, widely publicized in the French and foreign press, that there was "an ever increasing number of ill and stunted individuals, making army recruitment more and more difficult."[21] According to these accounts, not only was the number of recruits declining but their average height was smaller and their complexion paler, as well as there being more frequent manifestations of "general weakness." The causes cited included the growth of urban industrial centers at the expense of the rural areas, and a whole list of specific noxious causes ranging from "the eating of potatoes and abuse of tobacco and alcohol to universal misconduct." Broca, ever the positivist, took exactly the opposite view, claiming that "the French population is better nourished, better clothed, better housed and incidentally less ignorant than it has ever been before in any period."[22] Despite his protests, Broca's population figures and statistics on the height of army recruits could not sway the public mood nor match the impact and influence of popular literary characters such as Emile Zola's Rougon-Macquart family – the embodiment of decadence and degeneration.

It is not unusual for scientists to have difficulty competing with novelists for the attention of the public, but Zola's influence was extraordinary – even for a writer. As one scholar has said, Zola's novels were so widely read that for most of his contemporaries, "the mine of the 60s is *Germinal,* the condition of the proletariat is *L'Assomoir,* retail commerce is *Au bonheur des dames.*"[23] *L'Assomoir* went through thirty-eight printings in nine months, selling over 100,000 copies within five years of publication.[24] By extension, one may just as legitimately add that decadence and degeneration in turn-of-the-century France *was* the Rougon-Macquart family. The appeal of Zola's writing was not just the result of the lurid details of decadence, incest, and alcoholism, or the sheer length of the series – which eventually ran to twenty volumes. A key element was the scientific form and structure he used to tie the material together. Zola used the tools of his day, which themselves were transforming medicine from an art to a science.

While Zola was giving literary form to the idea of degeneration, medical and scientific work also continued on the problem. The physician most closely identified with the theory of degeneration was Bénédict-Augustin Morel, who first spelled out his ideas in the 1850s.[25] It is important to note that Morel was neither as pessimistic nor as broad in his application of the idea of degeneration as his followers were in subsequent years. For one thing, he considered it to be normal for humans to change and adapt to the environment; degeneration was only an "abnormal modification" that at least carried with it the resolution of the problem of preventing its spread to the rest of the population: sterility. In later years, however, the concept of degeneration proved to be too potent and attractive to be applied so narrowly. What began as a limited description by Morel of one example of evolutionary change became by the end of the century, as the biologist Etienne Rabaud described it,

blurred, taking shifting and confused outlines; it is frequently nothing more than a vague label which is attached, depending on need, to the most varied and notoriously incompatible phenomena, which engenders extreme interpretation, as removed from common sense as from reality.[26]

In the course of the nineteenth century, one influence that became increasingly associated with degeneration was the city. Though the dirt and stench of urban centers had been notorious since Roman times, the growth and overcrowding that accompanied the industrial revolution made the contrast between city and countryside much more striking by the second half of the nineteenth century. Numerous examples can be found in the work of the novelists of the day. Consider first this picturesque description of the markets in the Halles quarter of Paris at the beginning of the nineteenth century:

It has an abundance of everything, vegetables, market-garden produce and orchard fruit, sea and fresh-water fish; all that contributes to the comforts and luxuries of life . . . a market, a fair that never closes and a storehouse, garden and fishpond and the royal furniture repository. It is the most bustling and the wealthiest district on earth.[27]

By mid-century, Balzac described the same quarter as follows:

This unhealthy pile hemmed in on all sides by tall houses is the center of the black passages which meet here and join the quartier des Halles to the quartier Saint-Martin by the notorious rue Quincampoix, damp thoroughfares on which thronging people are stricken with rheumatics.[28]

In the second half of the nineteenth century, public health statistics added more information to the literary descriptions of Balzac, Eugène Sue, and Victor Hugo. Although some studies, such as those by Louis Villermé in the 1820s and 1830s, classifying the height and frequency of rejection of Parisian army recruits according to arrondissement, suggested that degeneration might be tied to poverty rather than the effect of the urban environment itself,[29] the idea persisted that all the inhabitants of Paris suffered from living in this largest of French urban agglomerations. Employers regularly showed a preference for hiring newcomers to the city over Parisian-born workers, whom they considered to be inferior in physical strength. This negative view of the urban environment was perhaps most graphically expressed in a variety of schemes that occasionally resulted in the creation of new factory-cities (*ville-usine*) such as Creusot and the mining centers of the north.[30] There is reason to be suspicious of the objectivity of these expressions of concern about urban degeneration. Although industrialists argued that these new towns would avoid the crowding and chaos of the older urban centers, employers would also benefit from the docility of the non-urban or newly arrived workforce with no tradition of organization or resistance to employers' demands. The ability to control workers better was a more compelling reason for the preferences of industrialists and employers.[31] Nonetheless, the employers' use of these negative views of the urban environment testifies to the currency of such ideas.

In England, Charles Booth and others developed this line of thought into an elaborate theory of "urban degeneration." As one scholar has put it, the poor represented no idle threat:

Herded into slums where religion, propriety and civilization were impossible, interspersed with criminals and prostitutes, deprived of light and air, craving drink and "cheap excitement," the "residuum" was large enough to engulf civilized London.[32]

In France, however, no such broad and elaborate theory was propounded, perhaps because there was no comparable urban investigative movement in the 1870s and 1880s that "rediscovered poverty." There was no French equivalent of Booth, or Alfred Marshall, or Llewellyn Smith. In addition, because of the revolutionary tradition in France, there was no lack of graphic examples – as in 1789, 1830, 1848, and most recently in the Commune of 1871 – of the urban residuum taking drastic action. But if the threat was more real, so too was its perception clearer. The Communards, after all, were defeated, and the surviving leaders exiled. Degeneration had a role in explaining the causes, but not in the vague sense of urban degeneration. The metaphor in France was still medical, but the analysis was more specific. It focused on crowd psychology and specific causes of irrational, criminal degenerative behavior. Of all the causes mentioned, the one receiving the earliest and most frequent attention was alcohol.

THE SOCIAL PLAGUES: ALCOHOL, TUBERCULOSIS, AND VENEREAL DISEASE

The credit for identifying alcohol as a medical problem is usually given to the Swedish doctor Magnus Huss in 1852. Although French doctors did not immediately follow his lead, the experience of the Commune sharply focused attention onto the question of the degenerative effects of alcohol.[33] Even before the declaration of the Commune, while Paris was under siege by German troops, a group of upper-class Parisians formed a "Patriotic Temperance Society" whose purpose was to curb the apparent increase in wine and spirit consumption they noticed when food became scarce.[34] After 1871, bourgeois opinion was quick to seize upon alcohol as an explanation for "working class irrationality" during the events of the Commune, and French physicians set up study commissions that were able to compile evidence from mental hospital admissions and the family trees of Communards that purported to show a link between drink and revolution. The oversimplification and self-contradiction of these explanations can be seen in the conclusion of one such study:

Now one can understand the bestial and savage faces of the workers in the uprising, the thefts, the massacres, and the arson; the insanity, imbecility and idiocy which affected such a large number of them; their vicious instincts, their lack of morality, their laziness, their tendency toward crime, and in the long run, their reproductive impotence. In short, it is not surprising to see that each new revolution brings an increase of atrocities and degeneration.[35]

These observations were accompanied by the creation of new organizations in France that attempted to correct the problem of alcohol. In 1872 a French Temperance Society was founded along the lines of the English and American movements. The organization was largely ineffective during the next two decades, but it did contribute to the passage of a law in 1873 prohibiting "public drunkenness." Although hardly striking at the root of the problem – its sponsors complained as much of having to share the streets with drunks as they did of alcohol's contribution to the Commune – the law was a first step toward government recognition of the problem, and by the mid-1880s public drunkenness had become the most frequently cited cause for arrest in Paris.[36]

The anti-alcohol movement generally failed to persuade the public that the Commune was anything but political in origin. Among physicians and psychiatrists, however, the Commune clearly marked the beginning of a long-term study of the problems of alcoholism. Moreover, in the next twenty years, these medical professionals broadened their perspective from seeing alcohol as a specific cause of working-class revolution to viewing it as a larger cause of the degeneration of the whole population.[37] They were aided in their task by the rising rates of admissions to insane asylums and the increasing numbers of suicides along with the arrests mentioned for public drunkenness. Paralleling these was a rising rate of alcohol consumption.[38]

Of all those studying the problem, no one gave it more scientific legitimacy than Valentin Magnan, head of admissions at the Sainte Anne mental asylum from 1867 until the First World War. Given his post, Magnan was in an ideal position to collect statistics, conduct tests, and publish the results of his work extensively. In the process he not only produced findings that became grist for the temperance movement's mill, but he sought to establish the central role of alcoholism in most cases of degeneration and mental illness. This latter work was not without larger significance to the history of psychiatry. In fact, Magnan has been credited with establishing a whole new paradigm of psychiatric diagnosis in the last quarter of the nineteenth century based on medical and biological disorder – thus replacing the "moral" model established by Philippe Pinel in the 1830s.[39]

One example of Magnan's work is the influential book *Les dégénérés,* written in 1885 with his pupil Paul-Marie Légrain, who shortly after became leader of the French temperance movement. The authors saw degeneration as part of the overall process of evolution that assumed that "normal" humans had developed in a range between a primitive "type A" and a perfect "type O." Human evolution could move in either a progressive or regressive direction along the line between the two types. Degeneration, however, according to this view, was a detour from the line toward a "type Z," which might be similar to the primitive A in some respects, but which ultimately ended in extinction and was not reversible. Thus, one of the major assumptions of this analytic framework was the distinction between the primitive and degenerate. Alcoholism was seen as a cause, along with poor nourishment and living conditions, for the detour from the normal evolutionary line. Much more vague was the role assigned by Magnan and Légrain to the hereditary predisposition to alcoholism, although they more clearly assumed a link between environment and heredity:

The hereditary influences are necessarily a complex product, formed by an accumulation of defects of diverse orders, acquired from ancestors during an indefinite series of generations. These defects would be, for example, misery, alcoholism, malaria, tuberculosis, insanity, etc.[40]

This view of degeneration makes clear how other noxious influences besides alcohol could be accommodated into the theory. Concern with problems such as venereal disease and tuberculosis generally developed later than the concern with alcohol. In the case of venereal disease, this was partly the result of the state of medical knowledge and partly the delicate questions raised by the means of transmitting venereal disease. Before the 1890s, discussion was confined to marginal and special segments of the population usually associated with the problem, such as prostitutes and military personnel. The discovery in 1879 of the bacterial cause of gonorrhea sparked a more general medical interest in the problem, but there was no equivalent of a Magnan for venereal disease in France until Alfred Fournier's work around the turn of the century.

Tuberculosis was even slower than venereal disease in arousing medical or public interest. One reason may have been that the disease was less widely reported; another was the general fatalism toward the problem. Alcoholism and venereal disease were seen as caused by a failure of will or morality; hence, they were seen by many as psychological problems that could be prevented by abstinence from drink or sexual activity. Tuberculosis, on the other hand, offered no such obvious course of remedial action. Thus, there was little the public could do while medical science searched for the cause and cure. One problem hampering this work was the difficulty in collecting data. There were no special dispensaries or clinics for tuberculosis until 1888, and the general apathetic acceptance of the disease resulted in the failure of many to seek treatment. One indication of the task facing the anti-tuberculosis leagues once they were established was that their first goal was the mandatory reporting of cases by doctors.

Even with better reporting of cases, the search for the cause of tuberculosis, let alone its cure, was not an easy one. For example, after Koch's discovery of the tuberculosis bacillus in 1882, the idea persisted that the organism grew better in the dark than the light. Hence, researchers saw the dark, damp corners of narrow twisting city streets or stair corridors of slum dwellings and tiny cramped rooms with no windows as the ideal breeding grounds for the disease. Statistics showing that the poor residents of slums had a higher incidence of tuberculosis than those of the more fashionable arrondissements of Paris lent support to this idea, and elaborate studies were done of room size, window openings, street width, and building height to supplement these findings.[41] A Paris study commission in 1906 recommended slum clearance of six "islands" where a significantly higher incidence of tuberculosis was found in the IVth, Vth, XIth, XIIth, XIVth, and XIXth arrondissements.

Although the recommendations were not carried out, the search for an environmental cure for tuberculosis – especially fresh air and sunshine – continued in France well into the twentieth century. At the same time, another line of inquiry attempted to show the hereditary cause of tuberculosis, as in a 1912 study by Charles Leroux and W. Grunberg of 442 working-class families. Their analysis of family trees suggested a much higher frequency of the disease in successive generations of the same family, thus adding the concept of heredo-tubercular to the already existing heredo-alcoholic and heredo-syphilitic.[42]

FROM DEGENERATION TO REGENERATION

The scientific and medical theory of degeneration was well developed by the end of the nineteenth century, even if it still lagged behind the literary and popular conceptions of degeneration. But as the scholarly studies and analyses compiled evidence that showed the extent of degeneration in graphic form, there was a shift in scientific and public sentiment that took a more optimistic view.[43] The reasons for the change in the public mood were many – ranging from specific and immediate diplomatic events such as the resolution of the Tangiers crisis of 1905, to century-long trends in social and economic development. There was, for example, the stubborn fact that the regime of the Third Republic refused to go away. Although more the product of convenience than design, the institutions created in the 1870s passed the tests of the ensuing decades. By the turn of the century the survival of the new republic had at least disproved one notion current in the 1870s: "If the Republic isn't the right system for France, the surest way to get rid of it is to establish it."[44] The fact that the Dreyfus affair produced the harshest criticism yet of the regime made its survival all the more significant.

Meanwhile, by the end of the 1890s the economy began to recover, and French trade, unemployment, and production figures greatly improved. Problem areas remained, and of course Germany and the United States continued to outdistance France economically, but the immediate concerns about economic decline were calmed as business revived in the late 1890s. In foreign affairs the shadow of the defeat by the Germans continued for a long time and reached into many areas of French life, but on the military and diplomatic level French leaders were able to offer at least some hope for redressing the imbalance when the Russian alliance was signed in 1894. Moreover, in another area of international politics the French could find additional clear-cut evidence of success: colonial expansion. In the 1880s and 1890s, large territories were acquired in north and west Africa as well as Madagascar and Indochina, holding out the promise of new economic resources, and at the same time demonstrating the ability of the military to conduct operations at great distances and under extraordinary circumstances.[45]

The revival was manifested perhaps most noticeably in nationalistic terms,[46] but there was also a significant change among intellectuals. Writers as diverse in background as Georges Sorel and Charles Péguy offered optimistic promises of regeneration in France by social or religious means. In addition, the 1900 World's Fair in Paris was a self-proclaimed turning-point in the shift of popular mood in the French capital. Held despite threats of boycott because of the Dreyfus affair, the exposition not only took place, it set attendance records that lasted until the 1960s. The exhibitions and displays were specifically designed to convince the public of the great strides that had been made over the course of the century. This included the standard technological marvels to be found at World's Fairs such as a moving sidewalk, public demonstrations of x-rays, extensive automobile exhibits, a Palace of Electricity, and the usual machine and manufacturing exhibits. Evidence of

French diplomatic progress was found in the particularly extravagant Russian exhibit, which included railroad cars from the Trans-Siberian Railway, a project under construction and largely financed by the French. Exhibits of colonial expansion occupied the whole of the Trocadero hillside across from the Eiffel Tower and were especially popular with the crowds, though as much from their exotic appearance as their educational appeal.[47] The fair even offered an opportunity for internationalists and social reformers to gather, congratulate themselves on the progress they had made, and plan for the future. International meetings in Paris during the fair year discussed problems from postal unions to public health, education to hypnotism, and photography to philately. There were 127 official international congresses in all, as well as meetings of many "unofficial" groups such as neo-Malthusians and several socialist organizations.[48]

The turn of the century also inspired many retrospective/prospective analyses of the state of humanity. One assessment more directly relevant to the question of decline was made a few years later when the Parisian journal *L'Européen* conducted an opinion survey on the question, "Is France decadent?" The editors' reasons for posing the question reveal much about the shifting mood of opinion about France in the previous years. The opening article of the series began:

For fifteen years dating from 1875 to 1890, a cloud of pessimism weighed heavily on France. Ideas, customs, the arts, all were affected. A literature was born from it. . . . All talk was of the decadence of the Latin race and that of France in particular.[49]

In the ten years following, the article continued,

things changed dramatically. The alliance with Russia, the visits of heads of state, two brilliant World's Fairs, colonial expansion, greater ministerial stability, and finally the recent treaties of intervention with neighboring powers, have restored a healthier outlook.

"Still," the article concluded, "the talk of decadence persists. Critics of the continuing low birth rate, those fearful of the spread of socialism and pacifism, and popular novels keep the concept before the public, most recently in a play with the very title *Decadence.*"

As a result, *L'Européen* sent the following question to 100 leading authorities:

Considering the preponderant place that France previously held in the world, many contemporaries consider that having fallen somewhat in rank, she has passed the peak in her evolutionary ascent, and since her period of glory is behind her, she can only continue to fall to the point where a people dies, much like an individual. Others, however, while admitting that from several points of view, especially economically, France has lost the top rank, contest the fact of decline and think that if other nations have surpassed her by accelerating their pace, she has not ceased to progress and can hope to regain in the future a new period of grandeur.

We have thought that it would be interesting to open the columns of a journal like *L'Européen* to an international inquiry. We have concluded it would be useful to know what people in other countries think of France and what some of her own representatives think of her.

We, therefore, pose to a certain number of people – politicians, thinkers, scholars, writers and artists – this question: Is France decadent?[50]

The journal aimed high in its selection of respondents, although not all of them took the inquiry seriously. George Bernard Shaw, for example, responded curtly, "Is France decadent? It must be, if the editors of its journals are beginning to pose such a stupid question."[51] Shaw's exasperation was the exception; most other responses, though brief, were to the point. Some were quite prophetic. Vilfredo Pareto ignored the question of decadence for lack of an adequate definition, and instead went on to predict a revolution in France "as violent and murderous as 1789" unless it was "impeded by some general European war."[52] Pacifist Frédéric Passy chose to describe France's status as one of relatively slower progress that only "seems to retreat the way a moving train appears to go backwards when next to a faster moving train." Passy's diagnosis of the cause of France's slower progress was, among other things, "the weight of the excessive demands of the armed peace," a problem for most other countries, he added, except perhaps the United States.[53]

Most of the other responses, both foreign and French, were positive, offering the familiar list of accomplishments in all aspects of French life. Yves Guyot, a deputy and former minister, found something positive to say about virtually everything in France:

Militarily – if I compare our army to others, I am reassured. Intellectually – compare the ignorance of the population thirty years ago to the number of people today who can read and write. Politically – she has undertaken an experiment which no other great European nation has dared to do. Economically – in spite of the protectionism and financial fantasies of her deputies, she remains the greatest reservoir of capital in the world.

Guyot's Pollyannaism sank to blatant chauvinism when he concluded, "I am very proud to be a Frenchman," citing as his reasons the elegance of French women, the quality of French food, and, in the end, "we always have Bordeaux, Burgundy, Champagne and Cognac which can never be rivaled in all the world."[54] The more serious foreign observer and expert on degeneration Max Nordau did not differ greatly from Guyot in his assessment:

France is in rapid ascension and is experiencing at this moment one of the most brilliant periods of its history. . . . Economically she enjoys a marvelous prosperity. . . . Politically she has regained the prestige of her most glorious days. . . . From the standpoint of territory she is as large and rich as the time when Napoleon was at the height of his power. Her colors fly over the most beautiful part of Asia, and her African empire . . . can only be compared to the Asiatic possessions of Russia in importance and facility of access. Morally and intellectually she is in the first rank of civilized people. Her science, her art, and her literature are superior to most of her emulators.[55]

The question of whether France experienced a revival prior to the First World War is not just another riddle such as resolving whether the half glass of water is half empty or half full. Perceptions of degeneration and hope for revival obviously could coexist. Logically, if pessimism were all-pervasive there would be no hope for regeneration; likewise, if all were well there would be no need for reform. If, as the evidence suggests, there was a turn in the mood toward a greater sense of progress in economic, social, and intellectual terms, it would make all the more glaring those elements in society that were not in step with the rest of the population. This was particularly true of the well-being of the population. Questions of taste and morality aside, those people considered to be criminal, poor, and unhealthy became relatively more "abnormal" as their numbers decreased compared with the prosperous, healthy remainder of society. They represented, in the words of one scholar, "a countercurrent in an age that became increasingly satisfied with itself."[56] These people thus were problems that were neither incorrigible nor to be ignored. Most important, they were generally seen as just that – "problems" – and as such they were to be corrected. Hence, eugenics and other proposals for reform and regeneration were precisely the product of the confidence and optimism that something could be done. Resignation and paralysis were not to be the responses to perceptions of decadence and degeneration.

BIOLOGICALLY BASED POLITICAL REFORM: EDMOND PERRIER AND SOLIDARISM

Although it is useful to separate degeneration and regeneration initially for analysis, the dichotomy between the two can be overemphasized. Most earlier criticisms, even by the Decadents, had been part of broader plans for reform that writers had in mind, if not from the start, then usually by the time they completed painting their gloomy pictures of society. Nietzsche had his superman, and Zola, after spending over twenty-five years and publishing twenty novels describing the misfortunes of the Rougon-Macquarts, promptly set off in a new series, the *Four gospels,* to present his view of the path to renewal and regeneration. Likewise, criticisms of French military and economic decline, population stagnation, or increased incidence of disease generally carried with them implicit, if not explicit, calls for reform and improvement. This is not to minimize the importance of the negative views in themselves, but rather to show that when eugenics emerged as a formula for regeneration, it was very much in line with other thinking of the day.

Eugenicists were very conscious of the broad range of these proposals, because their aim was to incorporate many of them into their own program. That there were more biologically inspired reform movements than eventually entered French eugenics is a testimony to the great impact of biology on social and political thought rather than to the limited scope of eugenics. For example, the sport and physical education movement, largely imported from England, developed separately from eugenics in France until the Vichy government's program of national regeneration in 1940.[57] Another example of the far reach of biologically inspired reform was the political doctrine of solidarism, which is worth examining further not only because of its substantial influence, but also because one of the major figures involved became a leader of French eugenics – the biologist Edmond Perrier.

Whether solidarism is seen as a shallow expedient to distract the masses from calls for more fundamental social revolution, or a genuine effort to find in science an alternative resolution to the class conflict presumed by both socialists and social Darwinists, most observers of France from the 1870s to World War One agree that solidarism merits the epithet that J.E.S. Hayward coined – "the official social philosophy of the French Third Republic."[58] Similar to Bismarck's state socialism in much of the legislation it called for – regulation of working conditions, establishment of insurance and pension programs, as well as the more radical but unsuccessful attempt to pass a progressive income tax – French solidarism was much more coherent than its German counterpart both in its theoretical justification as well as in the political spectrum from which it drew support. After all, social reform was much more compatible with a republican French government than an imperial German one. "No enemies on the left" hardly describes the policy of Bismarck and his successors. Yet this was the slogan coined by Léon Bourgeois, the politician most strongly identified with solidarism, who with this opening to the left swept into power with his Radical group in 1893. Bourgeois held various ministries over the next ten years, including prime minister in 1895–1896. In fact, for over twenty-five years Bourgeois exercised considerable influence both nationally and internationally. He refused the French presidency in 1902 and again in 1912, preferring to serve in the Senate and in international organizations such as the new World Court that he helped form. As will be seen, Bourgeois also became first honorary president of the French Eugenics Society in 1912.

Solidarism was an attempt to reconcile state intervention on behalf of social justice with classic liberal notions of individual freedom. Bourgeois drew heavily upon the writings of Alfred Fouillé, who had set out to create an alternative to the social Darwinist writings of the 1870s.[59] The doctrine was quickly applied to a variety of problems and programs, including the previously mentioned social reform legislation, mutual aid societies, public health laws, and the cooperative movement in economics.[60]

The most obvious appeal of solidarism was its emphasis on cooperation rather than competition or conflict in human affairs. It was this that Bourgeois offered, not in the socialist or Rousseauian sense of the communal general will superseding individual rights, but as an alternative to the rugged individualism of the social Darwinists. Obviously, Bourgeois did not need a scientific theory to justify this alternative, but given the scientific claims of social Darwinism that competition in nature not only extended to human affairs but was the motor that drove all progress, an alternate view of nature would be a great help in making the case for solidarism. Bourgeois found such a different view in the concept of "association" championed in France by Edmond Perrier and others. In one of the founding tracts of solidarism, Bourgeois repeated the following quote from Perrier to support the new doctrine:

In establishing in the living world whether competition is the precondition of progress, as has been so quickly learned by those who dream of social upheaval, progress has only been realized by the association of individual forces and their harmonious coordination. The natural sciences constitute not only the highest philosophy, but the only one capable of furnishing to governments the light necessary to clarify and heal the profound plagues of the present time.[61]

Perrier, who held the chair of anatomy/zoology at the Museum of Natural History, was obviously not shy about drawing broad general conclusions from his scientific research. More will be said later about the background of this biologist; for now, it is primarily of interest how he came to the theory of association which, like eugenics later, applied science to questions of social reform.[62]

Perrier's ideas stemmed from his research on hydra, coral, and other coelenterata – organisms that had fascinated biologists at least since the eighteenth century, when the regenerative capacity of polyps was studied in detail. Among nineteenth-century zoologists, Henri Milne-Edwards, one of Perrier's teachers at the Museum of Natural History, developed the idea of the physiological division of labor as an explanation of the growth and complexity of hydra.[63] Perrier went much further in developing a theory that not only explained the diversity but the formation of whole, new, more complex organisms. In fact, he claimed, "all higher organisms are nothing other than associations, or to use a scientific term, *colonies* of simpler organisms grouped diversely."[64] The implications of the theory for solidarism were made clearer in the two laws Perrier formulated to describe his ideas. The first, which he

called the "law of association," was based on Perrier's interpretation of cell theory and the process of division that he saw as resulting from the limits to the size of individual cells that had to
divide once they had grown to a certain point. The law of association was, therefore,

the forced consequence of the limitation of the size of protoplasmic masses.
Animals and plants are the societies formed often from innumerable individuals. The name *organism* is given to these societies. The individuals
who compose them, the *plastides,* are their *anatomical* elements. The organization results from their combination.[65]

One can see that Perrier was careful to underscore the integrity
of individual cells, presumably for scientific reasons, but with social implications as well. The role of the cells was spelled out in
the second law, called "the law of the independence of anatomical
elements," which explained the mechanism for change. Perrier
described their main features as follows:

Thanks to their aptitude for variance and their reciprocal independence,
these elements borne of one another have been able to modify themselves
in different ways, take diverse forms, acquire new functions and properties, augment accordingly the ability of these organisms to adapt to the
milieu and increase as a result their chances for survival. Each modification tested by an anatomical element is transmitted to its descendents.[66]

Thus, Perrier tied evolution up in a neat package, including explanations for the development of higher organisms as well as the
conservation of these changes. What was most important in the
theory for solidarism was the emphasis on cooperation without
sacrificing the individual integrity of the cells.

There is ample evidence that Perrier quickly realized the possible application of his theories to social doctrine; and in this he
was not alone. Alfred Espinas in France and earlier Rudolf Vir-
chow in Germany had used biological analogy, and in the case of
the Germans, cell theory, to support political ideologies.[67] It is
clear why Bourgeois and the other solidarists should turn to Perrier for scientific justification of their theories, which they claimed
were "only the expression at a higher level of the physical, biological and psychic laws according to which living and thinking beings
develop."[68] For his part, Perrier returned the favor in the preface
to the second edition of his *Colonies animales,* written in Novem-

ber 1897 shortly after the new formulation of solidarism became the rage of France. Although much of Perrier's lengthy preface described new work in the field and answered queries raised by critics, his concluding words were:

The natural sciences are themselves the highest, most important, most certain of philosophies. And this book will establish that they not only preach to us the struggle for existence; they also show us that this struggle – progress through strength – results from association. They teach us that in everything, association prospers. Associated elements, while keeping a freedom from one another which is the necessary condition of progress, remain united by constant compromises [*condescendances*], and confirm the place always held higher among the social virtues of the practice of *solidarism*.[69]

It is easy to see how the new ideas of eugenics at the turn of the century would appeal to Perrier. In 1900 he became director of the Natural History Museum, and with this added prestige he was the obvious choice to be the first president of the French Eugenics Society in 1912.

REGENERATION THROUGH BIRTH CONTROL

Of all the movements aimed at the regeneration of France at the turn of the century, none was written or talked about as much as birth control. One of the reasons is that two extremist groups developed diametrically opposed ideas about controlling births: natalists and neo-Malthusians. Although the term "birth control" is usually applied to neo-Malthusianism, it is important to note that both groups had similar responses to degeneration – "controlling" the quantity of the population; and both groups either ignored the question of quality or assumed it would naturally follow from the implemention of their programs. In a broad sense, therefore, both movements are examples of what Foucault identified as increasing bio-power in the modern world.[70] In a narrower sense, only by appreciating this similarity can one see that the crucial difference between the two movements was not *whether* to control reproduction but *who* was to control it. The neo-Malthusians wanted to permit couples to control (and presumably limit) family size. Natalists, on the other hand, were completely opposed to an uncontrolled, laissez-faire policy, which they blamed for the drop in the birthrate during the nineteenth century.[71] If steps were not taken to direct demographic trends, the natalists predicted, disaster would occur. Hence, they wished to control or manage the size of the population by guiding it toward an increase. As a result, natalists were not hesitant to call for all sorts of governmental means to encourage larger families, such as differential taxes, subsidies, marriage loans, and even a voting system based on family size. It is telling that the event that brought a temporary halt to the neo-Malthusian movement in France was a law passed by the Chamber of Deputies in 1920 banning sale and advertisement of birth control devices, a restriction of freedom of speech and commerce.

In addition to a common desire to increase control over human reproduction, the natalists, Malthusians, and eugenicists also shared a common concern about the degeneration and decline of France. Despite radically different backgrounds – the most vocal natalists claimed to be devout Catholics, whereas neo-Malthusians tended to be socialists or libertarians – both groups usually couched their programs in the broad terms of regeneration. This was the overall justification that natalists offered for the intervention they sanctioned in what had previously been a personal family matter – having children. And neo-Malthusians predicted regeneration rather than decline from families controlling the timing and number of children. Above all, these common goals and methods explain how in the history of eugenics in France there could be supporters who at the same or different times came from movements as apparently contrary as the natalists and neo-Malthusians.[72] Only by keeping this in mind can one understand the interrelationship between the three movements.

Though largely obscured by later developments, the French neo-Malthusian movement was among the most active in the world at the beginning of the twentieth century.[73] Its advocates mounted a national campaign, including lectures, publication of its own journals, and distribution of pamphlets in quantities that often exceeded 100,000. Some of the pamphlets written by Paul Robin, the founder of the French movement, give one a feel for the tone of the publications: *Libre amour, libre maternité; Pain, loisir, amour; Population et prudence procréatrice; Contre la nature; Malthus et les néo-Malthusiens; Vers régénération.* Similar examples could also be drawn from the writings of others in the movement, such as Senator Alfred

Naquet, Manuel Devaldes, and Gabriel Giroud.[74] The French neo-Malthusians sponsored the First International Birth Control Congress held in conjunction with the 1900 Paris World's Fair, but more typical of its propaganda efforts were small cards handed out on street corners with simple slogans such as "God blesses large families but does not feed them. Have fewer children!"

In contrast to neo-Malthusians in other countries who were usually middle class in origin, the French movement was working class in both its organizers and audience. The most crucial support came from grass roots union locals, which provided meeting places, contacts, publicity, and (most important) the audiences who came to hear the message from across the length and breadth of France. Such support was crucial because the union and socialist leadership in France was either indifferent or hostile to the neo-Malthusians.[75] Their socialist ideological position was generally that control of reproduction was an issue that must take a back seat to the revolution.

Throughout the nineteenth century, socialists had argued strongly against Malthus's idea that population growth brought poverty and misery. As counterexamples, the United States and Western Europe were cited as places that had seen both population growth and an increase in wealth during the century. Moreover, socialists could hardly be expected to blame the misery of the populace on demography rather than capitalism. To blame poverty on the fact of having too many children was to blame poverty on the poor. Finally, by the end of the nineteenth century the slowing down in the birthrate seemed to vindicate the socialist position, because poverty was apparently not disappearing. In fact, socialists began pointing to the declining birthrate as a symptom of wider problems. For example, an 1896 article in the *Revue socialiste* declared:

Capital uproots the wife from her role as spouse and mother. It imposes sterility on her.

Misery pushed to the extreme weakens the birthrate. The total absence of bread for children precludes their existence [*les retient dans le néant*]. This fact alone suffices to legitimize all the proletarian revolutions, all the insurrections of suffering, all the hunger revolts. The periods of great scarcity are most notable by their infertility. . . . The slowing of proliferation will be a constant until the day when revolution breaks new ground in the physical, intellectual, moral and emotional activity of people.[76]

It did not help the neo-Malthusians' standing with either the left leadership or the general French public that its founder and leader was Paul Robin, a maverick even by socialist standards. He had been nominated to the First Socialist International by no less a figure than Marx in 1870, and over the years had lived in England and New Zealand before returning to France where he was best-known as director of a school in Cempuis. There he used a coed-ucational approach to learning that also sought to give students instructions in the arts, physical exercise, and manual crafts as well as the traditional intellectual curriculum.[77] Robin was therefore outside the working-class tradition. Moreover, his personal life made him a lightning rod for criticism from the natalist move-ment, which was forming at the same time but with far greater resources at its disposal. One of the natalist founders, Jacques Ber-tillon, called Robin's work "criminal propaganda," attributing its origins at best to "the dreams that haunt this sick brain" and at worst suggesting its support "came from a country hostile to France."[78] At the same time, Bertillon did not minimize the effec-tiveness and the wide circulation that the ideas of Robin and his followers had achieved. A long chapter in Bertillon's most famous book, *The depopulation of France,* contained a detailed description that read like a legal brief, with charges and evidence against the neo-Malthusians. In fact, Bertillon took such great pains to docu-ment neo-Malthusian activity that one suspects him of overstating the strength of his opponents in order to make his own organiza-tion seem all the more necessary.

Bertillon's rhetoric ignored the fact that the neo-Malthusians were also concerned about the problem of decline at the end of the nineteenth century. Robin, for example, made it very clear that his goal was part of this broad movement by the name he chose for his organization – the League of Human Regeneration. The title of its journal was simply *Régénération.* The statutes of the league also illustrate this goal and the means to achieve it, at the same time revealing the potential for cooperation with eugenics. The leagues "founding principles," according to its statutes, main-tained

that the utility of the creation of a new human being is a very complex question involving considerations of time, place, people and public insti-tutions; that as much as it is desirable, from the family and social point of view, to have a sufficient number of adults healthy in body, strong, intelligent, agile, and good; it is little desirable to give birth to a great number of degenerate infants, destined for the most part to die prematurely, all to suffer much themselves and to impose suffering on their surrounding family and social group, to weigh heavily upon the always insufficient resources of public assistance and private charity at the expense of children of higher quality.[79]

As if to underscore the last statement, the statutes concluded, "The preoccupation of quality must always precede that of quantity."

The date of this document, 1896, was well before there was any organized movement calling itself "eugenics" in France; hence, the rationale can hardly have been a desire to curry favor with eugenicists. But the desire to use such an argument to broaden support from more established elements (which eugenicists were later to do) can be seen in a talk delivered by Robin to the Société d'anthropologie that same year.[80] Robin told the anthropologists that natural selection was no longer operating on humans to eliminate the weak; hence, artificial selection through contraception was necessary.[81] The members of the society were not very receptive to Robin, but after the turn of the century, when Adolphe Pinard began to popularize the idea of puericulture (the need to improve the quality as well as quantity of newborns), the editors of *Régénération* were quick to point out what they shared in common with the ideas of Pinard, the distinguished professor of obstetrics at the Ecole de médecine.[82] In 1902, a monthly column entitled "Practical puericulture" appeared in the journal and offered such folk wisdom as not having children in winter because it was too cold and harsh on the newborns. "April is the best month for birth and July the best for procreation," the editors advised.[83] A later article singled out a 1905 talk by Pinard at the Ecole des hautes études sociales on "Marriage aptitude," which called for "reasonable procreation," in part because, in Pinard's words, "after having produced children, one must be able to rear them."

Robin's league split in 1908, causing the disappearance of *Régénération* and its replacement by two other journals, one of which, *Le Malthusien,* edited by Albert Gros, sought to take even greater advantage of the potential appeal that eugenics might give to its program.[84] As a result, many articles appeared on eugenics that also drew on reports from English neo-Malthusians about the early activity of the eugenics movement in that country.[85] In fact, the journal was one of the only publications in France to use the word "eugenics" in any consistent way before the London Congress of 1912.

As the editors had done earlier in *Régénération*, Gros took special delight in following the pronouncements of Pinard and pointing out how they coincided with the position of *Le Malthusien*. One article used a March 1912 speech of Pinard's to poke fun at the natalists: "Our adversaries often seek to base themselves on the authority of Professor Pinard, member of the Academy of Medicine who is today the uncontested master of French gynecology." But the article then went on to show that Pinard had called for "conscientious and responsible procreation . . . upon which depends the conservation and improvement of the human race."[86] A few months later *Le Malthusien* gave extensive coverage to the London Eugenics Congress and the formation of a French Eugenics Society.[87] In fact, the subtitle of the journal was changed in September 1912 to *Le Malthusien: Revue eugéniste.*

Despite the strong support for eugenics by the neo-Malthusians, and the theoretical affinity of the two movements, the relationship was very one-sided. For although Pinard never openly repudiated his neo-Malthusian admirers, he certainly never returned the favor by showing any explicit support for them. In fact, Pinard continued to be publicly identified more closely with the natalists even though, as the quote in *Le Malthusien* suggested, he was critical of some of the "excesses" by those who totally ignored the question of quality.[88] As will be seen in the next chapter, although Pinard's early career and work on prenatal care and infant mortality justified this identification with the natalists, beginning in the late 1890s his new ideas on puericulture strained these ties. Instead, it was largely political and social rather than theoretical considerations that continued his link to natalists into the first decade of the twentieth century. Pinard could hardly be expected to throw in his lot with a group of radical socialist union hall organizers whom Bertillon had accused of "criminal propaganda." The resulting alliance between eugenicists and natalists was to have profound consequences for the history of French eugenics.

EUGENICS AND NATALISM

The association of eugenicists and natalists that occurred in France was not usually the case elsewhere.[89] Although the two movements were theoretically complementary – for example, eugenicists tended to concentrate on the causes of population decline, whereas the natalists looked at the effects – and both agreed that there were larger interests than those of the individual movements, the potential for disagreement was generally greater. Natalists argued that any eugenic measure of selection that might limit or inhibit procreation should be avoided, whereas eugenicists feared the growth of the inferior part of the population if it reproduced faster than the average rate of reproduction for the whole population. Hence, it was only in the case where so-called superior elements of the population limited births that eugenicists favored natalist calls for larger families. Conversely, to the extent that eugenicists thought that population control could slow the growth of undesirable elements, as was the case in the United States and Britain, they were in alliance with neo-Malthusian organizations.

France at the turn of the century was a clear exception to this rule, for it was the fear of depopulation, not overpopulation, that was most prevalent in the country.[90] Hence, there was no immediate or compelling reason for eugenicists and neo-Malthusians to join forces. Although such an alliance was eventually made, it was only done late, and hesitantly. This proved to be politically fortunate for the eugenicists because they were able to escape attack from the very powerful natalist organizations that developed at the beginning of the twentieth century.

The exact beginning of the natalist movement in France is difficult to date, in part because much activity occurred before formal organizations were created. Only in 1896 did the statistician Jacques Bertillon, the physiologist Charles Richet, the deputy André Honorrat, and two others found the Alliance nationale pour l'accroissement de la population française, which quickly became and remained the most important of the numerous natalist organizations that appeared in subsequent years. The very number of these groups is an indication of the widespread concern about the population problem that had been noted in France since the mid-nineteenth century.[91] As indicated earlier, one of the few quantifiable measures of decline (and implied decadence) was the size of the French population, whose growth during the course of the nineteenth century steadily slowed. In his 1867 article, "The supposed Degeneration of the French Population," Broca tried to separate the question of decadence from that of "disappearance" by

using the French word *depérissement* instead of *dépopulation,* the term
that became more popular toward the end of the century. Broca
traced the origins of concern with the problem to 1854, the first
year of recorded vital statistics in which deaths exceeded births
(992,779 to 923,461). He also noted a longer-range drop in fertility
from 3.4 infants per married couple in 1821–30 to 3.16 in 1856–
60. To explain these facts, however, Broca pointed out the unusual circumstances of 1854 – a year of grain shortage, cholera,
and the Crimean War. As for the drop in fertility, Broca claimed
it was more than counterbalanced by the falling death rate.[92]

By the 1890s there was little questioning of the existence of the
population problem in the scientific community. Although Broca
was correct in his observations about the death rate, which continued to drop enough to prevent another year of net population decline, natalists conveniently ignored it by focusing their attention
only on the yearly reports of births in France whose absolute number decreased every year, as it had done virtually throughout the
nineteenth century.[93] Jacques Bertillon, one of the founders of the
French natalist movement, was the most visible and vocal natalist
with training as a statistician. In an 1880 book entitled *Statistique
humaine* he showed his first interest in the field that his father,
Louis-Alphonse Bertillon, had helped create. Jacques' specific
concern with the birthrate was first expressed in an 1891 article for
the *Bulletin of the société d'anthropologie,* but the most complete
expression of his views was in the 1911 book, *La dépopulation de la
France.*[94] His fervent advocacy of natalism in response to the falling birthrate was by no means the only answer available to scientists studying the French population problem. As will be seen,
Lucien March, who was an even greater authority on French demography (he was head of the French Statistique générale), became a follower of the broader program of Pinard – puericulture
and eugenics. Charles Richet, a founder of the 1896 natalist alliance, also joined with his Ecole de médecine colleague Pinard to
create the French Eugenics Society in 1912.

As mentioned earlier, the population problem in France had not
always been seen as one of a declining birthrate. For most of the
first part of the nineteenth century the *growth* of the population
had been seen as a problem.[95] The slowing could therefore have
been welcomed as a long-sought solution to the overcrowding of
cities and unemployment. It took other events to make the level-

ing of population growth appear to be a problem, the most important being the unification of Germany in the 1860s and the Franco-Prussian War of 1870–71. The defeat itself was humiliating enough, but the ensuing national rivalry between France and a new German state with a larger population base and growth rate was more than enough to make many observers shift their view of French population trends. What might have been seen as finally relieving the pressures of population growth became instead a cause for new alarm at the nation's inability to match the military recruitment base of the new power to the east.

Despite the compelling logic of this explanation, it does not account for the twenty-five year delay in forming the first natalist organization in France. It is understandable that in the early years of the Third Republic there were more pressing concerns; hence, a two-part article by Charles Richet in the *Revue des deux mondes* in 1882, usually cited as one of the first statements of the problem in natalist terms, can be interpreted as a delayed reaction to the 1870 military debacle.[96] In reality, the article stands as an isolated example, because Richet's next article on the subject was not until fifteen years later, shortly after the founding of the natalist alliance in 1896. Because Bertillon's publications followed a similar pattern, this suggests that the Franco-Prussian War is at least insufficient as an explanation of the origin of the natalist movement, which burst on the literary and political scene as well as the scientific scene after 1895. It also reinforces the thesis that there was a coalescence of opinion in several countries around the turn of the century that included a perception of decline and degeneration, but also held out the promise that through science and government action these trends could be reversed.[97] Eugenics, natalism, and other movements calling for biological regeneration were the result. Of course, there was the added element of neo-Malthusian activity, which helped spark the natalists to organize themselves, but it was by no means a simple one-dimensional reaction. Richet's 1896 article on the population problem made no mention of neo-Malthusians, concentrating instead on a proposal for tax reform that would give incentives for large families.[98]

Once the French natalist movement was organized, it soon received wide exposure as having the answer to French national regeneration. One reflection of this can be found in French literature. Just as it offered a striking portrait of the view of decline and degeneration, so too the literature of the turn of the century presented solutions to these problems such as those found in the work of Zola. His *Four gospels* series, beginning with the novel *Fecondité* in 1899, was a deliberate outgrowth of the famous Rougon-Macquart series, which had been the most widely read depiction of decline in previous decades.[99] Zola's novel of regeneration by the founding of a large family on the frontier of France's newly acquired African colonies was hardly unique in its focus on the population problem. Eugène Brieux gave an equally didactic literary prescription in his controversial *Maternité*. Although the play was temporarily banned, the reason was its graphic depiction of the problem of childless couples and not the unpopularity of its natalist point of view.[100]

Another vein of potential support that natalists sought to exploit was in the political arena, largely because their program fit so well with traditional values and contemporary patriotic themes. Bertillon's charge that neo-Malthusian backing came from another country was one of the more subtle natalist appeals to French nationalism. Another French author, writing under the pseudonym Rommel, goaded his French readers by arguing that France could never win a war against Germany, whose growing population gave it both the means and justification for acquiring more French territory. Japanese newspapers were also quoted as claiming that the decline of the population doomed French colonization efforts in Asia to failure. But the most pointed of these statements was the quote attributed to von Moltke that France was losing a battle every day because of its declining birthrate.[101]

Despite this propaganda, the reforms of the natalist were not immediately adopted. For example, natalists were unsuccessful in passing any serious legislation before the First World War. Only in 1920, in the wake of the tremendous psychological and demographic shock of the fighting, was a law passed banning neo-Malthusian propaganda, but that was obviously more an indirect attack on a partial cause of the problem than a direct measure to encourage large families. It was not until 1939 that the first such laws were passed.[102] Despite the delays, natalists took advantage of numerous opportunities to state their case through sympathetic publicists and politicians such as Paul Strauss and Edme Piot. An example of this propaganda success but legislative failure can be seen in the earliest of these efforts – the Parliamentary Commission on Depopulation, created in January 1902.

The purpose of the commission was "to proceed with an overall study of the question of depopulation and the most practical means to combat it."[103] Despite the broad charge, it proved to be a great disappointment to the natalists. Following a policy of "out of sight, out of mind," the legislature generally ignored funding requests by the commission. Only three plenary sessions were held in seven years, and one scholar has suggested that the overall effect of the creation of the commission may have been to delay rather than hasten passage of any specific natalist proposals in the Senate or Chamber because these proposals were routinely referred to the depopulation study commission.[104]

The most significant work was done at the subcommittee level, where narrower parts of the problem were examined and, more importantly, the results published. For example, Bertillon and Honnorat prepared and published a report for the subcommittee on the "moral and sociological causes of depopulation" that argued that egotism and parents' ambitions for their children were major causes of the falling birthrate.[105] Pinard prepared a special report on puericulture that cited his and his student Charles Bachimont's study of birth weights for infants whose mothers were engaged in varying physical activities before childbirth; and Pinard and Richet published a report on the question, "Are there physiological causes that influence the decline in the birthrate?"[106]

Compared with the opinions expressed in political and literary circles, scientific opinion was more critical of the natalist position. Although statisticians and demographers raised few objections to some of the questionable population projections made by natalists, many in the medical profession disagreed with natalists, especially their unequivocal opposition to contraception. This was perhaps a reflection of medical practitioners' being in closer touch with the populace and hence more sympathetic to the conditions prompting decisions by parents to limit family size.[107] One example of medical opinion on the use of contraception can be found in the journal, *Chronique médical,* edited by Auguste Cabanès. While not a long-established or prestigious medical journal, *Chronique* was hardly a radical broadside like *Le Malthusien.* The tone and general appeal of the periodical was summarized in its subtitle, "Revue bimensuelle de médicine historique, littéraire et anecdotique." Serious medical practitioners could not have taken too dim a view of Cabanès' journal, because they regularly contributed to it and responded to questions on topics that he often used as the basis of articles claiming to represent a consensus of medical opinion.

It was for just such an article that Cabanès requested the opinions of readers in November 1904 on whether the use of contraception was justified. Specifically, he sought responses to an earlier article by a Dr. Klotz-Forest that maintained that pregnancy should be avoided.

whenever the pregnancy places the life or the health of the woman in peril; whenever the product of the conception would almost certainly be struck by degeneracy as a result of a hereditary defect of the parents; or [whenever] misery, "the worst of maladies," would condemn the innocent beings to a lamentable, precarious and sorrowful existence.

Among the authorities frequently cited in the article was Pinard, whose work was quoted in Klotz-Forest's conclusion:

Until now, the act of procreation has only been an instinctive act, such as it was in the age of the caveman. It is the only one of our instincts which has not been civilized. The greatest and highest of actions which man can undertake during his existence, upon which depends the conservation and improvement of the species, is done on the eve of the twentieth century as it was in the Stone Age.[108]

Cabanès' specific questions for his readers were:

1. Do you support or reject contraception?
2. If you accept it in principle, do you limit its application to medical cases, or, on the contrary, do you think that social or simply individual reasons could justify it?
3. In the event that you do not subscribe to [contraception], we would be grateful to you for specifying the reasons that make you reject it.

Three conclusions are worth noting about the responses printed in the February 1905 issue of the journal.[109] First is the size of the response. Cabanès printed forty-five letters, which he claimed "surpassed all our expectations." Second, thirty of those responding, or two-thirds, were physicians, hence they offer some measure of medical opinion on the question. Even the natalist Senator

Edme Piot had a staff member send a response, which is an indication of the attention Cabanès had attracted.

The third and most significant feature of the responses, however, was the strong support generally given for the practice of
contraception. Cabanès grouped the respondents into three categories: opponents of the use of contraception, supporters with some
reservations, and supporters without restrictions. Only eight of
the replies were from opponents, although they all were from
doctors (mostly provincial) with the exception of Senator Piot. A
slightly lower proportion of the respondents in the middle category were doctors (nine of thirteen). They most frequently cited
a danger to the life of the woman as justification for the use of
contraception or abortion, usually referring to personal experiences to illustrate the circumstances. Responses of note came from
Henri Cazalis, the poet and physician who had recently written a
book calling for legislation that would require a premarital examination, and from André Couvreur, an author in the style of Zola
and Brieux, whose novel *La graine* had earlier dramatized the disastrous consequences of venereal disease on offspring. More will
be said about these men in the next section on social hygiene, but
it is telling to find them in Cabanès' middle category of qualified
support because it reveals that they were essentially natalists who
wished to minimize the number of defectives that might be produced by a general rise in the birthrate. Widespread use of contraception would be counterproductive, they reasoned, insofar as it
would diminish the numbers of the fit as well.

No such fine distinctions were made by the majority of those
respondents who supported the unqualified use of contraception.
Virtually every one of the thirty responses called openly and strongly
for its use. "I would generalize it," said a Dr. L. Achard, chief of
a hospital staff in Algeria. "I approve without restriction," agreed
a lengthy letter from Dr. E. Callamand of Saint-Mande. The author Fernand Volney went even further, stating, "Not only do I
support the use of contraception, but I think that it should be taught
in public lectures." Dr. L. Maurice began his response, "Yes, one
hundred times yes, I absolutely welcome the principle of contraception."[110] These opinions were in addition to the expected responses of the leaders of the neo-Malthusian movement in France
such as Paul Robin and Nelly Roussel, or Odette Laguerre, editor
of the feminist journal *La fronde,* or Madame Severine, who had

earlier debated Charles Richet on the population question in the pages of *Revue philanthropique*.[111]

There were also responses of note in this group from three men who were also to become associated with the eugenics movement in France. One was the famous criminologist Alexandre Lacassagne, professor at the Collège de France and member of the organizing committee of the First International Eugenics Congress, who wrote a two-line response in support of contraception, saying, "it is justified above all for social and sometimes individual reasons."[112] Dr. Just Sicard de Plauzoles, already active in the Ligue des droits de l'homme and who later was to become one of the foremost leaders of the social hygiene movement in the late 1920s and 1930s as well as a strong advocate of eugenics, wrote, "contraception is a right of the woman who must remain free, even if married, to be or not to be a mother." He offered three instances when contraception was advised: "when the 'seed' is bad, when the health of the mother is threatened by pregnancy, and when misery awaits the child."[113] There was also a response from Edouard Toulouse, a psychiatrist whose Association of Sexological Studies led the revival of neo-Malthusianism in the 1930s and became one of the few institutional supports of eugenics in that decade. He cited his recently published book, *Conflits intersexuels et sociaux*, which maintained that

the choosing of motherhood has an immediately favorable consequence for the race. From the moment a wife is no longer blindly subject to the reproductive instinct and she chooses the most opportune moment and circumstances for herself, it is evident that the results obtained must be superior in quality. Children conceived in the best conditions and later better reared have the chance to be healthier and stronger.[114]

Cabanès' referendum thus shows not only the diversity of opinion on the population question, but the pervasive undercurrent of eugenic thought in France at the turn of the century. The strong support for the use of contraception and the potential alliance with those favoring the improvement of the species was to be delayed largely because another, less controversial means of improvement was proposed at the same time: social hygiene.

REGENERATION THROUGH SOCIAL HYGIENE

As if eugenic questions were not made complicated enough by the debate on the population problem, they also became entangled in the growing social hygiene movement at the end of the nineteenth century. Social hygiene grew out of a whole century of medical and public health measures whose scope was broader than concerns for the health of the individual.[115] The link to eugenics came from applying the concept of social hygiene to future generations which was inspired by the growing concern over degeneration in the 1890s.[116] Equally important in the advent of social hygiene was the influence of neo-Lamarckian hereditary ideas, which provided a theoretical explanation of how improvements in health would be passed to future generations. This concept will be discussed further in the next chapter. First it is necessary to examine the emergence of the new social hygiene movement that became closely allied with French eugenics.

Alcoholism

In its simplest sense, social hygiene was the combination of efforts on three major health problems considered separately in France before the turn of the century: alcoholism, tuberculosis, and venereal disease. Although work to combat each was different, they shared many similarities that ultimately permitted those in each field to join forces. One similarity was the view that the specific diseases were part of a general pattern of decline, with the assumption that treatment would bring regeneration. There was also the common view that those medical problems had to be treated in a broader context than that of the individual sufferer who, in the words of the Pasteurian Emile Duclaux,

has become a frightening being because of the millions of disease germs he creates and spreads about him. One must treat him humanely because he suffers, is not responsible and is only a part of the peril he represents. But one has the right to keep him from being a harm to the community.[117]

The medical profession had come to appreciate the need for a greater concern for society as a whole – not just for the individual patient.

Hence, the social hygiene movement, just as the birth control movements earlier, was another example of the call for increased intervention and control over individuals.

Of the three so-called social plagues, alcoholism was the most pervasive and the earliest to generate an organized opposition. As mentioned earlier, the founding of France's first sustained anti-alcoholic effort came shortly after the Franco-Prussian War and the Paris Commune. In 1872, the Association française contre l'abus des boissons alcooliques was created. It changed its rather awkward name the following year to Société française de tempérance.[118] Although the timing indicates political rather than medical reasons for the beginning of the organization, doctors were by far its most prominent constituents. A clear majority of its 500 members in 1878 were doctors, including Théophile Roussel and other such prominent names as Taine and Pasteur.[119] Despite this auspicious beginning, the organization proved to be more an official notice of the problem than the beginning of serious action by either scientists or the general public. An 1873 law against "public drunkenness" hardly struck at the cause of the problem. Another measure of the relative lack of attention is the far smaller number of medical theses dealing with alcoholism at the Ecole de médecine (only 149 between the years 1860 and 1913) than those on such topics as syphilis or tuberculosis.[120] By the early 1890s the Société française de tempérance was, in the words of one scholar, "in a state of moral and financial collapse, its twenty-five-year effort mocked by the rapidly increasing alcohol consumption statistics."[121]

The revival of the anti-alcohol movement at the turn of the century might simply be ascribed to the work of one man, Paul-Maurice Légrain, if the timing did not coincide so neatly with other regeneration movements of the day. Moreover, there are indications of additional interest in the alcohol problem, both in the Academy of Medicine, which formed an alcohol study commission in the late 1880s, and the temperance society itself, which created an annual prize for the best work written on alcoholism and heredity, thanks to a gift from the widow of Jules Lunier, a pioneer in the field of insanity and alcoholism.[122] Légrain, nonetheless, deserves credit for providing the impetus for bringing the alcohol question before the now much more receptive medical and public audiences of the late 1890s.[123]

Légrain's medical credentials were impressive. He was head of the Villejuif asylum, and later the Ville-Evrard asylum, which was the first to specialize in treatment of alcoholics. In 1889, his *Hérédité et l'alcoolisme* established, in his words, "the important consequences of the combination of those two pathogenic factors: alcoholism and heredity."[124] His next book, published in 1895 and entitled *Dégénérescence social et l'alcoolisme,* won the prize given by the temperance society for the best work on the question of "the descendants of alcoholics and the prevention of alcoholism," and marked the beginning of Légrain's new effort to reach a public he described as still "not convinced of the idea that alcoholism is an urgent evil to extinguish."[125] Légrain openly championed efforts to sway public opinion rather than calling for more medical work as the key to solving the problem, and he emphasized the difference in his approach by characterizing the work of the earlier temperance society as "an isolated effort on the problem by a few devotees who are not supported by the current of public opinion."[126]

In the same year that he published *Dégénérescence sociale,* Légrain founded a new temperance society, the Union française antialcoolique, which was much more successful than the earlier organization in reaching a broad audience. Thanks largely to Légrain's administrative and propaganda abilities, by 1905 there were 150 chapters and 40,000 members in the new organization. This success was not lost on some members of the older temperance society who worked to form the Union into an umbrella organization to coordinate the efforts of Légrain and other groups that had sprung up at the same time. In 1903 the Société française de tempérance was renamed the Ligue nationale contre l'alcoolisme, and by 1914 its constituent groups claimed over 125,000 members.[127] Thus, the efforts to combat alcoholism show a pattern of initial but limited activity in the 1870s, followed by a renewal of efforts in the 1890s both to reach a broader public and to cooperate with similar groups working on the problem. The next logical step was to join in efforts to combine an attack on all such social plagues after the turn of the century.

Tuberculosis

Tuberculosis, the second of the three plagues, was less publicized than alcoholism but probably of greater concern to medical practitioners at the end of the nineteenth century. Medical attention was initially aroused by Koch's isolation of the tuberculosis bacillus in the early 1880s, and concern mounted as reporting of the illness generally improved. By the end of the century, tuberculosis was recognized by the head of the Pasteur Institute as "the most widespread of all diseases."[128] In addition, the failure to find a cure was one reason that the disease was looked on with such fatalism by the public. With no simple solution such as abstinence, which was seen as the cure of alcoholism or syphilis, victims seemed to be faced with either quiet acceptance or self-delusion as a recourse. And the gradual decline in the victims' health only added to the feeling of hopelessness. At the same time it offered novelists little of the spectacular action that made patients with delirium tremens one of the mainstays of late nineteenth-century novels and plays about alcoholism.[129]

The nature of tuberculosis helps explain why there was no immediate call in the 1870s for public action against the disease as there had been against alcohol. In 1891, however, a Ligue contre la tuberculose en France was formed with the goal "of putting the question of tuberculosis on the agenda of public preoccupation."[130] As mentioned earlier, the distance members had to go in achieving their goal can be seen in the fact that their first efforts were simply to make declaration of the illness mandatory by doctors. Even this modest objective ran into resistance. For example, the 1900 International Congress of Hygiene in Paris debated at length whether to strengthen a guarded resolution calling for a declaration of tuberculosis in cases where "according to the different laws, it is possible to apply sanitary police measures in order to prohibit the propagation of the disease." In the end the delegates, all of whom were leading authorities on treating the disease, were only willing to vote that "open tuberculosis should be included among the diseases whose reporting is mandatory."[131] In 1903, Léon Bourgeois' new Commission de prophylaxie contre la tuberculose made a similar proposal specifically for France that met with a great deal of opposition from the medical community.

Although it was not until the First World War that there was any success even in a general plan for treatment of patients, the participation of so high ranking a politician as Bourgeois did much to raise public consciousness of the tuberculosis problem to the level of the other two scourges.[132]

Venereal disease

The campaign against the third of the social plagues, venereal disease, was similar in many ways to the campaign against tuberculosis. For example, the founding of an organization to combat syphilis came late (1901), as it did for tuberculosis. There were also a large number of unanswered medical questions about both diseases, in contrast to the small number of questions about alcoholism, which was generally thought to be the result of moral or psychological weakness. These questions directed attention to the medical aspects of venereal disease, and the obvious delicate nature of questions raised by the way it was transmitted hindered open public discussion of venereal disease even more than for tuberculosis.[133]

These problems notwithstanding, the mid-nineteenth century saw one of the earliest health campaigns, at least partly inspired by a desire to control venereal disease, when so-called *maisons de tolérance* were established to regulate prostitution.[134] A subsequent moral crusade against the houses in the 1870s undermined what little control the state could exercise over the health of prostitutes by ending the government's complicity in the "immoral" enterprise. By the time a neo-regulationist movement began pressing for new measures of control at the end of the century, it was part of both an international movement against venereal disease and the broader movement within France for regeneration through social hygiene.

In 1899, an international conference was held in Brussels on the "venereal peril," and included a sizable delegation from France. After many long sessions a new organization, the International Society for Sanitary and Moral Prophylaxis, was formed, with the goal of coordinating all efforts against the affliction. A direct outgrowth of the conference was the founding of a Société française pour la prophylaxie sanitaire et morale in 1901 under the leader-

ship of Alfred Fournier.[135] It would be wrong, however, to see
the origins solely as inspired from outside France. In the founding
statutes of the organization, acknowledgment was made of the
link to other social hygiene movements in France that had served
as models:

This organization is truly a league against syphilis, constituted on the
model of the two other leagues which today so valiantly combat alcoholism and tuberculosis for the benefit of all.[136]

The new anti-venereal organization was similar to the other organizations in its predominantly medical constituency – 75 percent of the 406 founding members were doctors, dentists, or phar-
macists, including many of the founders of the French eugenics
movement.[137] The influence of the organization through members' ties to other groups was considerable. In the words of a
chronicler of the society, it "was from its birth in touch with moral
societies, neo-regulationist medical societies and officials of the
prefectural police. Soon after, its members entered into contact
with the military hierarchy."[138] In fact, he concludes, it was not
just a pressure group for ending venereal disease but the beginning
of a whole new bourgeois attitude toward sex that began to popularize a new notion of "sex education."

The new organization was also helped from its start by the increasing publicity about the problem of syphilis at the turn of the
century in France. An example is *Science et mariage,* a book published in 1900 by the French poet and physician Henri Cazalis that
called for a mandatory medical examination before marriage to
prevent the transmission of tuberculosis and alcoholism as well as
venereal disease.[139] The book was significant in several respects,
but above all because it was timely, given the interest in degeneration and the founding of specific organizations to combat the social ills causing it. In addition, Cazalis, like the anti-venereal organizers, tied all three of the plagues together, one of the defining
elements of the new social hygiene movement. Finally, Cazalis's
idea was appealing in its simplicity; hence, it was easily grasped
by both the medical community and the general public. In June
1900, Pinard presented the book to the Academy of Medicine with
his wish that it could "be in the hands of everyone," especially
newlyweds, to serve as a kind of marriage manual.[140]

The publicity that Cazalis's book received was partly the motivation for Eugène Brieux's play, *Damaged goods* (French title: *Les avaries*), which became even better known and more controversial than the book that inspired it. The work was translated into several languages, with English-language writers such as Upton Sinclair and George Bernard Shaw among its greatest supporters.[141] In the work, which has been called "not a play but an interview with Doctor Fournier set on stage" (a doctor is the main character of the first and last of the three acts in the play), a young man contracts syphilis on the eve of his marriage to the daughter of a deputy. Although counseled to wait three years by his doctor, the man takes a quick cure elsewhere. When a syphilitic child is born to the couple, the deputy visits the original doctor, who suggests all kinds of laws that could be passed. These include creation of a public health office to combat syphilis, the prohibition of "the manufacture of poisonous liquors," and the elimination of tuberculosis by "paying sufficient wages and having unsanitary workmen's dwellings knocked down." In a not so subtle reference to Cazalis, Brieux has the deputy complain, "In this case it is for you to show the way. These are matters for scientific experts. You must begin by pointing out the necessary measures, and then . . ." But the doctor interrupts, "And then what? Ha! It is fifteen years since a scheme of this kind, worked out and approved unanimously by the Academy of Medicine, was submitted to the proper authorities. Since that day it has never been heard of again."[142]

Like Brieux's earlier play *Maternité, Damaged goods* was initially censored in France. It was written in 1901 but banned while in rehearsal. The following year it was staged in Belgium, where the controversy only added to its appeal.[143] By the time it was allowed back in France, the play had made such an impact that one contemporary noted, "It has done more by itself in three acts of the play than all the hygienists together in fifty years."[144]

The Brieux play stimulated discussion of venereal disease in medical journals as well as the general press. For example, the *Bulletin* of the Société de prophylaxie sanitaire et morale carried a running debate among its members about "Sanitary guarantees of marriage" in five of its seven issues from June to December 1903.[145] Brieux's work also inspired other writers to deal with similar subjects. In fact, something of a medico–social literary genre developed both in France and the United States, with such writers as André Couvreur, Michel Corday, and the Margueritte brothers "openly and enthusiastically acknowledging Brieux as a leader."[146] The most influential of these emulations was Couvreur's *La graine,* which had been the subject of one of Cabanès' surveys of opinion in the *Chronique médicale* in July 1903.[147]

Couvreur had already written other novels dramatizing certain effects of the social plagues on their victims, but in *La graine* he shifted his attention to tuberculosis, and, more significantly, he followed Brieux's example of showing the hereditary effects of the disease on subsequent generations. This time Cabanès sent questions to forty authors, doctors, and others about the general concept of responsibility in hereditary pathology and the specific suggestion of Cazalis that a premarital examination could solve the problem. On the latter question Cabanès asked, "What do you think of an inquiry about the health status of those intending to marry, and in what effective form could it be demanded of parents?" The responses indicated that all agreed there was parental responsibility for hereditary effects on future generations; but the question of a premarital exam drew a more mixed reaction. Ten responses strongly favored it by law, and an equal number was opposed (curiously enough including Couvreur himself), with the majority either raising practical objections, or expressing a preference for voluntary exams and better information being made available to couples.

CONCLUSION

More important than the specific results of Cabanès's inquiry was the increasing attention that was being paid to previously unrelated problems that were now seen to be part of a larger concern. Hence, social hygiene represented a frame of reference halfway between the narrow focus on specific diseases and the broad, vague concern with degeneration. In addition, there was now the beginning of debate on a remedy involving increased government monitoring of marriage and procreation. Serious consideration of these measures was to be delayed for twenty years before it was vigorously pursued by the French Eugenics Society, but the idea that the French population was threatened by several, similar biological disorders that menaced existing and future generations was more quickly institutionalized in a new social hygiene organization, the Alliance d'hygiene sociale.

Founding dates for such an eclectic movement are difficult to establish. Emile Duclaux, director of the Pasteur Institute, was among the earliest to give currency to the new concept of social hygiene in a series of lectures he delivered at the Ecole des hautes-études sociales in early 1902 that were published later that year as *Hygiène sociale*.[148] In January 1904, many of the participants in the recently founded leagues against the social plagues described here met at the Musée social in Paris to create a Social Hygiene Alliance whose founding statutes declared as its goal, "coordinating and seconding the efforts made in favor of social hygiene in France." The statutes went on to explain that the alliance "proposes to fight tuberculosis, alcoholism, infantile mortality, etc."[149] The organization began publishing a journal, and in July 1904 the first Social Hygiene Congress was held in Arras, followed by annual meetings before the war in such places as Montpellier, Nancy, and Lyons.[150]

There was much confusion at the start about what distinguished social hygiene from public health, a concept that had taken most of the nineteenth century to become established. It required some time before a neat theoretical distinction could be made such as the one offered at the Eleventh Social Hygiene Congress in 1921:

Public hygiene is the collection of measures in a country which aims at the general health and at the same time the defense of individuals and the collectivity against the risks of sickness and death. . . . Social hygiene has higher and further aims. Its objectives surpass the simple preservation of the race and extend to its constant improvement, to its perfection. It attacks, for example, diseases of a special order: tuberculosis, syphilis, and alcoholism which affect the individual and his descendents.[151]

The importance attributed to heredity will be shown later to be a reflection of the influence that eugenics had come to exercise on the social hygiene movement by the 1920s. But as this chapter has shown, social hygiene was only one of a variety of movements at the turn of the century that aimed at a biological regeneration of France. The natalists, neo-Malthusians, and even the solidarists also based their claims on biology, which made them potential allies of the eugenicists. The manner in which they became part of the eugenics movement, and especially the theoretical underpinnings that made it possible, will be examined in greater detail in the next chapter.

3

From puericulture to eugenics

Why was there a thirty to forty-year wait between Galton's first formulation of eugenic ideas and the creation of formal eugenics organizations? As Chapter 2 has shown, there was no lack of awareness that France faced many problems associated with decline and decadence at the end of the nineteenth century; and there were in fact many proposals to remedy them on a biological basis. Some proposals, such as the solidarism of Léon Bourgeois, soon moved away from their scientific origins to assume a more clearly political character, but others, such as the social hygiene movement, developed along strikingly similar lines to eugenics. As will be seen in this chapter, hereditarian ideas were also well enough known in these biologically based reform circles to produce several proposals of an explicit eugenic nature. For example, as early as 1862 Clémence Royer called in the preface to her translation of Darwin's *Origin of species* for allowing natural selection to do its job of eliminating "the weak, the infirm, the incurable, the wicked themselves and all the disgraces of nature."[1] The French also had available at an early date in their own language a contemporary study similar to Galton's *Hereditary genius,* thanks to the work of the Swiss botanist Alphonse Candolle, whose *Histoire des sciences et savants* appeared in 1873.[2]

The important point here is not the question of priority, but rather why it took so long in both the English and French-speaking worlds for these studies about the inheritance of superior intellectual qualities to inspire organized eugenic movements. The answer is not that it took time for people to see the logical connection between hereditary genius and the need for eugenic measures. In France there was widespread discussion, shortly after the appearance of both Galton's and Candolle's works, of elaborate eugenics proposals by Georges Vacher de Lapouge and others in

France who sought to make human evolution more rational by such measures as selective breeding.[3] In fact, discussion of eugenics in the period before 1900 was so common that when added to the public and social hygiene movements described in Chapter 2, it shows that there must have been other reasons for the delay in establishing eugenics movements. This chapter suggests that for France the answer lies in the marginal nature of the early proponents of eugenics and their lack of institutional support.

To underscore the importance of the question, it is worth noting that even in Germany and the Anglo-Saxon countries there was a delay before formal eugenics organizations were created – 1905 in Germany and 1908 in Galton's homeland, England. This suggests that there may have been something beyond the ebb and flow of confidence and despair in the public mood, or in the nature of hereditary theory (be it Lamarckian or Mendelian), that might explain the delay. For France, it appears that another difficulty was the very breadth of ideas subsumed under eugenics. For if its broad self-defined scope added to the potential appeal of eugenics, the movement also faced difficulties in drawing the diverse elements together. After all, one could work for the betterment of future generations without necessarily calling it eugenics. Nor was there any compelling reason for those in temperance societies to consult or identify with natalists, even though they shared some common assumptions and goals. Before considering how a eugenics theory that provided a common identity and framework for such activities was constructed, this chapter will examine the fate of Vacher de Lapouge and other precursors who anticipated many of the ideas of later eugenicists, but who lacked the position in society or the resources to put their ideas into effect. Their experience is a reminder that theory was not enough.

EUGENIC PRECURSORS

There is a certain irony in the fact that a woman, Clémence Royer, was among the first in France to describe what might be called the "eugenic" consequences of Darwinian evolution.[4] Women were obviously equals in the process of determining the quality of offspring (even more so according to some neo-Lamarckians), yet their social and political status was that of inferiors. Throughout the history of French eugenics, women participated only marginally in debates and discussions despite the fact that virtually all the proposals involved them intimately.[5] Royer was unusual in that she had a forum for expressing her ideas, thanks to her translation of Darwin's *Origin of species*. She was also a member of the Paris Anthropological Society, which gave her additional opportunities to discuss these questions, otherwise exclusively a male domain.

In the preface to Darwin's book, Royer observed that by society's protecting weak, infirm, and incurable individuals, "the evils they carry tend to perpetuate and multiply indefinitely." Meanwhile, the best elements are decimated by war, dangerous work, and daring exploits. What is worse, she went on,

while all the virile youth spends the most lively of its forces on prostitutes, it is the old men, sickly and exhausted, who found the new generations. They endow both sexes with the germ of the diseases which have struck them after having inherited them from their fathers who perhaps owe them to the vices of a youth passed breaking the laws of nature.[6]

Royer admitted that marriage involved selection, but for the wrong reasons. "The ideal man of the times is he who produces; the ideal woman is she who conserves and saves." The result of these choices, she concluded, "can only produce men of lucre and women of vanity." As a remedy, Royer proposed changes that were obviously based on her own experiences:

One should demand of women a part of what has until now only been demanded of men: that is, force united with beauty, intelligence combined with gentleness, and of men a little idealism combined with power of spirit and rigor of body.[7]

Despite the sharpness of her criticisms, Royer was in no position to rally followers around these proposals to control human evolution. This was not only because she was a woman in a male-dominated world, but also because her position as the earliest proponent of Darwinian evolution in France left her open to charges of being *plus royaliste que le roi*.[8] After Royer elaborated her ideas in an 1870 book, *L'Origine de l'homme et des sociétés*, Paul Broca attacked her position, especially the idea of eliminating the weak through a "struggle for existence." Referring to Royer by name, Broca admitted that she might be correct in her observation that "social selection" produced a lower average of humans than "natural selection," but he argued that the best elements would be superior. Moreover, he pointed out that the average of the species could only be raised in two ways – "either by eliminating the weak or by perfecting them. Nature followed the first procedure, civilization follows the second."[9] Hence, Broca's opposition undercut support from anthropologists for the radical proposals of Royer's.

Another example of eugenic ideas that failed to attract a following came from Ernest Tarbouriech, a law professor at the Collège des sciences sociales. In his book, *La cité future,* published in 1902, Tarbouriech called for sterilization of degenerates, mandatory reporting of pregnancy by women, and state support for rearing undesirable children.[10] These ideas, based on suggestions first made by Paolo Mantegazza in *L'anno 3000,* were largely ignored for three reasons. First, they were part of a much larger utopian scheme aimed at a scientific ordering of society to achieve social justice; hence, they were not expressed in a practical form for immediate implementation. Second, many of the elements were seen as excessively harsh. For example, although the neo-Malthusian journal *Régénération* welcomed Tarbouriech's rational approach to reproduction, its editors disliked the authoritarian flavor of the book.[11] Third, Tarbouriech was not a major social theorist with a large following, and he soon became occupied with his duties as secretary of the new Ligue des droits de l'homme. Although he was elected a socialist deputy in 1910, he died the following year at the age of forty-seven.

In the same category of marginal thinkers with eugenic schemes was an engineer from Bordeaux named Alfred Pichou who in 1896 proposed the creation of an organization to be called "The Elite." This "philanthropic association for the conservation of life and improvement of the human species" was a step beyond Royer's or Tarbouriech's ideas because of its highly structured organizational framework that perhaps reflected the engineer's mentality. This included provisions for local committees and cantonal representatives to select the Elite, as well as a board of directors in Paris to coordinate the work of the cantonal groups. Although Pichou's choice of language was extreme (he called for "a humanity absolutely regenerated"), his proposals were milder and more democratic than the name of the organization implied. Stripped of its rhetoric and elaborate organizational structure, Pichou's idea was simply to identify "those beings not yet afflicted with physical degeneration, hereditary defects, and transmissible illnesses," so that this part of the population could intermarry and "maintain its healthy state by a rational practice of hygiene."[12]

Pichou justified his division of humanity into two groups as a necessary evil because, in his words, "what retards the evolution of the mass is the stragglers – that is, those of weak constitution, the lazy." Potential conflict between the two would be mitigated by "the principle of solidarity between all beings who compose the human species [which] imposes duties for the Elected on behalf of the unfortunates separated from the Elite."[13] What is most significant about Pichou, however, is that after the turn of the century he managed to attract national attention with his ideas, both in Cabanès' *Chronique médicale* and in René Worms' *Revue internationale de sociologie*. Pichou's ideas and the attention they received were a signal of the broad interest in degeneration and the means of remedying it at the time, but they were not the inspiration for the beginning of an organized eugenics movement in France.[14]

The most extraordinary precursor to French eugenics was the work of Georges Vacher de Lapouge, a fascinating character who has recently received a great deal of attention from scholars.[15] Not only were his ideas controversial, but his active working life stretched over fifty years, giving him ample opportunity to influence French and other thinkers in the tumultuous years from the 1880s to the 1930s. Adding to the interest in Lapouge is the fact that his lavish praise of Aryans was picked up by European and American racists of the 1930s. As a result, he has usually been associated with the extreme right-wing of European politics that emerged at the end of the nineteenth century.[16]

Recent work has shown, however, that Lapouge's life and work were more complex than these long-held views suggest. His overt political activity, for example, was very limited – and for a time surprisingly left-wing. While at Montpellier in the late 1880s and early 1890s he joined the Parti ouvrier français of Paul Lafargue, and even ran for municipal office in 1888 and 1892, albeit unsuccessfully.[17] Only after the turn of the century did he give up his socialist self-identification, and he never again participated directly in politics.

Lapouge's active working life was spent as a librarian at Rennes

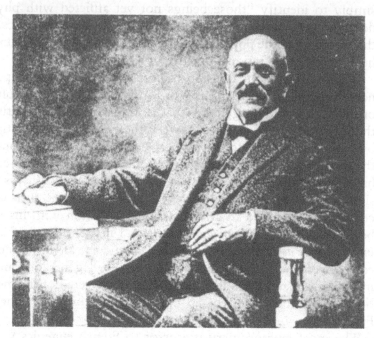

Figure 3.1   Georges Vacher de Lapouge, in a rare existing photo.
[Source: Jean Boissel, "Georges Vacher de Lapouge: un socialiste révolutionnaire darwinien," *Nouvelle école*, 38 (1982)]

and Poitiers as well as Montpellier, and like most provincial French
intellectuals, his greatest desire was to return to Paris with an academic appointment.[18] On one important occasion in his career,
Lapouge sought to dissociate himself from Drumont's extreme
anti-Semitism of the 1890s. This was only for the technical reason
that unlike Drumont, Lapouge considered Jews to be dolichocephalic (long-headed) – like the Aryans. In fact, he strongly opposed any mixing of the two groups, and was hardly flattering to
the Jews in his book, *L'aryen et son rôle social,* which appeared at
the height of the Dreyfus affair.[19]

   Although employed as a librarian and best known as a racist
ideologue, Lapouge considered himself, above all, a scientist. He
spent most of his free time at Montpellier and Poitiers collecting
skulls, studying human anatomy, and working on the most time-
consuming of his projects: a study of beetles, drawing on a collection that eventually reached 25,000 specimens collected over forty

years. Lapouge gave very concrete expression in 1909 to this self-image as a scholar, when he applied for a chair at the Museum of Natural History despite his limited formal training or connections with the anthropological or biological establishment. Moreover, he had hardly endeared himself to the political leaders of the Third Republic by the publication the same year of his book *Race et milieu* whose preface urged replacement of the national slogan "Liberty, Equality, Fraternity" with "Determinism, Inequality, Selection."[20]

What concerns us here is not Lapouge's political or scientific credentials but rather his eugenic ideas, which were among the earliest, most original, and at the time most elaborate of any proposed in France or elsewhere before the turn of the century. His proposals, beginning in the 1880s, also contained an appreciation of the possible far-reaching consequences of Darwin's and Galton's ideas on heredity and human selection. For example, in remarks to a *cours libre* he gave in 1886 at Montpellier on "Anthropology and Political Science," Lapouge made a promise:

To end the course I will reveal the theory of Mr. Galton on eugenics – the laws which regulate the production, the conservation and the propagation of superior families, the heart of any race – and which can, by a wise selection, permit the substitution of a superior humanity in the future for the humanity of today.[21]

As set forth in ensuing years, Lapouge's version of eugenics repeated some of the criticisms of dysgenic practices first identified by Clémence Royer. He listed no less than six different "social" selections that he claimed were causing the degeneration of the species by interfering with "natural" selection: military, political, religious, moral, legal, and economic.[22] Mixed in were borrowings from some of the common notions about degenerative influences mentioned in Chapter 2, such as the evils of alcohol, which Lapouge called "the most formidable of degenerative agents." He also issued an early warning of the pending depopulation of France.[23] If these ideas on degeneration were unoriginal, no less so were Lapouge's criteria for superiority, which amounted to little more than the Aryanism of Gobineau as manifested by the craniometric measures of Gall and Spurzheim. His simplistic use of the cephalic index, and reverence for "dolicho-blonds" of Germany, Scandinavia, England, and the United States, are of little intellectual interest except as an explanation for the unpopularity of his ideas in France and their later identification with Nazi raciologues.

The most original element of Lapouge's eugenics was not his identification of the causes of degeneration, nor his definition of the superior humanity for which he strove, but rather the means he proposed to achieve that superiority. The key to this part of his eugenics program, as described in *Sélections sociales,* was use of the technique of artificial insemination [*fécondation artificielle*], which Lapouge outlined as follows:

It would be the substitution of breeding and scientific reproduction for bestial and spontaneous reproduction, the definitive dissociation of three elements already in the process of separation: love, sensual pleasure and fertility. Operating under controlled conditions, a very small number of males of absolute perfection would suffice to inseminate all the females worthy of perpetuating the race, and the generation thus produced would be of a value proportional to the most rigorous choice of reproductive males. In fact, sperm can be diluted in several alkaline liquids without it losing its properties. One thousandth solution in an appropriate medium is effective in a dose of two cubic centimeters injected into the uterus. Minerva replacing Eros, a single reproducer in a good state of health would suffice to assure 200,000 births annually.[24]

Lapouge even claimed to have experimented with the procedure himself, indicating that sperm could be transported without harm. "I obtained at Montpellier," he indicated, "an insemination with sperm sent from Beziers by mail, and later even without the protection of a sterilizer." Jean Rostand has praised this work of Lapouge as the first experiment of "telegenesis" – that is, insemination at a distance.[25]

Lapouge's eugenics, in addition to the extent and originality of its measures, was also noteworthy in the short run because it attracted much more attention than the intermittent notice given by a few national journals to Pichou's ideas. Lapouge's articles appeared in the major French anthropological publications from the mid-1880s to the mid-1890s, as well as in new social science journals such as René Worms' *Revue international de sociologie,* Charles Gide's *Revue d'économie politique,* and Emile Durkheim's *Année sociologique.*[26]

Given this well-publicized eugenics program, it is a fair question to ask why it did not usher in a eugenics movement that would have preceded even those in Anglo-Saxon countries. The most obvious answer seems not to be the extreme nature of Lapouge's proposals. Although artificial insemination was hardly an idea calculated to win the hearts of the masses, equally radical measures were to enjoy a limited following throughout the entire history of the French Eugenics Society. A better and simpler explanation appears to be that the ideas were identified too closely with Lapouge himself. Thus, by the end of the 1890s, which was precisely the time when concern over degeneration and the search for regenerative measures were gaining wide currency, Lapouge had managed to make his position of outsider into one of persona non grata in French intellectual circles. Criticisms of Lapouge have been covered in some detail elsewhere.[27] Of note here is the fact that Lapouge fits the pattern of the classic outsider – despite the extent of his writings and the extraordinary publicity they received, his lack of resources and an official position was a crucial problem for him, as it was for the other precursors of eugenics in France before 1912. Lapouge could not be in more striking contrast to his contemporaries who were developing a different basis for a French eugenics movement. They were led by the least threatening of proponents – an obstetrician. The word they chose to describe their work was even different: not Galton's Greek-based term eugenics, meaning "well-born," but the Latin-based "puericulture," meaning childrearing.

PUERICULTURE BEFORE BIRTH

The word puericulture was coined by Alfred Caron, a Paris physician of the Second Empire whose interest in the health of newborns "from the point of view of improving the species" was first expressed in an 1858 paper read before the Société de médicine pratique. In 1865 he used the term puericulture in a short pamphlet and a course he was authorized to teach by the ministry of public instruction entitled "The education of young children and puericulture." A second, greatly expanded edition of the pamphlet appeared the following year. Despite the favorable climate of medical opinion – at this time the groundwork was being laid for the passage of the Roussel Law regulating wet-nursing in 1874 – Caron's new concept was not widely adopted.[28]

One indication of why Caron's idea failed to catch on can be seen in the refusal to allow him to speak on puericulture at a meeting in Paris of provincial learned societies in 1865. The presiding officer of the conference explained that he "could not open the floor to this question which would [only] provide hilarity at the meeting."[29] Other indications, however, are that the idea failed more from lack of interest than from the ridicule for applying agricultural terminology to human beings. For example, writing in 1906, Victor Wallich of the Ecole de médecine in Paris claimed that the sole copy of Caron's 1866 book in the library of the medical school had not only been judged unworthy of being bound, but the page galleys had not even been cut.[30] Although Littré included "puericulture" in his 1865 *Dictionnaire* (with the curt definition, "the art of raising children") the 1889 *Dictionnaire encyclopédique des sciences médicales* by Jaccoud and Dechambre ignored it, and there was no heading for the topic in the *Index catalogue* of the Library of the Surgeon General or *Index medicus* before the turn of the century. When Pinard revived the word in a talk at the Academy of Medicine in 1895, puericulture was thus only a distant memory that brought smiles to the faces of some older doctors in the audience.[31]

Adolphe Pinard came to the concept from his experience as head of the Baudelocque Clinic, a position he held simultaneously with his appointment to the chair of clinical obstetrics at the Ecole de médecine beginning in 1889. He began his work at a time of tremendous medical advance in the care of childbearing mothers and their newborns. For example, his mentor Etienne Tarnier had recently discovered antiseptic delivery as a means of preventing childbed fever, the leading cause of death in childbirth throughout most of the nineteenth century.[32] In fact, the high mortality rate of childbearing was the very reason that Wallich gave for the lack of interest in Caron's puericulture, because in the 1860s and 70s it was thought that there were too many fundamental problems of life and death to be solved before doctors could turn their attention to "the science of raising children." In addition to delivery procedures, palpitation in prenatal examinations for early diagnosis and more frequent use of cesarean delivery helped solve other problems of difficult pregnancies. The use of symphysiotomy also began to replace the more drastic embryotomy (dissection of the fetus) in difficult labor, and gastrointestinal problems in bottle-fed newborns were greatly reduced at the time by the use of sterilized bottles.[33] The adoption of these obstetric practices lowered the mortality rate of mothers in child delivery from between 10 and 15 percent during the first part of the nineteenth century, to between 2 and 3 percent at the end. At Baudelocque, Pinard boasted of only a 0.5 percent mortality rate in 1897.[34]

Because of these advances, it was much easier for Pinard – along with Tarnier's other celebrated pupil, Pierre Budin – to focus more attention on the conditions of the infant at the end of the century. Budin's efforts concentrated on improving the feeding of newborns,[35] and although part of Pinard's program included the encouragement of breast-feeding, his focus was to become much broader, eventually encompassing all possible elements affecting the health of the newborn.

One of the major effects of the work of Budin and Pinard, despite their different approaches, was a shift of attention away from the mother toward the child. This could take the form of advocating sacrifices by mothers, such as extending the period of breast-feeding and, as Pinard was to advocate, requiring a rest period for women during pregnancy. Some scholars have drawn the conclusion that this was the result of a negative view of women, a valid one in the sense that Pinard's ideas reflected traditional male attitudes of the day. For example, when Pinard first advocated a premarital exam, he assumed it would only be needed for men because they determined the moment of sexual intercourse. His call for mothers to stay with newborn infants as long as possible might also be interpreted in this manner, but it would be more accurate to describe this apparent lack of concern for the mother as overconcern for the infant. Pinard also provoked criticism because of certain features of his style of argument: his tendency to carry ideas to a logical conclusion, his single-mindedness, and his knack of expressing ideas in terms that all could understand. For example, one of the slogans he often repeated – "the mother's milk belongs to the infant" – was posted (along with others) on the walls of the Baudelocque Clinic. Pinard's concern with the health of infants was part of a general increase in attention to the infant that scholars such as Philip Ariés have found throughout European society during the nineteenth century. This may explain public receptivity of Pinard's ideas, but the timing of that increased attention by the medical community seems better explained by the advances in obstetrics than the vague waves of sentiment some authors describe as sweeping across Europe.[36]

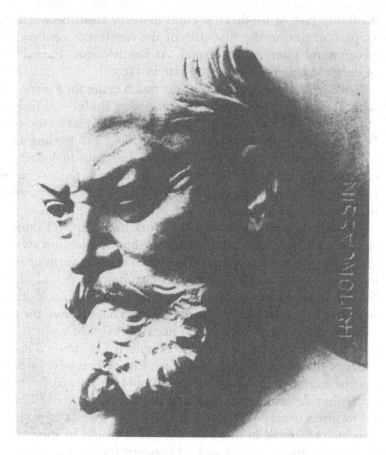

Figure 3.2   Marble bust of Adolphe Pinard, Amphitheater of Ecole de Puericulture. [Source: Roger Couvelaire, "Epigrammes familiales et violons imaginaires" (unpublished manuscript)]

It was not long after Pinard took over Baudelocque that he began to see childbirth from this different perspective. As he himself admitted, his initial goal was to make the conditions in the clinic as good as those in the Parisian hospitals, so that "there is not one method of child delivery for the rich and one method of child delivery for the poor."[37] By the end of 1890, however, he was already aware that there was a problem of availability as well as quality of care. He reported that more clinics were needed, and acknowledged the general principle that any pregnant woman had the right to medical care before and during childbirth. Pinard even went so far as to call for the construction of nurseries adjacent to the obstetrical clinics so that mothers could stay longer with their newborns under the care and supervision of medical personnel.[38]

Given Pinard's position and his published views, he soon made the acquaintance of influential Parisian philanthropists and reformers such as the natalist Paul Strauss and Marie Bequet de Vienne. The latter had founded a Society for Maternal Nursing, and in 1892 with Pinard's assistance she started a *maison maternelle* on the Avenue Maine as a "refuge or asylum for pregnant women." At the same time, Strauss convinced his fellow members on the Paris City Council to establish a similar refuge on the Rue Tolbiac.[39] These refuges were intended as a way station for women who had nowhere else to stay during pregnancy, but one unintended result of their operation was the discovery of information that directly inspired the revival of puericulture.

From the already established procedure of carefully weighing newborns, Pinard noticed a higher average birth weight for the children born of mothers who had stayed at the refuge. This was entirely counter to common expectations, because the whole point of the refuges was to help those women in the direst of circumstances. Accordingly, their babies were not expected to weigh as much as the babies of mothers who did not need assistance. Pinard attributed the difference to the fact that the women in the refuge were, of necessity, "rested and cared for" during a measurable period of time before delivery. He carefully selected a control group to test his hypothesis, and after three years of work he presented his findings to the Academy of Medicine. Pinard titled his report "Intrauterine Puericulture," and it compared the birth weights of 500 children born to women who had spent at least ten days at the refuge with the birth weights of 500 children born to women coming directly to Baudelocque who had worked until the onset of labor. Pinard found an average of 280 grams difference between the two.[40] Anticipating questions about the possible higher incidence of premature births as an explanation of the lower birth weight in the second group, he went further to attempt to determine the length of time children were carried before birth. In an imprecise measure, he estimated the length of time from the mother's last menstrual period, assuming that the chance for error was equal in both groups, and found that those who stayed in the refuge did carry children significantly longer. Over 66 percent of rested mothers carried babies more than 280 days compared with 48.2 percent for the other group. Likewise, there was almost double the chance of giving birth before 270 days (23.9 percent compared with 12.6 percent) for women working until the onset of delivery.

Today these findings seem almost banal, but they were a revelation at the time for Pinard, which directly inspired his revival of puericulture. In a November 1895 report to the Academy of Medicine, Pinard ended simply by stating, "This data indicates to us all that we must do if we want a strong and vigorous population," a conclusion that was not elaborated upon the following month when he presented the same findings to the Société de la médecine publique et l'hygiène professionelle.[41] But another report of the findings, written for his colleague Charles Richet's *Revue scientifique* early in 1896, revealed a significant change in Pinard's view of pregnancy and childbirth, when he concluded that

if the infants are bigger from the rested [women] than the overburdened, it is simply because their intra-uterine life was not troubled and their incubation was complete. They came out because they were ripe for extrauterine life. For the others, expulsed prematurely, the overwork is the wind that makes the unripened fruit fall.[42]

Pinard's agricultural allusions were obvious and deliberate, even though their clumsiness is part of the reason for the ridicule Caron's ideas had suffered earlier. This did not bother Pinard, who soon went on to expand his theory of puericulture into two stages – intrauterine and extrauterine – to describe the need for the care of both fetuses in utero and newborns. In addition to its obvious appeal to the nursing and infant care professions (which will be discussed later), the idea had great appeal to the medical and general public, particularly those concerned with problems of degeneration.[43] For example, when Pinard mentioned syphilis and alcohol as two particularly negative influences on newborns, he gave added ammunition to the new temperance and anti-venereal organizations described in Chapter 2. Puericulture also focused attention on the problem of infant mortality, and Pinard immediately became a hero in natalist circles. Paul Strauss quickly utilized the work of Pinard and his students at Baudelocque in a campaign for compulsory maternity leaves. A 1900 article by Strauss made clear how puericulture fit into the goals of the campaign:

It protects mothers from sickness, accidents and avoidable crimes, and it insures the child against the dangers and risks of its uncertain life. In the state of armed peace and the economic rivalry of nations, it constitutes the strongest and surest work for national defense.[44]

Now that it had become a patriotic cause, puericulture was quick to receive official governmental recognition when Pinard was named to the Senate Commission on Depopulation in 1902, where he was given the specific task of preparing a report on the causes of infant mortality. In 1906, Wallich claimed that "the word puericulture has by now entered common parlance. Everyone uses it; it is understood by all."[45]

The impact of puericulture also spread far beyond the borders of France through publications and international meetings. In 1900, Pinard and two others gave talks on puericulture at the Tenth International Congress on Health and Demography held in Paris in conjunction with the World's Fair; and Pinard presided over the meetings of a section on school education at the Third International Congress on School Hygiene in Paris in 1910. Although the impact appears to have been less on Anglo-Saxon countries – perhaps the translation of puericulture as "infant management" did not have the same ring – journals and eventually organizations of puericulture were founded in many French and Spanish-speaking countries. Belgium made the teaching of puericulture mandatory even before France; and the 1910 congress on school hygiene passed a resolution urging teachers to be trained in three aspects of puericulture so that the subject could be taught in all girls schools.[46] The 1909 *Index catalogue* of the Surgeon General listed several books and dozens of articles on puericulture in countries outside France, including Spain, Rumania, the United States, Belgium, Italy, and Mexico.[47]

PUERICULTURE AND HEREDITY

Despite its rapid and wide acceptance, puericulture would have been little more than a call for prenatal care and breast feeding without its hereditarian underpinnings. Producing healthy babies is a goal so obvious and uncontroversial as to be uninteresting. This is perhaps another reason why Caron's puericulture of the 1860's and Pinard's first mention of the concept made audiences smile. Pinard's puericulture, however, soon added the element of heredity, which connected the well-being of the infant not just to the health of the pregnant mother but to previous generations and those yet unborn. This made it far more complex and powerful than Caron's innocuous child-rearing platitudes. Pinard first mentioned heredity in 1899, when he advanced the idea of "puericulture before procreation," as an additional phase in the development of the infant that took into account "the dominant influence of the procreators."[48] Pinard understood heredity to be neo-Lamarckian – involving the hereditary transmission of acquired characteristics – which meant that newborns were subject to all sorts of environmental influences, both past and present. Thus, if infant health was the sympathetic focus drawing many diverse interests to puericulture, neo-Lamarckian heredity provided the theoretical link that held them together.

The most obvious reason why Pinard took heredity into consideration and Caron did not is that they lived in different times. The rising importance of theories of degeneration and debates sparked by Darwin's work made the 1890s quite different from the 1850s. This does not mean that there was universal agreement on exactly how heredity worked, but by the end of the century few ignored its importance.[49] The particular way in which the question of heredity was debated in France had a great influence on both puericulture and French eugenics. But in order to appreciate that influence, it is necessary to view the debate from a broad perspective so as not to miss the underlying inspirations for the ideas as well as their impact on society as a whole.

The fact is that by the end of the nineteenth century, intellectuals as well as the general public attached a great deal of importance to hereditarian ideas, which were not merely the subject of esoteric debates by men in overstuffed leather chairs, smoking cigars in learned societies, or the privileged topic of discussion in exclusive academies of medicine and science. Heredity had always been an everyday, commonsense idea about which all could have an opinion. After Darwin it was even better publicized, and a frequent subject of the literature and press of the day. When added to the wide current of opinion in France and Europe at the end of the nineteenth century that saw decadence and decline in biological terms, the question of inheritance became all the more important, despite disagreements on the exact nature of the hereditary mechanism.

Until the nineteenth century there had been little questioning of classical or folk explanations of inheritance.[50] The latter were usually based on limited personal observations of physical traits in successive generations – everyone has an opinion about whom a new baby resembles – as well as less tangible features such as intelligence and personality. Legal traditions concerning inheritance, such as primogeniture, were not based on any profound understanding of male versus female inheritance or the different predispositions of first-born versus later-born children. Instead, they were the result of practical economic or historical circumstances, patriarchal traditions, prowess in arms, or the necessity to keep landholdings intact.

Theoretical explanations until well into the nineteenth century were still largely based on tradition. Aristotle's idea that genital secretions were formed in each parent by emanations from the different organs of the body that were mixed in the uterus to produce the embryo was essentially the same as Darwin's, Galton's, and Haeckel's view of the hereditary mechanism, although each used different terminology. Galton probably made the most elaborate empirical refinement of these notions in the extensive calculations supporting his "law of ancestral heredity," which assumed a blending of equal proportions of characteristics from parents, grandparents, and other preceding generations.[51] Livestock and plant breeders may have had different experiences, but until the rediscovery of Mendel's work, no new theory was offered to explain their inductive results, which could be applied to human heredity.

Despite their common features, these ideas were still contradictory about what characteristics were inherited or how they might be modified. This, in turn, only added to the discussions about heredity. By far the best example of popular interest in the subject during the last half of the nineteenth century in France was the work of Emile Zola, mentioned in Chapter 2. His description of the pervasive decadence in the Rougon-Macquart series was crucially linked to hereditarian ideas. The major literary purpose served by Zola's depiction of heredity was as a broad plot device in the novels. Heredity not only provided a biological link for the characters of the various novels, but, like the Fates and gods of Greek mythology, it also determined much of these characters' destiny, which circumstances and human will could modify only within limits. This meant that certain of the characters' hereditary traits were fixed, even though it could not predict just when and where these traits would appear. This uncertainty added to the novels' literary appeal, but the lack of predictable hereditary laws was not purely Zola's choice. Rather, it reflected the lack of knowledge at the time about the workings of heredity.[52]

The outline Zola worked from was simple. He accepted Prosper Lucas's division of the laws of inheritance into a "law of innateness" and a "law of heredity." The law of innateness caused Zola the most trouble with his scientific critics because it presupposed a continuous element (foreshadowing August Weissmann's germ plasm), which was strongly attacked in France as being counter to the inheritance of acquired characteristics. The law of heredity was more in tune with this neo-Lamarckian view, and contained four facets: direct (resemblance to parents); indirect (resemblance to an aunt, uncle, or cousins) recapitulative (atavism); and heredity of influence.[53] As for the kinds of traits inherited, Zola included both physical and moral features. Other notions he accepted that were common in the mid-nineteenth century included preformation, and the tendency of sons to inherit physical traits from the father and moral traits from the mother. All kinds of dispositions and passions were presumed to be inheritable, such as alcoholism, sexual passion, propensity to crime, and mental illness (especially from the mother). For example, among the most important influences on heredity that was to become an important part of French eugenics was the physical and psychological state of the mother and the father at the time of conception, with drunkenness or physical coercion being two common causes of negative traits.[54]

If this description of the workings of heredity seems unclear, Zola's attempt to summarize things through his character of Dr. Pascal was even more confused.[55] Rather than faulting Zola, however, one should see in Pascal a reflection of the crosscurrents of scientific opinions of the day. The most influential presupposition about puericulture and eugenics in France was the neo-Lamarckian idea of the influence of environment on heredity.

Although it has become fashionable to fault the French for their attachment to the idea that acquired characteristics were inherited, at the turn of the century this represented by far the most widely held scientific and popular belief in Europe and the United States.[56] One reason for the predominance of neo-Lamarckism was its broad appeal. In many ways French society got the hereditary theory it desired. As will be seen, the inheritance of acquired characteristics was optimistic in its prospects for change, democratic in its assumptions of applicability, and supportive of work in health and social reform. Hence, it tied in well with the broader political and social ideas of the Third Republic (as was the case later with Lysenkoism in the Soviet Union). Thus, with reinforcement in the broader social and intellectual community, it became much more difficult to challenge neo-Lamarckism within the scientific community.[57]

NEO-LAMARCKIAN HEREDITY AND PUERICULTURE BEFORE PROCREATION

Pinard first addressed the question of heredity in an 1899 article in the *Bulletin médical* entitled "On the preservation and improvement of the species," which in turn was taken from his opening lecture to interns at the Baudelocque Clinic on November 7, 1898.[58] The title of the article referred to a proposal that Pinard claimed was nothing less than a new definition of the practice of obstetrics that was far broader than the traditional goal of "preserving women and children."[59] It was based on a new phase he added to the concept of infant development – Pinard called it "puericulture before procreation." Its focus was on the role of heredity in determining the well-being of the new child. Pinard admitted that disagreements existed between such eminent scientists as Darwin, Haeckel, Weismann, and Mathias-Duval over the exact workings of heredity, but this did not concern him. He simply assumed that it was

a known, capital fact, verified every day, both uncontested and incontestable: the dominant influence of the procreators, that is, the transmission from parents to children of their physical, psychological and moral qualities, physiologies and pathologies.[60]

Although he did not use the term neo-Lamarckism, Pinard gave examples of what he called "pathological heredity," by which he meant the hereditary transmission of negative characteristics acquired from parents in certain pathological states. This fit well with his earlier warnings about syphilis and alcoholism; but Pinard gave more specific evidence of his belief in the wide extent to which acquired negative characteristics could be transmitted. He analyzed 23 cases he observed at the clinic the previous year of "degenerate" infants born to parents who had previously produced normal healthy children. In 22 of the 23 cases, Pinard claimed, "I have been able to establish and certify that one of the two parents at the moment of procreation was either sick or convalescent." In half the cases the illness was typhoid fever, and in five cases, influenza.[61]

Although one might be tempted to see in this analysis a precursor of today's explanation of birth defects as a product of damage to otherwise normal reproductive cells, Pinard's idea involved more than that. In fact, it was closer to Darwin's "pangenesis," which saw hereditary transmission as determined by "the physical and psychic state of 'generators' at the moment of procreation." Elaborating on the inheritance of nonphysical characteristics as well, Pinard explained,

I am absolutely convinced today that every pathological state, every physical and moral depression, every physiological shortcoming of one or the other of the progenitors has a manifest influence on the product of conception and on its future development, because it is not only the constitutional heredity which is transmitted but also the state in which the cellular elements find themselves at the accidental moment of procreation.[62]

Pinard might just as well have been describing the *milieu intérieur* of Claude Bernard as the immediate environmental influence on heredity.

This was a very pessimistic view of the hereditary prospects for "preserving and improving the species," in the sense that every negative influence, every common cold, or every unsettled state of mind might take its toll on future generations. But in fact there was a brighter, more optimistic side to the picture, as indicated by Pinard's reference to the element of accident. If the current results of procreation were influenced, in Pinard's words, "too often, if not more, by the effect of chance," then a great improvement could be expected simply by making people aware of the consequences of their actions. Thus, if neo-Lamarckism warned of the increased possibility of negative influences on the quality of the population, it also held out the promise of improving it – and, more important, improving it quickly. Most immediately, Pinard predicted that

the syphilitic, the alcoholic, the sufferer from gout, the rheumatic, the convalescent, etc. would not hesitate to abstain from procreation if they knew that their progeniture would have all the chances of becoming degenerates if not worse.

As for himself, Pinard apparently practiced what he preached. Before having each of his own children, Pinard often told colleagues, he went to his country home in the Champagne region, read, relaxed, and drank nothing but milk.[63]

Pinard's recommendations went beyond treating specific ills such as tuberculosis, venereal disease, and alcoholism. People also had to be educated about the effects of these diseases on future generations. Hence, as noted in Chapter 2, Pinard presented Cazalis's *Science and marriage* to the Academy of Medicine in June of 1900 with the admonition, "I would like it in everyone's hands, and I hope it soon will be; because, in my opinion a revolution is necessary in our education. Ignorance is no longer synonymous with innocence, and too often ignorance is the worst enemy of innocence."[64] Pinard also joined Fournier's new Société de prophylaxie sanitaire et morale, and participated extensively in the 1903 debate on "sanitary guarantees of marriage." He called for the distribution of a *livret du mariage* instructing newlyweds on *maladies de la race* and marriage hygiene, although some critics argued that the couple might have better things to do on their wedding night than read the book. Pinard stopped short, however, of supporting at this time legislation requiring a premarital examination, because he still saw the problem as largely one of "changing customs by education."[65] This viewpoint made him welcome the publicity of the survey of opinion by the *Chronique médicale* on regulating marriage prompted by Couvreur's novel *La graine*. Pinard's answer to the question of responsibility in transmitting a hereditary illness was that it was "criminal" if done knowingly.[66]

Pinard did support limited, concrete government and private initiatives, such as a series of laws passed by the commune of Villiers-le-Duc (Côte-d'Or) that offered assistance to women who declared their pregnancy before the seventh month, and efforts by the Schneider industrial works at Creusot to improve housing conditions and the availability of medical assistance to workers. Although they were more closely related to puericulture after procreation and birth, both actions, Pinard noted, produced a drop in infant mortality.[67]

In a lecture to the Ecole des hautes études sociales in 1905 Pinard moved puericulture another step closer to eugenics when he outlined a general theory of "marriage aptitude from the physical, moral, and social point of view." This was the logical application of his puericulture before procreation to the most important selection process in human society. Echoing some of Clémence Royer's complaints of a generation earlier, Pinard began by noting that the choice of marriage partner was usually made for monetary or sentimental reasons rather than for purposes of reproduction. The similarities ended there, however, for according to Pinard's view of marriage, "the female being is simply a *seed bearer*. She is a jewel box enclosing the precious treasure transmitted by ancestors, the immortal elements which must constitute future generations."[68] Physiologically, he noted, the woman was fertile for 25 to 30 years beginning at age 12 to 16, and based on statistics there was no physical disadvantage to childbearing at the beginning of the period. Toward the end, however – after age 30 – he did note an increased risk of problems for both mother and child. The males showed no comparable risks with advancing age, except for the extended exposure to negative influences that could produce "disasters for the species which are too often the consequence of late marriage by men."[69] Pinard was referring to the vices of alcohol and prostitutes, which he evidently thought tempted only unmarried men.

Perhaps most significant about this lecture on marriage aptitude is what was not contained in it. Pinard presented no list of desirable physical or mental traits – such as blond hair, blue eyes, long-headed skulls, or even intelligence – that should be considered in choosing a spouse. Instead, he claimed that the condition of spouses and their ability to determine the time of procreation were the most important means of improving the quality of offspring. Pinard repeated his frequent complaint that at the moment, "children are the children of chance, and it is simply the satisfaction of sexual instinct that assures for better or worse – and how often for worse – the conservation of the species." In its place, Pinard insisted, should be "conscientious" procreation both on the part of the wife as well as the husband. He even admitted to being a "feminist" in the sense of advocating the freedom for a wife to choose when to have a child. Although this meant a wife's going against the legal obligation of obedience to her husband, Pinard insisted, "if circumstances place her in the presence of an epileptic or alcoholic spouse, she can refuse to procreate, knowing what the circumstances would be in these conditions." From the standpoint of positive action, Pinard recommended his own regimen of retreat and rest before conception, so that "the two procreators at the moment of procreation are at a maximum of eurythmy from the physical and moral point of view."[70]

Pinard realized that his ideas represented a revolution in the practice of having a family, but he claimed at least one indication of greater conscientiousness in recent French family patterns – the decline in the birthrate. His own studies for the Parliamentary Depopulation Commission had ruled out higher incidence of sterility or infant mortality as reasons for the relative decline of births in France. Pinard's conclusion was that it was the result of "the determined and conscious desire of spouses to have only a limited number of children."[71] In other words, parents realized that after having procreated children, it was necessary to raise them." Contrary to the natalists, Pinard welcomed this trend and chided them directly.

You demand that the wife procreate and you oblige her, in order to live, to work from morning until night and often at great distance from home. Frequently she must be separated from her child a few days after birth, and you wish to reduce infant mortality!

Begin by instituting the means to permit every mother to stay at home and raise her children. Make sure that every worker returning to his family can bring it the necessities of life, even if they are numerous. Only then will you be the true apostles of Repopulation.[72]

The neo-Malthusians were delighted with an apparent convert.

TOWARD EUGENICS IN FRANCE

Pinard could make fun of the natalists because of the security of his position as the most celebrated obstetrician in France. In fact, because of that reputation, the editors of the neo-Malthusian *Régénération* published his talk on marriage aptitude in their June 1906 issue and invited him to collaborate in their work.[73] Pinard, however, declined the invitation. This is not surprising, because despite the similarity of conclusions and Pinard's growing impatience with proponents of natalism, he did not share the larger ideological goals of the neo-Malthusians. Moreover, in spite of Pinard's criticisms, in the short run there was much more likelihood that his puericulture would be co-opted by the child care and natalist movement.

As mentioned earlier, the idea of puericulture from conception through childbirth (intrauterine and extrauterine puericulture) was very warmly welcomed, not just by natalists but by much of the nursing and educational establishment. In fact, the term puericulture soon became synonymous with all aspects of prenatal and postnatal care. For example, in the school year of 1902–03 Pinard was invited to give a series of talks to a class of girls in Paris aged ten to fourteen. Although Pinard offered little more than instructions on infant care (feeding, clothing, and bathing), the talks quickly attracted wider attention.[74] Among those who observed the classes was Louis Liard, vice-rector of the University of Paris and the head of primary education instruction for the ministry of education. The talks were published under the title *Puericulture du première âge,* and by 1909 30 percent of the departments in France had added it to the list of approved textbooks in primary school. The book went through six printings before 1913. At the same time, the subject of puericulture became part of the normal school curriculum for girls in 1905 and upper primary schools in 1909. The outline for teaching the subject recommended by the ministry of public instruction was a duplicate of the chapters in Pinard's book.[75]

Extra-uterine aspects of puericulture emphasized the care and feeding of newborns; hence, the audience it addressed was female. In fact, the followers of Pinard openly admitted that the lessons of puericulture after procreation were primarily for women, whereas those of puericulture before procreation were for men. The obstetrician Albert Fruhinsholz, who was also a son-in-law of Pinard, pointed out in a talk at the Third International Congress of School Hygiene, that "puericulture before procreation tends to be more the object of masculine teaching." A mixture of neo-Lamarckism

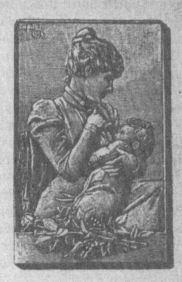

Figure 3.3   Cover of Pinard's *La puericulture*, 6th ed. (Paris: Armand Colin, 1913)

and male chauvinism was revealed in his call to confine such teaching to

post-primary school, lycées, normal schools, perhaps even army barracks. It is necessary for these young men to know "that they are the repositories of something sacred which they must respect as much as their honor, that they are responsible for the destiny of their race, and that it is in their power to annihilate, to diminish or, conversely, to assure the perpetuation and improvement of it."[76]

Fruhinsholz only mentioned puericulture before procreation, however, to indicate what did not concern him. His specific goal was to insure that girls were instructed in puericulture after procreation – that is, prenatal care during pregnancy and care of newborns. This was the main subject of his talk and the resolutions he introduced at the congress.

In this rush of support for puericulture after procreation, it is therefore by no means certain that puericulture would have developed into a French eugenics movement, because those elements of Pinard's ideas aimed at the hereditary improvement of the population could very easily have been lost in the emphasis on greater prenatal and infant care. The crucial, last step in the establishment of a viable eugenics movement involved appreciation of the importance of puericulture before procreation and its identification with eugenic work in other countries. Of necessity, this was done by Frenchmen more familiar with the previous work of Galton and new organizations in England, the United States, and Germany. One of these was Lucien March, head of the Statistique générale, who had worked with Pinard on the Commission on Depopulation. His statistical and demographic studies took him to many international meetings, and he was familiar with both Pearson's and Davenport's work. In fact, March translated Pearson's *Grammar of science* into French.[77]

In 1910, March wrote a lengthy article in the *Revue du mois* that compared puericulture before conception with the work of Ploetz's new International Society for Race Hygiene in Germany and the Eugenic Education Society in London.[78] This was among the earliest accounts in France of the new eugenics societies. Therefore, it is significant that these societies were immediately linked to Pinard's work. March's conclusion was that puericulture before conception deserved far more attention than the other two components of puericulture, which were largely being used to justify "the blind increase in births."[79] The growing awareness of Galtonian eugenics can also be seen in a February 1911 article by Georges Papillaut of the Ecole d'anthropologie entitled "Galton and biosociology," written on the occasion of Galton's death.[80] Although Papillaut was unfamiliar as yet with Pinard's work, his article was cited by Pinard the following year in his annual opening lecture at the Baudelocque Clinic, which marked the final step in the shift from puericulture to eugenics.

Pinard's 1912 talk at Baudelocque was a significant change in his thinking that reflected the influence of March and Papillaut, but even more so that of Charles Richet, his long-time friend and colleague on the faculty of the Ecole de médicine. Richet was a physiologist of international renown. He won the Nobel Prize in 1913 for his work on anaphylaxis, the body's immune reaction to poisoning, and he had broad interests ranging from aviation to metapsychism and pacifism. By 1912 he had also written the first draft of a book, *Sélection humaine,* which outlined a full-scale eugenics program from a Darwinian perspective. More will be said in the next chapter about the contents of this book, but its greatest immediate importance was that Richet's eugenics added the element of biology to Pinard's puericulture, which had grown out of obstetrics and pediatrics. The strong impression the new ideas had on Pinard is demonstrated by his opening statement to the audience at the Baudelocque Clinic in 1912: "In primitive life, says my eminent friend Prof. Charles Richet in a book treating the physiology of the species from the point of view of its perfectability, selection is the necessary consequence of the fierce struggle in which all beings are engaged." Apparently this was Pinard's first direct exposure to the work of Darwin, who had never been mentioned before in any of his writings on puericulture. Later in the article he referred to the *Descent of man* and Galton's *Hereditary genius,* but Pinard returned to Richet for a summary conclusion. "Civilization, which has done its best for the progress of the individual, has ended up degrading the species."[81]

The impact of this new perspective was even more obvious in Pinard's discussion of the specific means to be followed to improve the species. Whereas he had earlier talked about improving the state of body and mind of future parents at the time of procreation, Pinard now spoke about Galton's proposals for "the sterilization of physically or morally degenerate reproducers," as well as the encouragement of reproduction by those of sound body and mind. Though Pinard cautioned that "the demarcation line clearly separating human beings into *sterilizable* and *nonsterilizable* awaits some time before it can be drawn," he did note that Richet was in agreement with the use of sterilization.[82]

Pinard's reformulation of puericulture before procreation now reflected a concept more comparable to eugenics in other countries. He consciously reaffirmed the importance of heredity that he had already established in his notion of puericulture, but now he redirected attention toward the study of its influence on the quality of the species. Pinard even went so far as to coin the term *eugénnetique* to describe the study of the mechanism of degeneration. In so doing, he did not neglect his concern about syphilis, alcohol, and other agents as the primary causes of degeneration. But his goal was to find the intermediate process by which these agents worked, such as the one suggested by the work of August Forel on blastophthoria that Pinard hoped would offer an explanation of the general mechanism of germ cell deterioration as well as "the most favorable physiological moment for reproduction."[83]

CONCLUSION

What difference did it make that French eugenics grew out of puericulture rather than biology or anthropology? Most immediately it meant that it enjoyed a potentially broad base of support in French society. Generally it was more acceptable to call for having healthier babies rather than eliminating the unfit. And who was more trustworthy and respectable a proponent than the kindly baby doctor concerned with the health and welfare of the newborn? What more sober and objective authority than the census taker who gathered data on births, deaths, and occupational characteristics of the French population? In addition, puericulture gave the French eugenics movement a firm institutional base in the Ecole de médicine, where both Pinard and Richet held chairs. The identification with puericulture also gave French eugenicists alliances with those in social hygiene organizations fighting alcoholism, tuberculosis, and venereal diseases. At the same time it prevented conflict, at least initially, with the natalist movement and the Catholic church, who might otherwise have been opposed to a eugenics stressing the elimination of certain elements from the population. Finally, Pinard and his colleagues, as opposed to some early French proponents of eugenics, had a stature that made them visible and beyond criticism from the diverse groups concerned with questions of decline. While appealing to those wishing to use science for the improvement of the species, the founders of French eugenics also retained the confidence of the established elements of society who had little reason to suspect them of radically undermining its stability.

Did the influence of puericulture make for a substantive difference in eugenics as it was understood and practiced in France as opposed to other countries? Not in the overall goal of eugenics as the hereditary improvement of the human species. The major difference was in the means to be employed to achieve the goal. Puericulture stressed the positive measures that would improve the quality of infants, and deemphasized negative measures to eliminate "defectives." Crucial to this approach was the belief in neo-Lamarckian heredity, which assumed that the hereditary quality of all could be improved by bettering the conditions influencing conception and pregnancy. The most important consequence of this strategy, as seen in Pinard's advice on marriage aptitude, was to avoid spelling out which traits constituted improvement and which should be eliminated. But just because puericulteurs avoided this issue does not mean they were simply public health repopulators. In his June 1905 article on marriage aptitude, Pinard stressed that his goal was not just a blind increase in the French population. He and most other French eugenicists always insisted that their goal was improving the quality as well as the quantity of the population. Moreover, as will be seen in the next chapter, by 1912 there were Frenchmen such as Charles Richet who were quite willing to use negative eugenic measures to eliminate very specific traits from the population. Finally, despite its origins in puericulture, Pinard's concept by 1912 had been redefined to take into account work in other countries. Significantly, when a formal organization was created in December 1912, the name chosen was the French Eugenics Society. Puericulture had served its purpose and was now officially left behind.

4

The French Eugenics Society up to 1920

Despite the great amount of attention paid to eugenics and issues related to the biological regeneration of France, as late as 1910 there was still no formal eugenics organization in the country. Yet the debate, discussion, and creation of organizations with similar though more limited scope had done much to prepare the ground, as can be seen by how quickly the French Eugenics Society was established and the breadth of interest it inspired once certain key people were convinced of the need. The most prominent names in the organization were the leaders on questions of demography, health, and biological decline at the end of the nineteenth century and beginning of the twentieth century – Pinard, Richet, Perrier, and March.

The immediate inspiration for establishing a French eugenics society came from outside the country. But it was more than the example of already existing organizations in England, Germany, and the United States that prompted the French to form the society. The signal event was the holding of an international congress of eugenics in London in 1912. Those Frenchmen interested in the congress formed a Consultative Committee (Table 4.1) to represent their country; and it is a testimony to the interest in eugenics that despite the lack of a preexisting organization, the French committee was by far the largest one at the congress outside Britain. Forty-five individuals were listed for France, compared with ten or twelve each for such countries as Germany, the United States, and Italy.[1]

The background of individuals making up the French committee shows not only the broad appeal of eugenics, but people of considerable influence. Honorary presidents included two senators – Paul Doumer, who was a leader of the natalist movement and a future president of France, and Paul Strauss, who had been a member of the 1902 Senate Commission on Depopulation and was

Table 4.1. *French consultative committee to the First Eugenics Congress: London, 1912*

Title	Affiliation
Honorary presidents	
Charles Bouchard	Member, Academies of Science and Medicine
Henry Chéron	Minister of labor
Yves Delage	Member, Academy of Science
Paul Doumer	Senator
Achille de Foville	Secretary, Academy of Moral and Political Science
Louis Landouzy	Dean, Ecole de médecine (Paris)
Paul Strauss	Senator
President	
Edmond Perrier	Director, Museum of Natural History
Vice presidents	
Jules Déjérine	Professor, Ecole de médecine (Paris)
Charles Gide	Professor (economics), Paris Law School
Valentin Magnan	Head, Sainte Anne Asylum
Léonce Manouvrier	Secretary, Ecole d'anthropologie
Lucien March	Director, Statistique générale de France
Pierre Marie	Professor, Ecole de médecine (Paris)
Adolphe Pinard	Professor, Ecole de médecine (Paris)
Gaston Variot	Director, Institut de puericulture
Secretary	
Michel Huber	Statistician, Statistique générale de France
Members	
Félix Balzer	Member, Academy of Medicine
Jacques Bertillon	Statistician
Emile Borel	Mathematician
Paul Bureau	Professor (law), Institut catholique
Dr. Chevin	Director, Institut des begues
Albert Dastre	Physiologist
Amadée Doleris	Member, Academy of Medicine
Fernand Faure	Professor, Faculty of Law (Paris)
Gilbert Ballet	Professor, Ecole de médecine (Paris)
Eugene Gley	Professor, Collège de France

Table 4.1. *(Continued)*

Title	Affiliation
François Hallopeau	Professor, Ecole de médecine (Paris)
Félix Henneguy	Professor, Collège de France
Frédéric Houssay	Professor, Faculty of Science
Pierre Janet	Psychologist, Sorbonne
Alexandre Lacassagne	Professor, Collège de France
Adolphe Landry	Deputy
Paul-Maurice Legrain	Head, Asylum of the Seine
André Liesse	Economist
Dr. Maxwell	Staff, Procureur général
Albert Métin	Deputy
Georges Papillaut	Professor, Ecole d'anthropologie
Remy Perrier	Biologist
Jean Peyrot	Member, Academy of Medicine
Charles Porak	Member, Academy of Medicine
Joseph Reinach	Deputy
Jacques Roubinovitch	Psychiatrist, Salpiètre Hospital
Albert Viger	Deputy
René Worms	Editor, *Revue international de sociologie*

Source: Problems in eugenics: Papers communicated to the First International Eugenics Congress (London: Eugenics Education Society), 1912.

a prolific author on questions of public health and child care. Strauss later became a minister of health. Other honorary presidents represented the French academic elite – Louis Landouzy, dean of the Ecole de médecine, and Yves Delage, France's foremost biologist. The president of the Consultative Committee was Edmond Perrier, director of the Museum of Natural History, and the vice presidents included the physical anthropologist Léonce Manouvrier; Valentin Magnan, who had trained a generation of physicians studying the link between alcoholism and degeneration; and Lucien March, director of the French Statistique générale. Other members of the Consultative Committee were Fernand Faure, editor of the *Revue politique et parlementaire;* deputy of the National Assembly Joseph Reinach; and the statistician Jacques Bertillon, who was the most widely read writer of the French natalist movement.

As these last names indicate, the London conference was of interest to many outside the scientific community in France. One indication of the wide following was the daily coverage in the press.[2] The *Journal* engaged Cabanès as a correspondent to file reports on the congress for the newspaper's readers. Some of these reports were clearly aimed at instructing the general public about the new subject – "The eugenics congress studies the laws of heredity" and "What is eugenics?" were two of Cabanès' headlines – but most other coverage played on national pride by highlighting France's role at the congress. Paul Doumer's address at the opening banquet in which he expressed his hope that the next international meeting would be held in Paris was duly noted, as were the talks by Frenchmen who were active in the field.

The French participation at the congress indicates that the organizing committee was not just a paper creation for international prestige. The number of people who actually attended the congress and delivered papers indicates that the French were active participants as well. Eleven members of the Consultative Committee attended, six of them presenting papers; and they were joined by an additional seven Frenchmen not on the committee who also gave papers.[3] The subject matter of the papers illustrates one feature of French eugenics that was to continue throughout the movement's history – the large representation from medical and health professions. The widespread influence of neo-Lamarckian hereditary theory in France made eugenics especially appealing to those in medical professions. Quite simply, if the "environment" of disease could be ameliorated, it was thought that hereditary improvements could be passed to future generations. With the exception of Lucien March's presentation on social status and marriage fertility, all of the French papers delivered at the London congress were medical in nature. These ranged from Raoul Dupuy's and Frédéric Houssay's studies of retardation and birth defects (topics commonly studied in other countries) to those that were much more indicative of the neo-Lamarckian influence on French eugenic thought, such as Hallopeau's paper on the eugenic effects of syphilis, Magnan and Filassier's study of alcoholism and degeneration, and Adolphe Pinard's paper on his favorite subject, "Puericulture before procreation."

Houssay made clear early in his paper the need to "cling to the principles on which Lamarckian doctrines rest." As proof he cited the hereditary defects resulting from the "fundamental factors: alcoholism, syphilis and more generally all intoxications which arise either spontaneously or as a result of contagious disease."[4] François Hallopeau's paper was on the so-called hereditary-syphilitic. Magnan's student Filassier delivered their jointly authored paper on the hereditary effects of alcoholism, concluding ominously that "this population invaded by the poison is unfortunately not sterile."[5] Citing previous studies that showed that as many as three-fourths of the inmates of the asylums in the Department of the Seine were descendants of alcoholics, the authors observed:

The most distressing result of alcoholism is that not only does it profoundly transform the individual but it also transmits to his descendants the defects which produce the sick and criminals whose only contribution to society is a heavy burden or a danger.[6]

The French were not the only Lamarckians at the congress; in fact, some participants from other countries were very sympathetic to their viewpoint. For example, the Edinburgh physician C.W. Saleeby argued at the congress against the use of sterilization on the grounds that hereditary characteristics were acquired, hence they could be easily modified. Noting that Darwin himself had maintained such a position, Saleeby claimed that "biology after a period of exaggerated Weismannism was returning to that view." But he also clearly credited the French with being the major proponents, noting that "this congress is fortunate in listening to countrymen of the great Lamarck, from whom – a century after the publication of his *Philosophie zoologique* – we still could learn."[7]

Some French participants were wary about the government intervention in the lives of individuals that was advocated by many of the English eugenicists at the congress. Léonce Manouvrier, the anthropologist who had earlier done battle with the extreme hereditary determinism of Vacher de Lapouge and the "born criminal" idea of Lombroso, suggested during one discussion that the congress should be precise in its definition of eugenics, especially Galton's phrase, "agencies under social control," which were to be the means of achieving eugenic goals. Manouvrier was in favor of a broad definition of means, as long as the congress "could still distinguish between those which could and should be placed under social control and those which should be left up to individual choice." Though he argued that the former would include prevention of parenthood by epileptics, alcoholics, and the insane, the latter should leave the general choice of marriage partners up to the populace at large.[8] The next day, Georges Papillaut, a colleague of Manouvrier's at the Ecole d'anthropologie, seconded this view when the subject of sterilization came up for discussion again. Acknowledging that the costs of maintaining "defective" offspring were high to society, Papillaut was nonetheless of the opinion that "the measures by which the state could interfere with family hygiene and individual selection were detrimental to personal liberty and responsibility, and this was worse than the expenditure."[9]

Not all Frenchmen at the congress (or in subsequent years) shared the anthropologists' limited view of the scope of eugenics. Frédéric Houssay, a future vice president of the French Eugenics Society, stated in a paper at the London congress that sterilization "ought assuredly to be taken into account as a valuable contributor to the improvement of the human species as a whole." To those, such as Papillaut, who objected to this action in the name of individual rights, Houssay continued:

Enforced sterilization, if its value for social preservation is sufficiently established, is only one particular aspect of the right to punish. This is, in fact, neither an act of revenge or retaliation. Its legitimacy rests entirely on the primordial need of society to preserve itself and to eliminate all centers of contamination whose spread and extension would imperil higher civilization and social life itself.[10]

As will be seen, this broad range of differing opinion was one of the distinctive features of the early years of French eugenics.

THE FOUNDING OF THE FRENCH EUGENICS SOCIETY

On their return to France, many of those who had attended the London congress decided to create an organization analogous to the societies already in existence in Germany, Sweden, England, and the United States. At the initiative of Lucien March, the group decided to call a meeting, presided over by Edmond Perrier, of those individuals who might be interested in founding a "French society for the study of questions relative to the amelioration of future generations."[11] This meeting was held on December 22, 1912, at the amphitheater of the Ecole de médecine in Paris. The honorary presidency was accepted by Léon Bourgeois, the former president of the Conseil des ministres and at the time minister of labor, whose solidarism movement fit quite well with the underlying views of eugenicists. After speeches by Paul Doumer, Louis Landouzy, and Edmond Perrier, the statutes for the society were presented by Eugène Apert, a pediatrician whose specialty was hereditary childhood diseases. Discussion and voting on the statutes were postponed, however, until another meeting at the medical school the following month.

These organizational activities plus the election of officers took place on January 29, 1913. Perrier was elected president; Pinard, Landouzy, and Frédéric Houssay became vice presidents; the pediatrician Eugène Apert was elected secretary general and Lucien March the treasurer. The fact that all of these officers had been prominent on the Consultative Committee at the London congress indicates that the new society did not differ greatly in composition from the group representing France at London. The statutes reveal both the international perspective of the founders and the particular circumstances that had defined French eugenics from the start.

Of the four stated goals of the society, the first is most telling of the influence of neo-Lamarckism:

Research and application of knowledge useful to the reproduction, preservation, and improvement of the species; in particular, it [the society] studies questions of heredity and selection in their application to the human species, and questions relative to the influence of milieu, economic status, legislation, and customs on the value of successive generations and on their physical, intellectual, and moral aptitudes.[12]

There had been some debate about the naming of the society during the organizational meetings, with Pinard and proponents of the term "puericulture" losing out to those who favored "eugenics" because, in the words of March, "it has become current in English-language countries . . . is an accomplished fact, and no other [term] appears to us able to replace it."[13] Equally important to note is the omission of references to Galton's phrase "agencies under social control" that would be used to achieve the eugenic goals. Hence, Manouvrier and others at the London conference who had wished to respect individual choice apparently carried the day.

The second goal, "encouragement and development of sciences which are applicable to the studies of the [eugenics] society," is less specific, but in other sections of the statutes it is clear that this refers to encouraging research by such means as publishing a journal, holding regular meetings for presentations of papers, and discussions. This encouragement also foresaw the establishment of a research facility comparable to the Eugenics Laboratory of Karl Pearson at the University of London or the Eugenics Record Office of Charles Davenport at Cold Spring Harbor on Long Island.[14] Lucien March, in particular, strongly advocated the need for such an institution, having visited the Eugenics Record Office on a recent trip to the United States. He even translated and published a facsimile of the form used by Davenport to document family histories of patients in hospitals and inmates at insane asylums and prisons. In fact, March went further, urging that similar studies be done of normal families. He reasoned:

In noble families, genealogical tables of ancestral lines are carefully preserved; breeders possess the same hereditary histories of their principal concerns. Why should every individual in democratic societies not have an equal concern to furnish the principal characteristics of his origins to his descendents?[15]

Despite these hopes, no such laboratory was created in France, at least in March's lifetime. Nor was the third goal of the French Eugenics Society, which envisaged "the eventual formation of local societies having the same purposes," ever achieved. As will be seen, events soon dictated a change in strategies that either modified these goals or made them subservient to the final goal of "publicizing ideas favorable to the improvement of successive generations." There was, nonetheless, an initial drive to recruit members for the organization.

Considering the fact that its founders deferred the formation of a grass roots, mass organization, the French Eugenics Society's initial membership appeal was impressive. Over 100 people became founding members. This included only half of those who attended the London congress, which can be taken as an indication that many, such as Magnan, Bertillon, and the backer of natalist legislation in the Chamber Henry Chéron, did not find in eugenics the support they sought for their plan to revitalize France. No doubt Bertillon and Chéron had been shocked by the English and

American talk of sterilization and birth control. But the fact that others joined to fill the ranks of the French Eugenics Society can be interpreted as an indication of the initial wide appeal of eugenics in France. It was not a small dedicated group of zealots who went to London, but individuals with a broad range of backgrounds and interests. Many found what they were looking for at the congress.

An analysis of the background of these and others who made up the founding membership shows the diversity of these interests. This is not surprising because the formal definition of the French Eugenics Society was broad enough to accommodate people from many different fields. In particular, the lack of reference to how the eugenics research would be "applied," and the neo-Lamarckian presumptions about the influence of environment, meant that virtually all those interested in improving the human condition could be considered eugenicists if they thought that improvements were passed hereditarily to subsequent generations. This view was particularly appealing to physicians, as can be seen in Table 4.2 showing the background of the founding members of the French Eugenics Society. Data from the United States, Britain, Germany, and Japan are added for comparison.

As the table shows, over half the founding members of the French Eugenics Society were physicians. No other occupational group comes anywhere near that number. Two provisos should be made about the predominance of doctors in French eugenics. First, figures for other countries show that France was not the only country in which doctors took an interest in eugenics. In both the German and Japanese societies, physicians were also the largest single occupational category. Doctors were also well in evidence among eugenicists both on the council of the English Eugenics Education Society and the American Eugenics Society.[16] In fact, these figures suggest that the British and American eugenics movements, heretofore thought of as the models for eugenics, may themselves have been unusual in that their memberships included large numbers of biologists and social scientists. These figures are sketchy, but they indicate the need for more comparative study of eugenics.

One explanation for the high proportion of doctors in eugenics is that even a strict Mendelian view of heredity did not exclude the importance of environment in achieving the potential development of genetic characteristics. In other words, no matter how good the chromosomes, the offspring produced by them could

Table 4.2. *Occupations of eugenicists*

Occupation	France[a] No.	%	England[b] No.	%	United States[c] No.	%	Germany[d] No.	%	Japan[e] No.	%
Politician	7	6.7	2	5	5	3.3	2	0.5	–	–
Scientist[f]	5	4.8	13	32.5	46	30.0	17	4.2	4	5.4
Physician	54	51.9	9	22.5	30	19.6	136	33.4	53	70.7
Businessman	4	3.8	2	5	–	–	29	7.1	–	–
Lawyer	4	3.8	4	10	–	–	13	3.2	–	–
Administrator[g]	9	8.6	1	2.5	–	–	5	1.2	–	–
Anthropologist	6	5.8	–	–	5	3.3	7	1.7	–	–
Clergy	–	–	1	2.5	4	2.6	–	–	–	–
Educator[h]	4	3.8	1	2.5	41	26.8	36	8.8	2	2.7
Other[i]	11	10.6	7	17.5	22	14.4	165	40.5	16	21.6
Total	104		40		153		410		75	

[a] Founding members of French Eugenics Society, from *Eugénique,* 1(1913), 54–60.

[b] Elected council members of Eugenics Education Society for 1914, from Donald MacKenzie, "Eugenics in Britain," *Social Studies in Science,* 6(1976), 504–05, which also supports Farrall's earlier study.

[c] Board members and Advisory Council of American Eugenics Society, 1923–35, analyzed by Barry Mehler (Ph.D. dissertation, University of Illinois, 1987).

[d] Members of German Society for Race Hygiene, December 31, 1913.

[e] Founders of the Japanese Eugenics Association (1925), from Zenji Suzuki, "Genetics and the eugenics movement in Japan," *Japanese studies in the history of science,* 14(1975),161.

[f] For England, this category combines MacKenzie's "university teachers and researchers" and "nonacademic scientists"; for Japan, there are only biologists; for the United States, it includes biologists, zoologists, and geneticists.

[g] Government as well as private social welfare agencies.

[h] This does not include physicians or scientists with university appointments. For the United States, three-quarters were psychologists and sociologists.

[i] For Germany, 40 percent of this category were wives of men in the other categories.

not improve the race if they were not properly nourished and guarded from disease. The second reason why physicians stand out in French eugenics is the relatively even distribution of eugenicists from other occupations. Because of the breadth of interest, no other group, such as anthropologists, lawyers, or politicians, rivaled the physicians. This is in contrast to England and the United States where scientists and educators rivaled and even surpassed physicians in numbers. Finally, it is worth noting that there was almost a total lack of female founders of the French Eugenics Society, an irony in that French puericulture paid so much attention to motherhood. This was not unusual by comparison with other national societies, with the exception of the German Race Hygiene Society, which had many female members in 1913. One reason for this exception is that the German organization sought a broader, popular base; in addition, most of the women (13.8 percent of the total membership), were wives of male members.[17] This conjugal membership had been the practice from the beginning of the German society. A 1909 membership list shows eight of ten women (out of a total of forty-seven members) listed as wives of members.

THE FRENCH EUGENICS SOCIETY: PATTERN OF MEMBERSHIP, FINANCING, AND ACTIVITIES

The history of the French Eugenics Society can for convenience be divided into three periods: prewar, 1920 to 1926, and 1927 to 1941. The First World War is an obvious break, because the society simply suspended operation. No meetings were held, and the journal of the society, *Eugénique,* ceased publication. Moreover, the war had a great impact on the concerns of members of the society after its meetings and publication of its journal resumed in 1920. The next break, 1926/1927, occurred when the French Eugenics Society decided to merge with the Eugenics Section of the French Office of the International Institute of Anthropology (IIA). More will be said later about this organization, but the most obvious change resulting from the merger was that publications of the Eugenics Society thereafter appeared in *Revue anthropologique,* the journal of the Ecole d'anthropologie, which also published the proceedings and other papers of the IIA. The last break is 1941. There was no formal termination of the society, but the last recorded meeting was on December 5, 1941, when the German eugenicist Eugen Fischer gave his address entitled "Problems of race and racial legislation in Germany." At the same time, *Revue anthropologique* and the Ecole d'anthropologie were suppressed by the Nazi occupiers.[18]

The first period of the French Eugenics Society, though the briefest, was the one of most intense activity. Meetings of the society were held monthly at the Ecole de médecine, and usually consisted of presentations and discussions of original works of research both by society members and guest speakers. *Eugénique* also appeared monthly through June 1914, and in a major publicity campaign, the society printed and distributed three thousand copies of the first issue containing the statutes of the society and the list of founding members.[19]

Postwar meetings of the French Eugenics Society never reached the frequency of the prewar meetings, yet they show a remarkable regularity and continuity. They were held twice a year, usually in May and December, with no year missed throughout the 1920s. In fact, interest was so steady to the end of the decade that it is tempting to make the case that a better ending point for the second period of the society's activities might be 1931/1932, when a sharp decline in activity of the French Eugenics Society (although not the work of all eugenicists) coincided with other changes such as the onset of the Depression and the takeover of the International Eugenics Federation by Germany and the Scandinavian countries. French reactions to these developments will be considered later, but from the standpoint of internal organization, the 1926/1927 date is more significant as the end of the second period.

Although meetings in the second period were less frequent, attendance on the whole was higher than in the first period. The increase is largely explained by the presence of interested visitors and new members. Although no regular meeting had more than twenty recorded in attendance, of greater significance in the attempt to reach more people was the sponsorship of larger conferences by the society on special topics of more general interest. Among these was a series of meetings in 1920–21 on the eugenic consequences of the world war. The activities of the French Eugenics Society in the 1920s also expanded to encourage the founding of other organizations pursuing similar goals, although not exactly as envisioned in the founding statutes. This began in December 1922 when the society announced the formation of a Comité d'union contre le péril vénérien.[20] As will be seen, however, the new organizations proved to be less the herald of a new network of suborganizations than an indication of fragmenting of support for the Society, because these new groups soon split off from the parent eugenics organization.

The third period in the society's history began with the campaign for passage of a law requiring a medical examination before marriage. This marked a major shift in tactics that accompanied the merger of the society with the IIA and *Revue anthropologique*. By the end of the decade, meetings of the society were held less frequently, especially after the campaign for a premarital exam bogged down in the legislature. Other activities of French eugenicists continued in the 1930s, but they were independent of the French Eugenics Society, whose work consisted of meeting irregularly and publishing occasional articles in *Revue anthropologique*.

Financing of the French Eugenics Society throughout its existence was closely linked to membership, because dues were the principal source of revenue. Treasurers' reports for the first two periods show only a few exceptions to this dependence on membership dues for revenue.[21] One exception came at the very beginning of the society's life when money was most needed to cover expenses until dues could be collected. The society was aided by donations, the largest of which was 500 francs from Juliette Reinach, a member of a prominent Jewish family with interests in politics and publishing.[22] The other exceptional income came in 1923 when the society began to receive royalties from the publication of papers given at the 1920 conference on the eugenic effects of the war.[23] But royalties were a declining source of income, and as membership and dues began to drop off the following years, treasurer Lucien March, noted in his budget report, "new efforts are necessary to augment the resources of our society."[24]

The most striking feature of the budgets of the society was their small size: from 2,000 to 4,500 francs per year. These sums are dwarfed by comparison with expenditures of other organizations in France working on related matters. For example, the portion of the budget of the French labor and health ministry devoted only to the prevention of venereal disease in 1925 was 500,000 francs.[25] Given the small size of its budget, the French Eugenics Society could only afford to pay the printing costs of *Eugénique,* the rent

Table 4.3. *French Eugenics Society members, 1913–25*

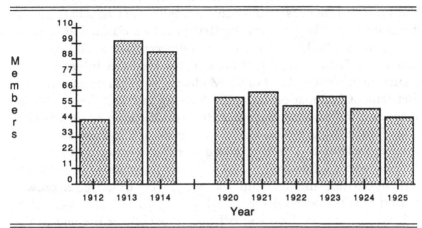

Source: Eugénique, (1913–26).

on its offices, and dues for memberships in international organizations. Budget restrictions were largely the reason that no other
wide-scale propaganda efforts were undertaken after 1913. The
printing and mailing of the 3,000 copies of *Eugénique* cost the society 2,000 francs, or roughly half its total budget that year.[26] In
fact, one must conclude, albeit indirectly, that budgetary considerations prompted the merger of the French Eugenics Society in
1927 with the IIA. As a result, the society gained access to the
resources of the Ecole d'anthropologie, including use of its journal.

Budget reports also offer at least a conservative estimate of the
size of membership in the society. The dues remained constant at
20 francs per year. Therefore the number of dues-paying members
can easily be determined from yearly dues receipts. Although using this source has the advantage of guarding against self-serving
or inflated membership statistics – only those who actually paid
money are counted – these reports are better as a relative measure
of interest in the organization from year to year than the absolute
count of all who attended meetings or otherwise showed an interest in the work of the society. Most likely, far more attended than
paid dues. The pattern of membership is shown in Table 4.3.

The budget and membership figures of the French Eugenics Society (even allowing for nondues-paying participants) clearly in-

dicate that it was no mass organization, nor even a central parent society with local chapters, as called for in its statutes. By contrast, the English Eugenics Education Society in 1911 had branches in Birmingham, Glasgow, and Belfast. In 1914 it claimed over 1,000 members. In the United States a more decentralized approach resulted in a Galton Society of New York; Eugenics Education Societies of Chicago, St. Louis, Madison, and Minnesota; a Race Betterment Foundation set up by Kellogg in Battle Creek, Michigan; and the original Eugenics Record Office on Long Island.[27] The French organization was much more of a learned society of doctors, scientists, scholars, and government officials attempting to gain wider influence by reaching decision-makers in France.[28] The fluctuating membership was the largest in the brief prewar period. Yet the postwar membership showed a remarkable stability, with numbers dropping off only gradually at the end of the 1920s.

The members' background did not change greatly from the prewar period. If anything, there was increased interest from physicians during the 1920s when social hygiene and the passage of the premarital examination law were the society's chief concerns. There was a shift, however, in the subspecialties of medicine represented, with public health replacing obstetrics and pediatrics as the most common practice of the new physicians coming to eugenics. The interest of anthropologists continued and even increased, thanks to the closer ties with the Ecole d'anthropologie, and occasionally a lawyer or deputy would appear at meetings of the society to speak on legal aspects of divorce or the premarital exam. Generally, however, the participation of politicians dropped off after the war. One exception was the senator and cabinet minister Justin Godart, who helped start a series of public lectures at the Sorbonne on social hygiene in the late 1920s and who sponsored revised legislation for the premarital examination law in 1932. The other exception was Pinard, who began a post-retirement political career in 1918 at the age of 74, when he ran as a candidate for deputy in the National Assembly. His election has been described as largely honorary; but Pinard served for ten years, and used his position as president of the Chamber (an office determined by age) to introduce the first bill for a premarital exam in 1926.[29]

LEADERS OF THE FRENCH EUGENICS MOVEMENT

Only a handful of men held the principal offices of the French Eugenics Society throughout its existence. In 1912, Edmond Perrier began as president, with Frédéric Houssay, Louis Landouzy, and Adolphe Pinard serving as vice presidents. Eugène Apert was secretary general, and Lucien March was treasurer. When Landouzy died during the war, he was replaced as vice president by Charles Richet. When Houssay died in 1920, Apert replaced him as vice president, and the public health pediatrician Georges Schreiber filled Apert's old office of secretary general. The following year, Perrier died and Pinard moved up to president.[30] That was the last change of officers until Pinard stepped down from the presidency in 1927 and was replaced by Apert. In almost every case promotion was not only from within the society, but from previous officers. Schreiber and Richet were the only people to become officers who were not already officers at the founding of the society in 1912.

A closer look at the background and interests of these leaders gives one a better idea of what kind of Frenchmen became members of organized eugenics and reveals certain common features about them. For example, they generally had a background in medicine, enjoyed a prominent standing in their fields, had a neo-Lamarckian view of heredity, and displayed general interests beyond their own area of expertise. In other words, they were concerned with larger social questions of the day. Perrier, Pinard, Landouzy, Richet, and March represent a good selection of leaders to examine because of their importance to French eugenics.

Edmond Perrier (1844–1921), the first president of the French Eugenics Society from 1912 to 1920, had achieved great fame as a research biologist long before he came to eugenics. His two decades of teaching and writing about biology were formally acknowledged in 1892 when he was elected to the Academy of Sciences, taking the anatomy/zoology seat of Armand de Quatrefages. In 1900 he became head of the Museum of Natural History. One indication that his activity in eugenics at least did no harm to his standing among his colleagues was that in 1913 he was elected vice president of the Academy of Sciences, and in 1915 president.[31] In 1920, Perrier was even elected president of the Syndicat d'initiative of Paris, the main tourist organization for the French capital!

Perrier's training was in biology, not medicine; but as has been seen in Chapter 2 he was definitely a Lamarckian. In fact, he was one of the most influential neo-Lamarckian theorists at the end of the nineteenth century.[32] Perrier was a native of Tulle (Departement of Corrèze) in the Massif-Central. The son of a school principal, he was accepted both to the Ecole polytechnique and the Ecole normale supérieure (ENS) in Paris. At the suggestion of no less a figure than Pasteur, Perrier decided to study science at the ENS. There he was a student of Lacaze-Duthiers, who secured him an appointment at the Museum of Natural History as an assistant (*aide-naturaliste*). His dissertation on the spines of starfish and sea urchins began an interest in marine biology that continued throughout his career. From 1881 to 1883, Perrier participated in oceanographic expeditions to the Mediterranean and Atlantic; and in 1887 he established a marine biology laboratory for the Museum of Natural History at Sainte-Vaast-la Hougue on the Normandy coast. The latter responsibility reflected Perrier's advancement at the museum, beginning with his appointment as professor in 1876 and culminating in 1900 with his succession to Milne-Edwards as head of the museum.

That Perrier was concerned with subjects beyond his research on marine animals was demonstrated by his early interest in Darwin's ideas on evolution. Although cautious by nature, in 1879 Perrier was convinced of the transformation (the French term for evolution) of species, and announced it in dramatic fashion before an audience at the Museum of Natural History.[33] Thereafter, he became one of the most outspoken supporters of evolutionary theory in France. His interest in Lamarck soon followed and, as has been shown, served as a scientific basis for the political doctrine of solidarism. Eugenic improvement of the human species was simply the next logical step for Perrier to take beyond the bounds of his academic interests. Another side of Perrier indicating his broad interest was his role as scientific popularizer. Not only was he a frequent contributor to such journals as *Revue scientifique* (beginning in 1870) and *Nouvelle revue,* but after the turn of the century Perrier wrote a regular column for the newspaper *Le temps* on subjects ranging from "Months without 'R', oysters and the masculine sex" to "Is the earth alive" and "Sleep." Three collections of these articles were published as books.[34]

The work of Adolphe Pinard has already been described in some detail, especially in the puericulture movement and as a deputy in the National Assembly. He and Budin were the leading obstetricians of the day, both having been the most successful students of Etienne Tarnier, the dean of nineteenth-century French obstetricians.[35] Pinard organized and ran the maternity clinic of the Paris Medical School at Baudelocque for twenty-five years after its founding in 1889. Albert Fruhinsholz, one of Pinard's most celebrated students as well as his son-in-law, placed him "at the head of [a list of the greatest] obstetricians of all time" in France.[36] His championing of puericulture not only reoriented the focus of French obstetrics back on the child, but made Pinard's reputation international. This stretched from Latin American countries, where puericulture was very warmly received, to Russia, where Pinard was summoned for a consultation with the Czarina in 1904 when she became pregnant with the future Czarevitch.[37] Pinard's success in parliamentary and governmental service was clearly built upon his reputation and renown in medicine.

The medical accomplishments and neo-Lamarckism of Pinard need little further elaboration; but a look at his background and training is of interest.[38] His beginnings were the most modest of all the leaders of French eugenics. The son of a small landholder and part-time textile worker from Méry-sur-Seine in Champagne, Pinard had only a primary school education when he left for Paris at the age of eighteen to become an apprentice to a pharmacist. He continued to work while completing his studies, then entered medical school, where he was brought under the tutelage of Tarnier and Alfred Richet, father of Pinard's later colleague Charles. He began teaching at the Ecole de médecine in 1878 and became an *accoucheur des hôpitaux* in 1882, and when Tarnier created a second chair of clinical obstetrics in 1889, Pinard was selected over Budin to fill it and direct the Baudelocque Clinic, which went along with the appointment.

It was this appointment that put Pinard in a position to make his greatest impact on the practice of obstetrics in France. For besides shifting attention away from the mother toward the child, Pinard employed a method of research based on observations at

the clinic that gave weight to his own proposals and set the pattern
for research methodology in twentieth-century obstetric medicine. Each year, Pinard would have one of his interns compile and
publish the results of cases handled at Baudelocque. One of his
students, Bachimont, wrote his medical thesis based on 4,455 cases
from 1889 to 1898. It was from such data that Pinard showed a
difference of 300 grams in the average weight of full-term infants
born to mothers in stand-up occupations who worked until delivery compared with those who were able to rest during the last
three months of pregnancy.[39] As mentioned earlier, it was also
from this clinical experience that Pinard came to his neo-Lamarckian view of influences on newborns.

Perhaps the best explanation of what led Pinard to eugenics was
his persistence in following his convictions beyond the narrow
confines of his training and practice. For example, in 1891 he realized that his goal of improving infant health through prenatal
and postnatal care would require intervention on a broad social
scale. The very concept of puericulture that he announced (or revived) in 1895 in front of the Academy of Medicine was revolutionary in its broader view of both obstetrics and child care; and
Pinard was not reluctant to utilize new means to achieve the results he desired. Hence, his participation in eugenics was only one
example of many activities he pursued outside the classroom and
clinic. To summarize, in 1892 he joined Madame Becquet in setting up an asylum with both private and government support for
displaced expectant mothers. In the 1902–1903 school year, Pinard
gave a series of talks at a girls primary school in Paris on "La
puericulture du premier âge" that were published the following
year and reprinted several times.[40] In 1902, Pinard also served on
the Senate Commission on Depopulation, for which he and Richet
prepared a subcommission report on infant mortality.

During the First World War, when a state of emergency was
declared in Paris and a military government ran the city, Pinard
was made vice president of a Committee for the Protection of
Mothers and Children. He saw it as an opportunity to use the
extraordinary powers created by the war to institute his "program
of social, legal, and medical protection for mothers and newborns." In fact, his zeal to protect pregnant women and new mothers
was only checked by the competing needs of the war. His proposal "to forbid absolutely the access to work in factories by all

women either carrying children, nursing a child, or having given birth within six months" was not warmly received by military authorities anxious to use the female workforce to meet labor shortages in munitions factories.[41] Pinard's involvement in eugenics, not to mention his eight years of service in the Chamber of Deputies after the war, are thus best seen as a reflection of the lengths to which he would venture outside the normal activities of his medical practice in order to achieve his goals. Given this unswerving devotion to the cause, plus his prestige and position in the Chamber, Pinard was a natural choice as successor to Perrier in 1921 as president of the French Eugenics Society.

If Pinard's background was the story of the small-town artisan's son who came to Paris to make his fame and fortune, Charles Richet's life followed a very different course.[42] Born to the family of a professor of surgery at the Ecole de medécine, Richet's grandfather had been *Procureur général* of the High Court of Justice during the Second Republic.[43] Given such family connections, it is therefore not surprising to find Richet moving quickly up the hierarchy of the medical profession.

His credentials as a researcher were first established by work on animal body temperature. It was Richet who showed that dogs cooled themselves by panting. His most important discovery was a phenomenon he called anaphylaxis, the increased sensitivity of the body to moderate doses of some poisons that produce fatal reactions to even the slightest subsequent injections rather than building up immunity. Anaphylactic shock was not only helpful in explaining the mechanism of poisoning; its similarities to infection led Richet to suggest it as a key to understanding the general action of disease – that is, by the creation of poisons within the body. Richet was named to the chair of physiology at the Ecole de médecine early in his career, in fact while his father was still on the faculty; and in 1913 he received the Nobel Prize for physiology. When he died in 1935 it was noted in scientific journals as well as throughout the French press, from establishment newspapers such as *Le Temps* to worker dailies such as *Le Populaire* and *Le Peuple,* which ran a front-page obituary with his photograph.[44]

Richet's stature, therefore, equaled if not exceeded Pinard's; and the way he came to eugenics was similar to that of the obstetrician – from a willingness to pursue activities beyond his immediate research interests.[45] For Richet, however, this was not unusual,

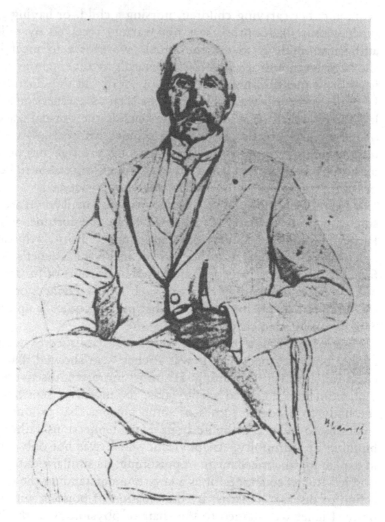

Figure 4.4   Charles Richet. [Source: "Charles Richet: autobiographie," *Les biographies médicales,* P. Busquet and Maurice Genty, eds. (Paris: J.-B. Ballière, 1932)]

because his interests had always been broad, whereas Pinard's eugenics stemmed directly from his overriding goal of raising better children. For example, one of the most controversial of Richet's interests was psychic phenomena. His first experience was at age sixteen, when he and his sister succeeded in hypnotizing one of her girlfriends. He studied psychic phenomena in more detail during medical school despite a warning from his father; and his first publication on a medical subject concerned work on somnambulism, based on hypnotic experiments he continued while an intern in the 1870s.[46] According to Richet, he became even more deeply involved in these phenomena after a visit by the Russian psychologist Aksakov in 1884. The Russian told him of an Italian medium named Eusapia whom Richet not only visited but invited to his Mediterranean island home for three months. There she was studied by such visitors as the English writer Frederick Myers and fellow physiologist Arsène d'Arsonval.[47] During the following year, Richet, the Englishman William Crookes, and others founded the Society for Psychical Research, with Richet as the first president. He retained an active interest in the subject for the next thirty years.

Not surprisingly, the scientific obituaries of Richet played down this aspect of his work. One article called his parapsychology "as yet uncertain and debatable," and another otherwise laudatory eulogy called the interest "a chimera," one of Richet's "secretly cultivated gardens" of interest.[48] This is clearly wrong in the sense that Richet's work in parapsychology was widely known and typical of the kind of subject that would spread his reputation among the general public. In fact, Richet wrote his first novel *Possession* in an attempt to describe psychism outside the constraints of scientific or even general interest nonfiction publications.[49] This and another of his novels, *Soeur Marthe,* were later performed on the stage with Sarah Bernhardt in the lead. These were not Richet's only ventures into the literary world. He published poetry as early as 1874 with a friend Paul Fournier under the pseudonym Charles Epheyre (the last name being the French pronunciation of the letters "F" and "R").

Richet's literary ventures were typical of a curiosity that led him to indulge a wide variety of interests. A trip to Egypt, Palestine, and Syria in 1876 spawned a lifelong interest in Egyptology. Another example of Richet's broad interests was his participation in the development of French aviation. Richet met Victor Tatin while both were working in the laboratory of the physiologist Jules Marey; and from the late 1880s to the time of the Wright brothers' flight in 1904, he and Tatin experimented with the construction of heavier-than-air craft. His interest continued thereafter, thanks to a close family friendship with Louis and Jacques Breguet, who were among the most successful leaders of French aviation after the First World War.

One of Richet's interests that, along with his work in psychology and intelligence, helps explain his attraction to eugenics, was his study of history and participation in the pacifist movement at the turn of the century. As Richet told it, in the early 1880s the English pacifist Hodgson-Pratt convinced him to become more active in the movement, and thereafter he gave numerous talks and wrote articles and even books on the subject. Richet eventually became president of the French Peace League and served on the International Committee for the Arbitration of Disputes. A friend of Carnegie's and other world pacifist leaders, Richet's proudest contribution to the effort was the book *Le passé de la guerre et l'avenir de la paix,* published in 1907. In fact, when Richet received his Nobel Prize for physiology, Bertha von Suttner wrote him that he should have been awarded the Peace Prize instead.[50] Thus, Richet was already preoccupied by the largest concerns of mankind – past, future, and present – when eugenics, demography, and hereditarian thought began to receive more attention in France around the turn of the century.

As mentioned in Chapter 2 Richet was active in the natalist movement from the start; but as will be seen, his work and interest in physiology and psychology was important in shaping a very independent line of eugenic thought. Richet's unique background and ideosyncratic approach to eugenics make his participation in the French eugenics movement with men such as Pinard all the more striking. In addition, his stature as a Nobel laureate, member of the Academy of Science, and editor of *Revue scientifique* meant that when he became vice president of the French Eugenics Society, it added much to the legitimacy of the organization.

The background of men such as Louis Landouzy and Lucien March is less well documented than that of Perrier, Pinard, or Richet, but they were also important figures of the day. Landouzy, like Richet, came from a well-connected medical family, both his father and grandfather having been physicians. He became professor at the Ecole de medécine in 1880 and dean of the faculty in 1901. One reason for Landouzy's interest in eugenics was his work on diseases such as syphilis and tuberculosis. For example, he delivered a talk at the 1902 International Congress of Tuberculosis on the role of social factors in the etiology of tuberculosis, and in 1905 he published *l'Enquête sur l'alimentation d'une centaine d'ouvriers et d'employés parisiens,* which reflected a concern with the broader influences associated with the illnesses.[51] These professional reasons for Landouzy's interest in eugenics must have been reinforced by the fact that he had ample opportunity to discuss the subject after he married the sister of Charles Richet.

Lucien March, head of the Statistique générale, was attracted to eugenics by his work on the French birthrate, the most closely watched of all statistics in France at the turn of the century. His pioneering studies on fecundity and mortality for different regions and occupations in France were unusual in their broad view of the population problem in France.[52] Both his government affiliation and facility with figures made March a natural choice as secretary-treasurer of the French Eugenics Society, a position he held for the entire active life of the organization.

This survey of eugenics leaders shows them also to have been reactionary, not in the ideological sense but in their being motivated by the well-publicized perceptions of decline and degeneration at the turn of the century. Their eugenics was inspired much more by a reaction to decline than any strong desire to advance or perfect the human species. Perhaps this was the result of their limited expectations, which made them skeptical of the eugenic promises of their German or American counterparts. It was not necessarily the result of any kinder feeling toward the lower classes, whom they saw increasingly falling prey to degenerative influences. In the end, there is nothing surprising in the fact that these comfortable, successful, bourgeois doctors and professors should place more emphasis on preserving rather than improving society. After all, they had the most to lose.

FRENCH EUGENICS ON THE EVE OF THE FIRST WORLD WAR

As shown earlier, the work of the French Eugenics Society in this initial period was the most intense and varied of any time in the organization's history. Meetings were held monthly, and the journal *Eugénique* appeared with almost the same frequency. A membership drive was conducted, and overall the society functioned as an active, full-fledged organizational focus of eugenics in France in a manner that was never repeated after the war. A closer look at the substance as well as the organization of prewar French eugenics is therefore important not only for its own sake but also in order to appreciate how much the war changed it. French eugenics was comparable to the movement in England, Germany, and the United States at this time, both in its level of activity and in the broad range of ideas and opinions it encompassed. Only by understanding the breadth of activity before the war can one appreciate how dramatically the First World War narrowed the focus of French eugenics.

It took a few months in 1913 before the French Eugenics Society was meeting on a regular monthly basis as its founders envisaged, but by May of that year both the meetings and the journal were monthly affairs. This continued through May of 1914 (excluding a summer break, which was to be expected of any organization of academics in France), so that in all some fourteen meetings of the society took place in the year and a half before the outbreak of the war. In that same period, ten issues of *Eugénique* appeared.

Although meetings included the usual organizational business of introducing new members, giving treasurers' reports, and the like, their main focus was the presentation of papers by members and invited guests. Topics covered a surprising variety of subjects. Some were of interest to the many Lamarckians in the society, such as the eugenic effects of alcoholism, the hereditary transmission of psychological traits, and a call for mandatory reporting of syphilis. But other talks considered Mendel's laws, the phenomenon of "hereditary return to type," and the normal and pathological morphology of dentures. Equally surprising was the great interest shown in eugenics movements in other countries, as manifested by talks at meetings and material published in *Eugénique*. For example, for the fifteen talks given at the society, five were reports of activities outside France on topics such as the passage of the English Mental Deficiency Act of 1913 and the organization of a permanent international eugenics committee. In addition, two other talks were given by foreigners themselves – the Swiss Ladome's paper on alcoholism in December 1913, and a paper by the English neo-Lamarckian eugenicist C. W. Saleeby in January 1914 on the "Progress of eugenics."[53]

Eugénique was usually divided into four or five sections, the longest of which was a reprinting of the papers presented at meetings. The minutes and treasurer's reports were another regular feature, as was a section of analysis and review of published literature on eugenics. A final section was called "The eugenics movement," covering activities in France and other countries.

Perhaps the most important characteristic about French eugenics in this early period was its breadth of scope. Although the French were eventually to be identified primarily with the milder, neo-Lamarckian eugenics, this was by no means clear at the outset. For example, natalists such as Adolphe Landry were definitely Lamarckian in their assumptions about what was necessary to "preserve and improve the species," but men such as Frédéric Houssay, J. Laumonnier, and Charles Richet had other notions of the best means of "diminishing the number of bad elements" – which would have been welcomed by any Anglo-Saxon Mendelian eugenicist. All members of the French Eugenics Society could find common ground in their perception of degeneration, which manifested itself in many ways, but from the start they were far from agreement on programs to be followed in order to remedy the problem. Hence, Landry wrote an article early in 1913 for the general interest periodical *Revue bleu* answering the question "What is eugenics?" with the flat statement that sterilization and marriage restriction for individuals with certain defects were "repugnant to our need for liberty and our delicate individualism." Instead, he argued for an emphasis on the positive goal of trying to improve these unhealthy elements as well as "fortifying elements of mediocre quality and preserving from evil those that are healthy."[54]

In contrast, Laumonnier had written an article for *Larousse mensuel* a few months earlier that placed the first emphasis on eliminating the undesirables. And although Laumonnier agreed that the healthy elements should be encouraged to reproduce through programs that Landry and Pinard championed – puericulture before and after birth, the work of temperance societies, and construction of better housing – he placed most of his hope in negative measures based on precedents such as "military service, quarantines or mandatory vaccinations which entail certain restrictions on individual liberty."[55] Among these measures he included control of immigration, marriage restriction, and sterilization.

This viewpoint can also be found in the book by Charles Richet, *Sélection humaine,* published in 1919 but written before the war in

1912. This work merits closer examination for several reasons besides the fact that it helps define the boundaries of French eugenics. As mentioned in Chapter 3, an early draft of the book was instrumental in converting Pinard from the concept of puericulture to eugenics.[56] In addition, the book's significance was enhanced by the stature of Richet, the Nobel laureate, editor of *Revue scientifique* and frequent contributor on science to the most influential general interest magazines such as *Revue des deux mondes*. Richet's prestige and role as a popularizer of science thus gave his eugenics writings access to the wider French reading public. Nor was Richet merely a peripheral figure of the organized movement who happened to use the word "eugenics" to describe his views. Though not a founding member, Richet soon joined the French Eugenics Society and became a vice president after the war. He also gave his share of time to the movement by attending meetings and giving public talks.

Given the author's prestige, *Sélection humaine* was an influential book from the start. It was reviewed by the major publications of the day, and even those who disagreed with Richet's ideas could ill afford to treat the author's views lightly. Opponents of eugenics also recognized the importance of the book and mentioned it frequently in their attacks.[57] Finally, the form of the work added to its significance, because it was one of the few book-length treatments of eugenics as a whole program.

Of greatest interest were the ideas contained in the book that differed markedly from the mild, positive eugenics of baby doctors and museum directors. From the beginning, Richet, like Laumonnier, demonstrated little concern with the short-sighted eugenic goals of French natalists and patriots. His major concerns were closer to those of eugenicists in Anglo-Saxon countries. For example, Richet complained,

Nothing is more extraordinary than our indifference to human selection. One could laugh if it was not so sad. We improve breeds of chickens, ducks, horses, pigs, lambs, even species of cauliflower, beets, strawberries and violets! Man improves and perfects everything except man himself.[58]

Painting as bleak a picture of the struggle for existence as any social Darwinist, Richet bluntly stated that in nature "the weak are crushed. . . . The individual is nothing, the species is everything."

He then pointed out that only humans have introduced the concept of individual personality and the sentiment of tenderness that
"brings aid to the sick, even when their malady is more or less
incurable." Likewise, the sick, the deaf and the blind are cared for,
invalids are protected, and even criminals are given "delicate attention." Thus, man went against the law of nature.

On the question of the workings of heredity, Richet also offered
an unexpected view for a Frenchman: that the influence of the environment was small. "In the long run, perhaps," he conceded,
"and at the end of several centuries, the environment modifies
individuals and their descendants. But when it is a matter of four
or five generations, the influence of milieu is negligible."[59] Richet
was obviously not in the camp of the neo-Lamarckians; and his
view of the nature of heredity led him to propose a different means
of improving the race, based not on improving the environment
but by selecting mates for breeding. As he argued,

If one wishes to create a human race of great height, it would suffice to
choose (as the father of Frederick the Great did) men and women of great
height, marry them and in two, three or four generations, to have their
children marry, having eliminated those who on reaching adulthood were
not sufficiently tall. Thus would be created artificially a human race of
great height.[60]

The list of characteristics that Richet considered inheritable was
quite long, beginning with the obvious physical features of height,
hair, and eye color, but also including such things as muscular
strength, resistance to disease, and fecundity. Indeed, at times Richet wrote of heredity in anthropomorphic terms:

Suppose that all human beings were at the disposition of a very wise
observer, given tyrannical power and having before him several centuries to experiment. He could fashion human races with whatever physical characters, vigor, height, color, longevity and fecundity that he wished
to give them. Heredity dominates everything.[61]

Of all the inheritable traits, however, Richet was most concerned with intelligence. His reasoning was quite simple. His strong
positivist philosophy tied progress to science. In fact the opening
chapter of *Sélection humaine* was entitled "Progress and science."
For Richet, science meant intelligence. Although he saw intelligence as "essential for human progress," Richet admitted that

"vigor, health, beauty, and sexual attraction" were necessary to maintain physiological functions and insure reproduction[62]; but he made it very clear that they were subservient to the fostering of intelligence. Four whole chapters of the book dealt with different aspects of intelligence, its moral dimensions, and its application to invention and assimilation. One feature of Richet's preoccupation with intelligence as a eugenic selection criterion is that despite this similarity to the American eugenicists, he never advocated the use of intelligence testing or IQ measures of the population.

There were many features of Richet's definition of superiority and inferiority in human selection that he shared with other French eugenicists. For example, like most Frenchmen of his day, Richet saw whites as superior to Africans or Asians, and he opposed race mixing. More will be said in Chapter 8 about this view of racial hierarchy, but of note here is a link to eugenics harking back to the ideas of Vacher de Lapouge. Richet also opposed the evil triumvirate that was the scourge of all social hygienists – alcoholism, tuberculosis, and venereal disease – but he proposed the elimination of these evils in a manner that reflected his different view of heredity. Rather than concentrating attention on treating the afflicted, Richet called for "banishment of all those with the maladies to islands" such as Corsica, Sardinia, Ireland, Crete, Ceylon, or the Phillipines.[63]

The drastic nature of his proposed measures to improve the species was another striking feature of Richet's eugenics that set him apart from many of the French eugenicists of his time. Although one might quarrel with his lack of sensitivity, one can hardly accuse Richet of vagueness in describing his program to improve the human race. For example, he was quite explicit in advocating the prohibition of marriage between Europeans and "inferior races."[64] Another measure called for "the elimination of the mentally deficient," a goal that followed logically from his views on intelligence and heredity. For these *anormaux* ("deaf mutes, idiots, rachitics, and hydrocephalics") Richet suggested that

at the least the state should not take part in the care of these poor creatures. Nature has condemned them, and it is no good to go against an irrevocable judgement which nature has pronounced. Leave these unfortunates in the care of their families, and you can be sure at the end of a few years they will be no more.[65]

Richet also described the necessity of preventing these people from procreating; and considering the two most obvious means available – sterilization and marriage prohibition – Richet opted for the latter, not on moral grounds but as a practical expedient, until such time as society had developed the means and the sentiment to make sterilization more acceptable. For those who objected that this would be a violation of personal liberty, he argued that the precedent was already set by the state's right to regulate marriage. Richet claimed that he was merely extending the process. Moreover, he did not see the right of procreation in absolute terms.

No sentimental ranting will make me acknowledge the right of unfortunate individuals to bring into the world children as unfortunate as they: epileptics, alcoholics, degenerates, neurasthenics, criminals, tuberculars, the feeble, the ugly, rachitics and the deformed.[66]

Eventually this was to become the position of the French Eugenics Society when it advocated a premarital examination law in the 1920s, but at the time Richet was clearly in opposition to the views of those such as Manouvrier and Papillaut who did not wish to use agencies under social control to limit the individual's right to procreate. Richet's position was simply that "no person has the right to perpetuate illness and misery in the human race."

It would be wrong simply to make Richet into a cold-hearted ogre who anticipated the worst eugenic excesses of the Nazis in later years. For one thing, his method had a logic, even if it was based on false assumptions. For another, certain of his ideas were progressive and democratic – his program of developing intelligence, which consciously cut across sex and class boundaries. He urged, for example, that education be mandatory beyond the primary level and open to all so that those with the highest intelligence could benefit regardless of social or economic status. Nor did he consign the less intelligent to some dark reaches of society where they might anonymously serve their superiors. On the contrary, Richet called for all to be able to develop their intellectual faculties to the fullest. He singled out women, for example, as a potential resource that "suffers from the effects of an intellectual torpor perpetuated from generation to generation . . . , the fatal result of the miserable regimen to which they have been subjected."[67] As for the mass of young working men and peasants,

Richet offered another proposal that drew on his pacifist views –
converting the two years obligatory military service into something more meaningful. "Suppose," the Nobel laureate and pacifist wrote,

that instead of preparing young men for wars which will not take place
[this was written in 1912], they are made to pursue a series of scientific,
artistic and literary studies. Suppose that instead of putting them in barracks, they are kept in schools. Suppose that instead of teaching them a
small number of useless things, they are taught a great number of useful
things. Then one would keep the intellectual faculties of the peasant and
worker from atrophying after leaving primary school.[68]

The purpose of this extended consideration of *Sélection humaine*
has not been to suggest that Richet represented all French eugenicists. On the contrary, in many ways he was not typical. For example, in his chapter "Elimination of abnormals," Richet anticipated that his views might seem a "contradiction of what we have
said on different occasions about French natalism." To this he responded,

There are already enough humans on the face of the earth. In the near
future it is a plethora rather than a scarcity of people which is to be
feared. The growth of the French population is of the utmost importance
for France, but only for France.[69]

The conclusion he drew from this reasoning was very different
from what the natalists were accustomed to hearing: "We must
devote ourselves to the quality more than the quantity of our children."

Richet's book demonstrates quite graphically that there was a
diversity of opinion in French eugenics in the period before the
First World War. Hence, it would be inaccurate to oversimplify
French eugenics by considering it only as a neo-Lamarckian populationist movement. Just as these strains of thought can be found
in other countries, so too can many of the harsher, Mendelian-
based eugenics ideas be found in France. French eugenics covered
a broad spectrum of opinion, but this in turn makes the role of the
First World War all the more crucial in its influence on French
eugenics in the 1920s. For there is no question that the war losses
and heightened patriotism resulting from the war brought French
eugenicists squarely back to the question of population decline,

and at least for the first half of the 1920s made social hygiene the first item on the agenda of the French Eugenics Society. Harsher, negative proposals such as Richet's would have to await a later time when different conditions made them more acceptable to the public.

5

Postwar eugenics and social hygiene

The First World War cut short the initial phase of vigorous activity by the organized eugenics movement in France. Begun as a learned society with nearly regular monthly meetings and publication of a review, the French Eugenics Society attracted a wide range of interested parties and ideas. The society was in close touch with eugenicists in other countries, and exchanged visits with major proponents in both England and the United States. In fact, the French participation in the international movement was such that the Second International Eugenics Congress was scheduled to be held in Paris in 1915.

All of this was changed, of course, by the First World War. Meetings and publications of the French Eugenics Society were immediately suspended, and not resumed until after the war. Only occasional articles appeared on eugenics in other French journals, as the war completely absorbed the attention of the nation. The most far-reaching result of the war for eugenicists, as for most others, came from the loss of life that made the fear of depopulation an even greater concern than it had been at the turn of the century. In one sense, this heightened awareness of the population problem made people generally more open to the ideas eugenicists had talked about before the war. This is reflected in the many private initiatives begun after 1920 that, when added to the sharp increase in government involvement in everyday life that carried over from the war, blurred the distinction between private and public spheres that had made some people wary of eugenics before the war. But such subtleties were overwhelmed by the immediate effect of the war – to heighten the fear of depopulation. This in turn directed eugenic thought more than ever toward positive eugenics – that is, measures to ensure larger numbers of the fit. Hence, the broad and diverse range of eugenic ideas discussed and proposed before the war was quickly narrowed to focus on the neo-Lamarckian improvement of the population. In the years after the war, virtually all ideas aimed at eliminating the birth of "dysgenics" were ignored. Now the watchword of the French Eugenics Society became "social hygiene."

As mentioned in Chapter 2 the concept of social hygiene had a long prewar history dating back at least to the last quarter of the nineteenth century.[1] The concept was vague, however, and applied in many different contexts. In fact, the most frequent definitions were phrased simply in terms of the diseases combatted, especially tuberculosis, alcoholism, and venereal disease. For example, the 1904 founding statutes of the Alliance d'hygiène sociale gave precisely this definition, and as late as 1930 the *Larousse* defined social hygiene as "the most appropriate methods to limit the ravages of social diseases such as tuberculosis, cancer, and syphilis, and to combat plagues such as alcoholism."[2] One of the earliest to lend scientific credibility to the idea of social hygiene was Emile Duclaux, director of the Pasteur Institute, who argued in a 1902 book that there was a broader theoretical dimension implied by the term that

envisages illnesses not in themselves but from the social viewpoint; that is, from the point of view of their repercussions on society and the ability of society more or less to preserve itself and fight them.[3]

Here was the medical equivalent of the eugenic view of human biology – not from the viewpoint of individual health (or individual heredity, in the case of eugenics) but from the overall health of society (just as eugenics looked to the hereditary prospects for the whole species). Neo-Lamarckism had already provided the common ground for social hygiene and eugenics in France before the war to the extent that diseases were seen as hereditary. The First World War made such an association even more logical by its emphasis on the subservience of the individual to society as a whole.

EUGENICS AND WAR

It would be difficult to exaggerate the effect of the First World War on all aspects of French life. Although the appropriateness of calling it the first "world" war has been questioned by some, the description of it as a "total" war is accurate, not so much because it describes the number of countries or the proportion of the world's surface that became involved, but because it aptly reflects the fact that all levels of society were mobilized in the war effort.[4] France managed to escape the dramatic upheavals that literally remade the political and ideological map of Central and Eastern Europe, but the battleground of the Western Front was northeastern France, thus making it the West European country most directly affected by the war. Indeed, the impact is so obvious and far-reaching that the task here is not to show that eugenics was affected by the war, but rather to sort out the eugenics and related questions as they emerged in postwar years.

Undoubtedly, the single most important development in the war (as far as eugenics is concerned) was the loss of life involved.[5] The cold figures for French soldiers killed – over 1.3 million – are chilling enough, but when considered on an individual basis, the losses had a devastating psychological impact. For example, although the leaders of the French Eugenics Society were too old to enlist, the war came home to them in many ways. Charles Richet described the teaching atmosphere during the war at the Ecole de médecine as follows:

I gave my physiology course in the summer of 1915 without great enthusiasm. My class of young girls and boy students too young [for combat] and of old doctors was only lightly attended. I conducted no physiological experiments either during the course or at my laboratory.[6]

Both Richet and Pinard lost sons in battle. Pinard's was his firstborn, already marked to follow his father's career in medicine. When he was informed of the loss, Pinard is reported to have said, "Vive la France!" The death of Richet's son Albert was all the more tragic because it came in the closing days of the war. Even worse, the death of Albert, a much-decorated flying ace who had survived years of dangerous missions, came in a tragic mixup at the hands of a fellow French pilot. His father took small comfort from the fact that he had five other sons or sons-in-law who survived the war. As his memoirs record,

If I were God, I could perhaps forgive him (the other pilot), because perhaps there was no moral error. But I am not God! I am not even a judge! I am only a poor man whom the death of a courageous, noble and hardy son has placed in irrevocable mourning; and I do not forgive! I will never forgive![7]

These losses, coming after the fear of depopulation in prewar years, led to a further anxiety about the French birthrate – and with good reason. The combination of the war losses and the removal of almost all able-bodied males to the front – eventually 7.9 million out of 8.5 million males from ages 18 to 46 were mobilized – cut the birthrate in half from its prewar level of 18.2 per 1,000 to 9.5 for 1916, the lowest in French history. By 1919 the rate had only recovered to 12.6.[8]

Questions about possible neo-Lamarckian effects on the survivors (mutilations, psychological stress, wartime diseases) combined with shock at the loss of life to make the population problem such an overriding concern that it stifled other eugenic discussions in the immediate postwar years. The result was to narrow the range of eugenic ideas and produce the general strategy of supporting positive eugenics in the form of a social hygiene program. There was another reason for such an approach – it also reflected the sobering intellectual shock of the war to the positivist prewar eugenicists, who had sought to remake the world and the humans in it. The more limited objective of simply trying to improve the existing population biologically through social hygiene measures was much more compatible with the postwar spirit of rebuilding, both physically and psychologically. As one member of the French Eugenics Society described this mood,

The concrete, living world does not obey the fantasies of reformers. It has strict and even hard laws upon whose discovery we must try to focus our efforts. The truth is, it is the only way to be useful to our country and the generations that follow. Do not begin in another form the humanitarian dreams of 1914. They are too costly![9]

Support for such a social hygiene/eugenics program was very widespread. Ample evidence of the concern with the population and health questions can be found in a variety of initiatives both public and private. The first government actions were taken by the 1919 "blue horizon" Chamber, elected at the beginning of the postwar era. The election campaign itself reflected the public concern with population questions, as candidates added *père de famille* to their titles or the number of their children to their campaign literature.[10] Although the new Chamber stopped short of passing some of the more radical measures proposed (such as the family vote), a number of laws that lived up to the electoral promises *were*

passed. These ranged from the first organized system of paying
bonuses for large families, to reductions on train fares and schooling.[11]

One of the best known of these actions was the so-called Law
of July 31, 1920 against abortion and the advertising and sale of
contraceptives.[12] Attempts to pass such legislation before the war
had been unsuccessful, but in the postwar mood it was a different
story. Attached as a rider to a package of compromise bills already
voted by the Senate at the end of the 1920 session, the anti-
Malthusian legislation was introduced with these words:

In the aftermath of the war, where almost one and one-half million
Frenchmen sacrificed their lives so that France could have the right to
live in independence and honor, it cannot be tolerated that other French
have the right to make a livelihood from the spread of abortion and Malthusian propaganda.[13]

The proposition passed with an overwhelming majority, and although it did not solve the problem of the declining birthrate, the
new law was successful in eliminating, at least temporarily, an
organized birth control movement in France.

Other government actions revealing the mood of the times included the creation of the first cabinet-level health ministry in 1920
– the Ministère de l'hygiène, de l'assistance et de la prévoyance
sociale. It grew out of an undersecretariat of the ministry of labor
created during the war entitled *Service de santé militaire*. Given the
numerous measures passed during the war, the creation of this
ministry was only the next logical step in the government's increased participation in social hygiene matters.[14] For example,
several laws passed during the war sought to restrict the production and sale of alcohol. Although these were difficult to enforce
among civilians in wartime, the military was able to prohibit soldiers, draftees, and eventually those in civilian war production from
frequenting cafes and restaurants except at mealtimes.[15] Another
measure that focused more on treatment than on prevention was
the opening of outpatient centers for venereal disease. By the end
of 1917 there were sixty-five centers in fifty departments offering
consultation and treatment.[16]

The most important new measures taken by the government in
the health field were to combat tuberculosis. Medical examinations at the time of conscription turned up large numbers of would-

be recruits with the disease, and rather than sending them back to civilian life in this condition, Léon Bourgeois, with the backing of Landouzy, pushed a measure through the National Assembly to provide treatment for the recruits along with soldiers who were discharged because of tuberculosis. By the end of 1917 there were seventeen new sanatoriums designated for this purpose, plus fifty hospitals under military control and another forty under the ministry of the interior.[17] In fact, as will be seen, it was because the French government had shown so much interest in the tuberculosis problem that the American Red Cross and the Rockefeller Foundation decided to contribute to the effort.

The new health ministry was first headed by Jean-Louis Bréton, a leading natalist whose appointment shows very clearly how these health problems were connected to concerns about the French birthrate. Bréton had been a deputy since 1898, and made his reputation as a natalist before the war with such proposals as exempting fathers of large families from military service and a call for the family vote.[18] Bréton was not the only postwar cabinet member who had been active in the natalist movement. Auguste Isaac, a Lyon businessman who had been outspoken on French population problems before the war and president of the first Natalist Congress held in Nancy, became minister of commerce in 1919. In addition, André Honnorat became head of public works and Adolphe Landry minister of the navy.[19]

Among Bréton's actions was the creation of a permanent Conseil supérieur de la natalité suggested in the prewar years by Bertillon, and to which he named Isaac as president and Pinard and Richet as vice presidents.[20] Bréton also created the Institut d'hygiène to be administered and directed by the Ecole de médecine, which became a new center of research and instruction in social hygiene and other health fields.[21] Among those on the first administrative council of the Institut were Pinard, Richet, Alexandre Couvelaire (Pinard's son-in-law, who had succeeded him at the Ecole de médecine), and Edouard Jeanselme, an expert on venereal disease who was later to join the French Eugenics Society. Finally, Bréton created a Comité nationale de propagande d'hygiène sociale et d'education prophylactique.[22] Although it was severely hampered by lack of funds for the four years of its existence, the committee was a direct forerunner of the much more important National Social Hygiene Office.

In the postwar years, Pinard's ideas about puericulture were also given renewed emphasis and official sanction. Even before his retirement from the Ecole de médecine in 1914, Pinard had overseen the creation of a chair of Hygiène de la première enfance, whose first occupant, Antoni-Bernard Marfan, quickly set about to create a separate institution to teach puericulture. With the aid of Pinard, these efforts resulted in the founding of the Ecole de puericulture in the postwar years.[23] In 1923 the teaching of puericulture was made mandatory for all French schoolgirls.[24] Twice a month they were to be taught childcare lessons in feeding, bathing, and diapering infants. Puericulture also entered the textbooks of both public and Catholic schools by the 1930s.[25] The popularity of puericulture was so great that in 1924 the Chamber of Deputies attempted to create a new chair of puericulture at the Ecole de médecine without even consulting the faculty. Upset at the precedent it might set and suspicious that the real motive of the Chamber had been to create a chair for Benjamin Weil-Hallé who was to be director of the Ecole de puericulture (the statutes required the director to be a member of the faculty), the professors voted 30 to 1 against creation of the new chair, arguing that it was not necessary because Marfan's chair already existed.[26]

PRIVATE INITIATIVES

The founding of the Ecole de puericulture did not come from a French government initiative. It was originally the idea of the American Red Cross, which had helped with war relief and wished to donate $100,000 for a more permanent institution to help the children of France. After initial discussion with the dean of the faculty of medicine, the Red Cross was directed to Pinard, who became head of a Franco-American Foundation that eventually sponsored a project jointly with the French government (represented by the Ecole de médecine) to create the Ecole de puericulture.[27] A similar approach had been used by the International Health Board of the Rockefeller Foundation to fight tuberculosis in France during the war and, as will be seen later, another joint effort between Rockefeller and the French government in the area of social hygiene was to have important consequences for French eugenics later in the 1920s.

These and other private French efforts to improve the health

and population of the country reveal the depth of support for social hygiene and biological regeneration after the war. Of all the
initiatives concerning the well-being of the French population that
were inspired by the war, however, the most touching and indicative of the times were the various prizes and gifts established to
encourage large families. To be sure, some of these predated the
war, such as the Prix Bernard established in 1912 by the Abbé
Bernard of Rouen and awarded to families with four to five children.[28] But during the conflict the number of such prizes increased
dramatically, often as commemorative acts by families who had
lost sons in battle. A Prix Barnoud was established in July 1916,
providing five awards of 300 francs each for "modest but not in-
digent families" in rural cantons around Lyon; and when the
youngest of his seven sons was killed, Auguste Isaac created a prize
of 500 francs to be given each year to a family in his home department of Rhône-et-Loire with seven living sons.[29] Much more substantial, and also telling of the fact that presuppositions about
"quality" often underlay the natalists' efforts to encourage the
"quantity" of the population, was the Prix Lamy named after
Etienne Lamy, perpetual secretary of the Académie française in
1916. Based on an initial donation of 500,000 francs, prizes of 25,000
francs were awarded by the academy to two families annually who
were "French, Catholic, and peasant." The size of the prizes stimulated a great deal of interest, so to guide the judges, criteria were
established that stipulated further that the families chosen must be
"among the poorest, largest in size, the most Christian in belief,
and of the highest morality."[30]

Along similar lines was the best-known of all these private natalist initiatives: the Cognacq-Jay prizes. The money for these
awards came from the owner of the Samaritaine department store
and his wife. Two kinds of prizes, also administered by the Académie française, were created. First, there were annual awards of
25,000 francs for every department of France, given to families
with nine living children whose parents were both under forty-
five years of age. Second, there were 200 awards of 10,000 francs
to families with five living children whose parents were under thirty-
five. Although the terms of the Cognacq-Jay gift made clear that
"political or religious questions must not exercise any influence in
the awarding of the prizes," the amount of money involved was
so great (about 5 million francs awarded annually) that criteria had

to be established to screen the large number of nominations for the awards. Once again, a natalist initiative was forced to consider the question of quality. In this case, the parents had to be of French birth and show financial need; moreover, each family nominated was required to have an affidavit from the mayor of its commune plus other notables who could comment on the "reputation, life, and morals of the family."[31] One can see in these efforts not only the degree of interest in population questions, but also why there continued to be a basis of cooperation between natalists and eugenicists after the war. Both groups found it difficult to separate the questions of quantity and quality.

A different kind of private initiative that also mixed eugenic and natalist ideas was the establishment of a housing development outside Strasbourg called Ungemach Gardens. This project was begun in the 1920s, and eventually saw the construction of 140 houses whose occupants were drawn from "young married couples in good health, desiring to have children and raise them under favorable conditions of hygiene and morality."[32] The Strasbourg project was widely reported in French and foreign publications of the day. The American eugenicists Paul Popenoe and Roswell Johnson described it in their book *Applied eugenics* (1933 ed.) as the only garden city "planned definitely as a eugenic experiment."[33]

The namesake and benefactor of the garden city was Léon Ungemach, owner of a large Alsatian candy factory, who entered politics in the early 1900s at the end of his career, becoming wartime and postwar mayor of Strasbourg. The motivation for building the housing was not entirely philanthropic, as the source of money Ungemach donated was 2.5 million marks he had invested during the war in overseas securities as a hedge against the depreciation of the German currency. Because the funds were considered war profiteering, the money was subject to confiscation, but Ungemach proposed a different way of "returning the money to the community." According to an agreement signed in January 1920, a private foundation was created to build housing that would "encourage the development of large families." To make the dwellings available to all, rents were to be set at 25 percent below comparable accommodations elsewhere. The city of Strasbourg would donate the land for the project with the proviso that both land and dwellings would be given to the city in thirty years.

Starting with an initial capital of 6.5 million francs, the Ungemach Foundation held a design competition for the houses and then began selection of occupants. The first forty houses were ready by the end of 1924, and 242 applications were received from families well before the completion date.[34] Given this interest, the council of the foundation was quickly forced to come to grips with how to comply with the terms of the charter agreement in choosing occupants. It was easy enough to eliminate older couples without children or to establish a measure for income limits, but with so many applicants and the prospect of even more in the future (the following year there were 663 requests for the next 65 houses), a more rigorous system of evaluation was needed.[35]

What the foundation eventually devised is revealing about both the overriding concern with the population question and the impracticality of applying eugenic ideas to the real world. For although the decisions on applicants were based on what the foundation council called "eugenic information" compiled on each family, the basis for the decisions was largely a consideration of the existing or prospective quantity rather than quality of the family members. Specifically, a formula that awarded points in various categories was used. Most important, twenty points were given for each child, the total of which was divided by the number of years the parents were married. Hence, there was a rather heavy weighting toward family size and the youth of the couple. An additional point was given for each brother or sister of the parents, implying a belief in a predisposition (either biological or behavioral) toward fecundity. To reflect financial need, there was a reduction of one point for each 1,000 francs of yearly income over 18,000 francs; and another six points was deducted for each 1,000 francs of income from interest above 3,000 francs per year. Evidently, making a living from one's own labor was considered eugenically preferable to living too much on one's investments. The one additional consideration that may have reflected either eugenic or practical concerns was a mandatory visit to the home of each applicant. A rating of one to ten was given for "order and cleanliness," with a minimum score of six but more typically a seven required for approval.[36]

Ungemach Gardens was not unique in its attempt to provide better housing for the working-class populace. The idea first gained currency during the Second Empire of Louis Napoleon, but garden city and workers housing movements became more strongly

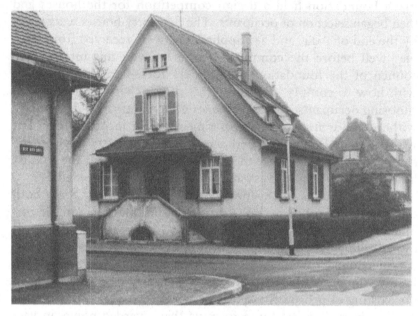

Figure 5.1   Houses at Ungemach Gardens (Strasbourg)

established in Germany, England, and the United States after the turn of the century. France had thus fallen well behind other countries by 1914.[37] The German rule of Alsace-Lorraine from 1870 to 1918 would seem to explain Strasbourg's position in the vanguard of planned housing, except that the eastern provinces of France had been the centers of such progressive reform in France since the middle of the nineteenth century. Mulhouse, for example, built its first workers' housing in 1853, and the leaders of the Musée social, Jules Siegfried and Georges Risler, both came from the Alsatian textile region of France.[38]

Ungemach Gardens was not particularly deserving of its title as a "eugenic experiment." Despite the claims of Popenoe and others, it was hardly in the same tradition as the Nazi *Lebensborn* program, which encouraged SS officers to mate with blond-haired, blue-eyed "Aryan" women.[39] Indeed, the lack of physical or even nationality screening at Ungemach Gardens is perhaps the most telling feature of the experiment. Yet, potential fecundity was a goal and an important consideration in choosing occupants, and success in this respect was reflected in the statistics frequently cited

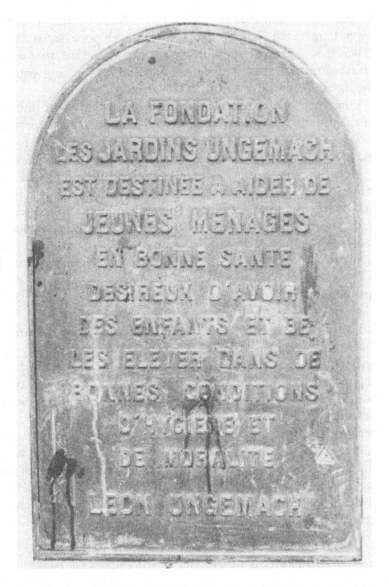

Figure 5.2 Commemorative marker, Ungemach Gardens (Strasbourg). "The Ungemach Gardens Foundation was created to help healthy young married couples wishing to start families and raise children under sound conditions of hygiene and morality." [Léon Ungemach]

by the foundation that showed a much higher birthrate for families in Ungemach Gardens than for the French populace as a whole.[40] It was this concern with biological goals, therefore, that made the Strasbourg experiment different from other housing projects of the day that typically had social or economic goals.

Ungemach Gardens is thus a striking example of the importance of the population question in postwar France, with its pretentions to serving eugenic ends. Yet, despite the publicity of its founders, the Strasbourg experiment went unnoticed by the members of the French Eugenics Society. There is quite simply no record of their interest in or even awareness of Ungemach Gardens. It is true that Strasbourg is a long way from Paris, even longer in the sense that Parisians notoriously ignored developments in the provinces. The reverse, however, may also have been true. Popenoe and Johnson claim that the idea for Ungemach Gardens originally came from Alfred Dachert, an employee of Ungemach's who had read the first edition of *Applied eugenics*.[41] Dachert became the first and only director of the gardens throughout its entire existence.

If it is true that the idea for Ungemach Gardens came from Dachert, it means that Dachert was as ignorant of French eugenic writers as they were of him. In 1949, when Dachert tried to find support for keeping the project from reverting to the city of Strasbourg, he looked outside France to England and the United Nations for help.[42] But another explanation for the lack of contact between Dachert and French eugenic writers lies in the particular course of action chosen by French eugenicists after the war that aimed at instituting more familiar social hygiene measures and using the national government as the enforcer. This will become clear upon closer examination of the activities of the French Eugenics Society after the war.

THE FRENCH EUGENICS SOCIETY AFTER 1920

After the war it required time for the French Eugenics Society to reconstitute itself. When it did, however, the society's activities in some ways went far beyond those of prewar years. Breadth and variety of ideas were sacrificed, but by narrowing its focus of attention, the society was able to concentrate its efforts more effectively. This explains in part why the French Eugenics Society was able to mount a legislative campaign for a premarital examination in the late 1920s (discussed in more detail in the next chapter). In the meantime, there were obstacles to be overcome before the society was organizationally or ideologically ready for such an undertaking.

There was, first, reluctance by some eugenicists to become closely identified with the natalist cause. Naturally, Richet was most outspoken in reminding his colleagues that eugenics societies "have another purpose which is also very noble but quite different: that is, to assure not a numerous posterity but an elite one. It is not a question of quantity for us but of quality."[43] Another society member, de Pulligny, agreed that "official repopulators" were so eager to encourage more births by all that they ignored questions of "inheritable defects, either mental or physical, and living conditions which are often incompatible with a minimum necessary for a rational puericulture."[44] Pinard, the father of puericulture, asked the National Assembly in his speech to the opening session of 1924, "Is raising the birthrate all there is to do? No. That is only half the task. Quantity is not enough. In addition and above all quality is necessary."[45] These reluctant natalist voices never went so far as to suggest that repopulation efforts might actually be dysgenic (that did not come until the 1930s), nor were there heated debates in the eugenics society's meetings over quality versus quantity. It was always assumed that both goals could be accomplished by a policy of positive eugenics. The concern was that the question of quality might be ignored altogether.

The first activities of the French Eugenics Society after the war show both the emphasis on positive eugenics and the adoption of new means to carry out the program. It is clear that the wartime experience was uppermost in the minds of eugenicists by the decision made at the first postwar meeting of the eugenics society in May 1920 to hold a series of conferences the next winter entitled "The eugenic consequences of the war." The idea was partly an effort to carry out a decision that had been made before the war to hold a conference on eugenics jointly with the Ecole des haute etudes sociales in the winter of 1914–15. Holding the conferences in 1920–21 was thus a way for the eugenics society to show continuity, at the same time examining the subject of greatest concern to all in France – the effects of the war.

These conferences were important in several respects besides indicating that the French Eugenics Society had resumed its work.

First, the format of the conferences reflected a change in the organization and strategy of the society. During the prewar years it had functioned as a learned society, holding regular monthly meetings at which business was transacted and scholarly papers were read. After the war, however, the eugenics society conducted its business less frequently but often in conjunction with larger conferences it sponsored for a wider public. To be sure, these were hardly meetings for a mass, general audience; but there is evidence that the lectures, conferences and *cours libres* did reach the intellectual, scientific, and political decision makers of France. For example, the series of talks given on the eugenic effects of the war were published as a book in 1922, and although no exact sales figures are available, royalties were a significant source of income for the French Eugenics Society in subsequent years.[46] In addition to the conference on the war, other topics covered by such meetings included social hygiene, the study of twins, and premarital examination laws. It is difficult to assess the overall effectiveness of the new strategy, but many of the visitors in attendance later helped replenish the membership ranks of the eugenics society in the postwar years.

Second, the 1920–21 conferences also signaled, in addition to organizational changes, the increased emphasis by the society on positive eugenics and social hygiene. That the results of the war should lead to an emphasis on positive eugenics was not by any means inevitable; in fact, eugenicists in other countries came to quite different conclusions about the results of the war. For example, English and American eugenicists (and even some French) saw the war as having greatly increased the number of dysgenic elements in the population. They argued that contrary to the social Darwinian assumption that war would accelerate the struggle for existence and survival of the fittest, the war had selected the best male specimens of the population for mass slaughter; hence, society was permanently deprived of their desirable traits, which would not be passed to subsequent generations.[47] In France as early as 1896, Vacher de Lapouge had expressed such a view, and it was repeated by Charles Richet in his prewar pacifist book, *The passing of war and the future of peace*. Richet maintained that war

produces a veritable counter-selection, and it leads to the impoverishment of the race. First, the sick and feeble are exempted from service. Invalids, deaf-mutes, the blind, one-armed, legless, hare-lips, the rachitic, tubercular, the insane, idiots, the feebleminded and the impotent are

well protected by military laws. None of these unfortunates risk death
on the battlefield. They are kept in the rear and spared. Those who are
chosen to disappear are the most fit and able. Young, robust men who
are the hope of future generations are the ones declared fit for service and
fit for death.[48]

According to this reasoning, any eugenics program after such a
catastrophe as the First World War would have to deal with the
problem of increased numbers of these dysgenics as well as how
best to foster the birth of the physically fit.

  Such negative questions, however, were never directly considered at the postwar eugenics conferences in France. Perhaps it
was too awful a conclusion for the French to contemplate, although the influence of neo-Lamarckian hereditary thought had
always been more optimistic about the prospect of improving the
species. The speakers at the 1920–21 conferences on the eugenic
consequences of the war repeatedly emphasized the positive role
eugenics could play in rebuilding and improving both the existing
population of France and future generations. For example, in Edmond Perrier's keynote address to the opening session entitled
"Eugenics and biology," he offered this modified definition of the
goals of the French Eugenics Society: "To research, define and
spread the means of perfecting the human races by indicating the
conditions which each individual, each couple must strive to fulfill
in order to have healthy and beautiful babies."[49] Perrier was equally
clear in his opposition to the negative measures that eugenicists in
other countries employed, because in his words, "in a civilized
country, one would not dream of suppressing individuals afflicted
with hereditary defects nor forbid them from reproducing. We
must try to remedy the imperfections of their progeny in their
earliest years." Hence, the long-range solution to the effects of the
war, according to Perrier:

The environment itself must cease to be a cause of degradation. National
vices like alcoholism, lack of personal care which propagates contagion,
and overindulgence of all kinds must be unmercifully proscribed. Homes
and cities, all that touches communal life must be the object of carefully
coordinated attention.[50]

Other speakers insisted that such a program was even more urgent because the war had generally worsened the health of the
country. This was the other side of the neo-Lamarckian coin; for
if improved hereditary characteristics could be acquired, so too

could negative ones from the effects of war. But these acquired hereditary defects were described in a very different manner from the more permanent results Richet had warned of in 1907. Eugène Apert's paper at the postwar conference entitled "Eugenics and national health" described these neo–Lamarckian effects of the war as stemming from the serious increase in disease, especially a rise in the incidence of syphilis and tuberculosis, the latter among women and children on the home front. As for the direct effects of the war itself, Apert noted in children born during the war "a regrettable rise in frequency of certain defects, and in particular nervous defects which are explained by the fact of conception and pregnancy in the midst of fear, sorrow, anguish, air raids and bombardments."[51]

Apert was less concerned about the extent of neo-Lamarckian influences from the battle front, telling the audience that not all of what soldiers had suffered would be passed to their children. "As to wounds, amputations, ankylosis, serious scars and fractures, reproductive capacity is not diminished nor is there a danger of transmission to future generations."[52] The other developments were bad enough, said Apert, and when added to the effects of wartime malnutrition on young children and the increase of disease among adults, his conclusion was that "the population after the war is in such a condition as to make more necessary than ever the health measures that have already been called for before the war."[53]

Apert's program for improving the hereditary health of France was similar in outline to Perrier's but much more specific. In addition to calling for campaigns against alcoholism, syphilis, and tuberculosis, he also spoke of the need for better housing, especially for workers, to be located outside congested cities.[54] Apert even advocated the construction of a transportation system to carry workers to their jobs. At the same time, he lamented the spread of the eight-hour work day, because although it was beneficial to manual laborers and professional classes, for the rest of the working class it only "increased the time spent in bars and unhealthy lodgings." Finally, Apert called for campaigns to increase the birthrate and decrease the infant mortality rate. The latter, he noted, could most easily be done by following the advice of fellow eugenicist Adolphe Pinard, whose puericulture had long called for "leaving children with their mothers and giving them all the facilities necessary to continue breastfeeding."[55]

Other talks at the postwar conferences included Lucien March's analysis "Birthrate and eugenics" and Georges Papillaut's "Psycho-social consequences of the last war from the viewpoint of eugenics." March's paper is worth noting, for he sought to answer the concerns of eugenicists in other countries that population growth would result in a general lowering of the quality of the population because the lower classes had higher birthrates. March argued that although the birthrates in France varied widely among the populace, they did not follow a pattern according to income. There were variations that followed regional and occupational lines, but no simple correlations between wealth and family size. For example, according to March's prewar studies, the birthrate was "higher among farmers, sailors, fishermen, coal miners of the North and the heads of large industries than among the middle classes, workers and especially salaried employees."[56] In addition, March argued, "nothing permits the conclusion that innate abilities, as opposed to acquired abilities, are lower in poor families than in rich families, especially if one adds all categories of the population: cities and countryside, intellectuals and artisans." Hence, March, like most of the other conference speakers, did not hesitate to call for support of programs to increase the population of France.

The only talk that mentioned the need for negative eugenic measures was Georges Schreiber's "Eugenics and marriage." Noting that screening was required before entering the army, he asked, "Why is it less important when it comes to marriage?" Schreiber also claimed that such a screening was more necessary than ever because of the dysgenic effects of war that Richet had described. Schreiber proposed a physical examination before marriage – a practice already in use or under discussion in several American states and European countries. He was not very specific about sanctions for failure to be examined, nor did he go into detail about what was to be done with the results of the exams. His proposal was only a first suggestion for establishing a screening process. Moreover, his overall goal was not very different from that of his colleagues: eliminating the "hereditary" diseases of tuberculosis, syphilis, and alcoholism, as well as some others, such as cancer and mental illness.[57]

Significantly, even Schreiber's mild suggestion was not followed. Instead, the French Eugenics Society began to support other organizations in France that were combatting one or another of the so-called hereditary diseases mentioned at the conference. Individual members of the eugenics society were already doing this by their participation in the multitude of institutions and organizations alluded to before, such as the Ecole de puericulture, the Institut d'hygiène, and the Conseil supérieur de la natalité. Reciprocal relations were established as members of other organizations joined the French Eugenics Society. These included Just Sicard de Plauzoles and Edouard Jeanselme of the Ligue nationale contre le péril vénérien, Emile Leredde of the Comité d'union contre le péril vénérien, André Honnorat, a senator and frequent cabinet minister who participated in several social hygiene organizations, and Georges Risler, president of the Musée social.[58] Publicity and financial support were given to these organizations, with activities of the French Eugenics Society ranging from production of a film on venereal disease to radio broadcasts and sponsorship of an annual lecture series on social hygiene at the Sorbonne.

It should be noted that the eugenics society's policy of working with other organizations was more than a knee-jerk response to postwar political and psychological conditions. There had been some movement in this direction before the war, as shown by plans to hold a joint conference with the Ecole des hautes études in 1914–15. In addition, the French Eugenics Society was closely involved in creating another important new organization after the war: the International Institute of Anthropology (IIA). Inspired by the shock of the war to the European scholars who had studied human society, the institute's four divisions included one devoted to eugenics. Although the primary purpose of the organization was international cooperation, the French office of the IIA helped sponsor conferences and meetings in France on eugenics in the early 1920s, and, as will be seen, later replaced the French Eugenics Society itself as the institutional home of eugenics in France.

THE NATIONAL OFFICE OF SOCIAL HYGIENE

Given the wide support for social hygiene in France, it is legitimate to ask what went wrong with the strategy of the French Eugenics Society to pursue such a program. French eugenicists presented their new ideas at the 1920–21 conferences on the war and established contact with many of the organizations working on similar and related problems. The beginning of a powerful co-alition seemed at hand. Indeed, by the end of the 1920s such a coordinated effort was a reality, but the French Eugenics Society was not at its center. The most important reason for this development was the breadth of the appeal of social hygiene, which proved to have its drawbacks as well as its advantages. This had been pointed out by one eugenics society member, Georges Papillaut, as early as a 1921 meeting.

The definitions given for eugenics in England as in France are very vague, and could be applied perfectly well to all questions of individual and social hygiene. . . . A flock of societies have crowded in the way, and the zeal of their members is far from exhausting the humanitarian sentiments they display. I hope that the eugenics society does not become confused with the latter.[59]

In other words, not only could eugenics work with social hygiene, but so too could virtually every health organization in France. It was because of this broad definition that the ideas of the postwar eugenics conferences, the propaganda efforts, and the society's joint organizational ventures elicited such a strong response in government circles, private organizations, and among the general public. In fact, so many other groups were involved that the eugenics society had no chance to control the social hygiene movement and keep it in line with even the neo-Lamarckian goals of the society. Cordial relations were kept with the more important organizations that helped the French Eugenics Society in later campaigns, but by the end of the 1920s, social hygiene in France had become virtually indistinguishable from public health. Instrumental in this change was the creation in 1924 of a new institution with the resources and backing that could direct the movement: the National Office of Social Hygiene. The establishment of this new office reveals yet another facet of the postwar organizational politics of health and social reform in France that affected the eugenics society.

The social hygiene office owed its origins to the same postwar conditions that affected the French Eugenics Society. It grew out of a privately organized campaign against one of the social plagues in France: the First World War tuberculosis program funded by the Rockefeller Foundation.[60] The tuberculosis project was part of the general war relief effort of the foundation, based on the specific recommendation in July 1916 of Warwick Greene, director of the Rockefeller War Relief Commission in Berne. He was convinced that an opportunity existed for the foundation to help in France not just because of the increased incidence of tuberculosis during the war, but also because the French government was becoming increasingly aware of the problem and ready to take action.[61]

The tuberculosis problem had already been recognized as acute in France by many prewar observers, particularly in comparison with other Western countries. For example, of 692,768 deaths in France in 1912, 83,783 were attributed to tuberculosis, most of them (69,731) to tuberculosis of the lungs. This figure – over 10 percent of all deaths were due to pulmonary tuberculosis – was significantly higher than for other countries. In Germany it was 8.3 percent, in England 7.2 percent, and in Belgium only 6.2 percent.[62] As early as 1903, a Commission de prophylaxie contre la tuberculose, under the leadership of Léon Bourgeois, had been established but one of its first goals (calling for the mandatory reporting of cases of tuberculosis) met strong resistance from the medical community on grounds of professional confidentiality. Shortly after the outbreak of war, the French government was forced to become involved with the problem because of the high incidence of tuberculosis among recruits and soldiers. In November 1915 a commission was appointed to study the problem, and in March 1916 a permanent Comité d'assistance aux militaires tuberculeux de guerre was created. The next month the so-called Bourgeois Law was passed creating "dispensaries of social hygiene and preservation against tuberculosis." And in September a system of treatment in sanatoriums was organized for soldiers with tuberculosis before their discharge from the army.[63] As expenditures on hospital facilities and loss of manpower increased, the French government was naturally eager for help as well as for ideas about broader measures to deal with the problem.

In the view of the Rockefeller Foundation's field staff, the French government's measures were lacking in two respects: they ignored the civilian populace, and concentrated only on treatment and not prevention. As a result, the foundation proposed a program that would supplement French efforts and take a broader, long-range approach to the question of prevention, a luxury that a private organization could afford because it was not subject to immediate military and political pressures as the French government was. The

Rockefeller program was accepted, and eventually consisted of two distinct parts. First, there was a national publicity campaign to educate the French populace about the causes and means of preventing tuberculosis. This included the latest techniques utilizing motion pictures, posters, brochures, lectures and, for the first time in France, tuberculosis stamps, which were the forerunner of today's Christmas Seals. Much of the language and style of the propaganda was influenced by that used in the war effort, some of it not very subtle. For example, one poster depicted a dead Prussian eagle with a sword through its heart and the words announcing, "The German eagle will be defeated, so too must tuberculosis." Another poster carried the heading, "The other peril," and the explanation, "We must not rest on our laurels. Tuberculosis threatens us. It must be defeated."[64] Mobile publicity teams were equipped and sent around the French countryside to carry the message against tuberculosis. The scene when the delegation arrived in a town was described by a reporter for *Le Matin* in the following manner:

A delegate arrives. He pays a visit to all the newspapers and to the municipal, military, prefectoral, and religious authorities. . . . The mayor offers a free hall to the impresario – I mean the delegate. After the hall has been obtained, the delegate covers the city with posters. And such posters! Barnum and Bailey would not be ashamed of them. . . . The legends and designs make people laugh. They gather in a circle, they are amused, and instructed.[65]

The second part of the Rockefeller program focused both on treatment and what the Americans called "team play against tuberculosis." In the words of the foundation, this approach required the establishment of

a complete organization which permits the tracking down of tuberculosis cases as early as possible, to be able to observe and treat them for the entire life of the individual either until he is well or until the illness ends in death, and after the death of the individual to continue observation of the family.[66]

The Department of Eure-et-Loire was chosen to be the primary demonstration site for the project because it was close enough to Paris and endowed with enough facilities. A smaller demonstration was also conducted in the XIXth arrondissement of Paris to obtain results in an urban setting. Some financial assistance from

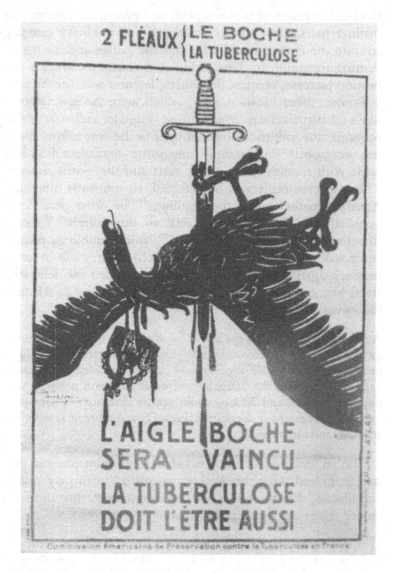

Figure 5.3   Poster for the Rockefeller tuberculosis campaign. [Source: Alexandre Bruno, *Contre la tuberculose: La mission Rockefeller en France et l'effort français* (Paris: Villages sanatoriums des hautes altitudes, 1925)]

the American Red Cross and the French government helped relieve the lack of dispensaries and sanatoriums, but a greater deficiency was found in the general lack of nurses to make home visits. To solve this problem, a whole system of education for visiting
nurses had to be established to train the necessary personnel.[67]

This was obviously no small undertaking, even by Rockefeller
standards. The first 5 years of the tuberculosis campaign and related nursing education program cost over 2.5 million dollars, or
more than one-quarter of all the expenditures by the foundation's
International Health Board in these postwar years.[68] Given this
investment, it is not surprising that the foundation was interested
in seeing the establishment of a more permanent and broader institution in France that could build on the lessons of the tuberculosis project. This was to be the National Office of Social Hygiene.

The idea for the office grew specifically out of the propaganda
and statistical work of the tuberculosis program, both of which
had greatly impressed the French. The appeal to French health
professionals of gathering statistics on the population is understandable, but the impact of the propaganda effort on the general
public was even more profound. The reporter for *Le matin* was
quite frank in his assessment of how the Rockefeller program was
different from other health programs of the French.

The directors of the "International Department of Hygiene" of the
Rockefeller Foundation are aware that even the best article does not sell
unless you "hit the nail on the head." Possessors of that excellent though
neglected commodity known as the truth, they find that public education
is necessary in spreading it, and that this, after all, consists of nothing
more than applying the art of advertising to the facts of science. This is
their harangue to us by posters and cinema:

> No one, Frenchmen, has excelled you in the scientific study of tu-
> berculosis. But it is not enough that your scientists combat this dis-
> ease; each one of you must take part in the battle, must benefit from
> the knowledge acquired, and perform in his turn the office of edu-
> cator. . . . Why do you give your patronage to charlatans? Because
> they advertise. We have taken advertising away from them and use
> it in the interest of science.[69]

When the tuberculosis program was turned over to the French
in 1924, the head of what had been the Rockefeller Foundation

tuberculosis project, Selskar M. Gunn (a public health specialist from Massachusetts), stayed on as head of the Paris office of the International Health Board.[70] It was Gunn who arranged for the Rockefeller support that created the social hygiene office, but there is ample evidence that the Americans had the idea in mind well before the tuberculosis program ended. In March 1922, for example, Linsly R. Williams, then director of the tuberculosis program, sent his superiors a nineteen-page "Memoire on hygiene in France," which described a broad program that could result, he claimed, in "saving 200,000 lives annually" within ten years.[71] It included no less than fourteen different organizations to be created or coordinated. Among them were propaganda and documentation centers, offices to monitor tuberculosis and venereal disease as well as nursing establishments and hospitals, plus new offices of industrial hygiene, food and drugs, and sanitary engineering. So complete was the memo that Williams even included a list of potential French personnel and a projected budget of 7.75 million francs. Nor was this simply an internal Rockefeller document meant only for New York. It was presented to no less a figure than the French minister of health, who responded positively and in detail.[72]

Implementation of the idea, however, was hampered by the complications of French cabinet politics. Already in October 1922, steps had been taken that would result in abolishing the ministry of health and merging its functions with those of the ministries of interior and labor. Moreover, cabinet changes were so frequent that it was difficult for the Americans to arrange meetings with ministers, let alone exchange ideas. For example, between February and June of 1924 Gunn attempted to present his ideas for an overall coordinating health agency to three different heads of the health or labor and health ministries. It was not until September that he finally saw Justin Godart, minister of labor and health, the man who would establish the program.

Godart was one of the major social reformers of the Third Republic. Elected a deputy from Lyons before the turn of the century, he went on to become a senator and hold several different cabinet ministries. Health reform had long been one of his primary concerns, and in fact it was Godart who headed the wartime Service de santé militaire, which had been the forerunner of the health ministry. In addition to being favorably disposed to Gunn's ideas, Godart was well connected politically and stayed in office long enough to put the project into motion. His first step was to commission Gunn to make a general study of health organizations in France. Then he formally presented the cabinet with a proposed decree to create a "National Office of Social Hygiene" to replace an office with a similar name that Bréton had created in 1920 but that had been handicapped all along by insufficient funding. The new office was to have an initial budget of 443,600 francs, of which the Rockefeller Foundation was to provide 300,000 francs.[73]

The importance of the American money in the creation of the office is obvious. Although Gunn made clear the foundation's expectations that French government support would increase, it was slow in coming. Not until 1928 did French contributions exceed those of the Americans. The foundation's directors were sensitive to the extent of Rockefeller funding of the office, as indicated by the following memo of George Vincent, chairman of the International Health Board. Responding to a report by Gunn at the end of 1925 that included a financial chart of the social hygiene office's operations, Vincent wrote,

I wonder if it might not be wise to suggest to SMG [Selskar M. Gunn] that in future editions of the chart we do not appear as part of the organization. There is a certain humor in our status of co-ordinating equality with the French Chamber of Deputies. It is possible, however, that it might be interpreted in another way.[74]

SOCIAL HYGIENE IN PRACTICE

With the establishment of the social hygiene office, it remained to be seen whether and how its functions would serve the interests of French eugenics. Theoretically, the stated goals of the office fit well within the idea of social hygiene as eugenicists understood it in postwar France. Although the first goal and last goals were vaguely stated as the collection of documentation on social hygiene, and the "coordination of all efforts being made on behalf of protecting public health," the second goal was specifically to provide information to medical and health personnel on "hygiene, social diseases, and their prevention." The third was even closer to the goals of the eugenicists:

The establishment in France and in the colonies of a continuous and methodical propaganda to the public, in order to make known the hygiene and prophylactic measures necessary for the maintenance of health, the fight against social diseases, and the preservation of the race.[75]

Many of those associated with French eugenics were named to the organizational council of the new office, including Honorrat (who was named president), Couvelaire, Jeanselme, Sicard de Plauzoles, and of course Pinard. With the exception of Pinard, however, all were recent members of the French Eugenics Society, and none came from the inner circle of officers.

The chances of the social hygiene office's coming under the sway of French eugenicists were diminished even more in the long run because of the scope of the organization and the size of its budget. As for the latter, from its inception the budget of the National Office of Social Hygiene was so large that there was no way for the French Eugenics Society to compete with it as coordinator of social hygiene work in France. As mentioned earlier, Rockefeller money continued at a steady 300,000 francs per year to the end of the decade, whereas French government funds slowly increased. In fact, after surpassing the American contribution in 1928, the French money increased rapidly, so that by 1930 it was triple the Rockefeller funds.[76] At the same time, the initial influence of eugenicists in the office diminished as additional services were added or expanded that tended to be specialized and serve the particular interests of organizations already established and working on specific health problems, such as venereal disease, tuberculosis, and alcoholism, or the recently created organizations working on cancer, mental health, typhoid fever, and diphtheria. This meant that from the standpoint of size alone, no one group could control the office's operations. A few examples of the organizational evolution of the National Social Hygiene Office will illustrate how quickly its size and diversity grew.

When the social hygiene office began, its internal organization reflected a fairly balanced effort to meet its four goals. For documentation, a central office was created to collect general information and respond to outside requests. Additional information was gathered by a separate section charged with conducting a systematic survey of public and social hygiene in every department; and all the data was to be organized by a statistical section modeled after the one used in the Rockefeller tuberculosis program. For outreach, a liaison office was created to work with existing organizations, but even more important in the long run was a propaganda service that was also copied from the tuberculosis program.[77] In addition, the social hygiene office was given two existing services that continued to function with relative autonomy: the Venereal Disease Prevention Service, which included over 200 treatment centers in hospitals, clinics, and dispensaries, as well as inspection services at ports; and the Central Nursing Bureau, which ran the schools for visiting nurses created by the Rockefeller Foundation and continued to receive separate funding from the foundation.

In the next seven years, almost all of these programs expanded, and at least one new major division was added to the social hygiene office: the Colonial Social Hygiene Service. By 1931 the documentation service was responding to nearly 2,000 requests for information annually, but the largest and most active program (with the exception of the quasi-independent venereal disease protection service, whose budget had grown from 3 million to 20 million francs) was the propaganda service. One indication of the size and scope of its work is the wide variety of techniques it used and the size of the audiences it reached. For example, following the model of the traveling tuberculosis medicine show, nine mobile teams circulated throughout France in 1931 and presented more than 2,000 conferences and films to a total audience of over 1 million people. Almost 7 million pamphlets, leaflets, and other printed materials were distributed. The service broadcast 975 radio programs and presented 142 performances of two plays entitled *Mortel baiser* (on venereal disease) and *Vivre* (on tuberculosis). Among the films produced were: *Le voile sacré* (the veil referred to in the title was that of the visiting nurse), a new film first shown at the Grand Amphitheatre of the Sorbonne and introduced by Alexandre Couvelaire; *Maternité* (a film on puericulture shown to 420,000 viewers during the year); *A l'ancien chauffeur* (a film on alcoholism); *Le baiser qui tue* (a film for the military on venereal disease); *Un grand fleau social, le cancer; La diphterie; La source* (a film about typhoid fever); and *Ames d'enfants* (subtitled "The slums").[78]

The wide variety of subjects dealt with in these films indicates that the number of problems covered by social hygiene had grown considerably from the old trio of tuberculosis, alcohol, and venereal disease. This is only natural given the vagueness of social hygiene's definition and the relatively large amount of funds at its

144 Quality and quantity

disposal. The office soon became involved with almost every health organization in the country.[79] For the year 1931, no less than fourteen specific national campaigns were being supported by the National Social Hygiene Office. Besides those working against the traditional social plagues, the office supported efforts against other diseases such as cancer, diphtheria, and typhoid fever, as well as more general problems such as infant mortality and mental illness. Other campaigns in 1931 and subsequent years were conducted against slums and rats and in favor of pure drinking water, milk, dental hygiene, and the preservation of eyesight.[80] Two other campaigns indicate that although the scope and size of the social hygiene office placed it beyond the control of eugenicists and their allies, they could still avail themselves of the resources of the office. One campaign supported every year was in favor of increasing the birthrate, jointly sponsored by the Conseil supérieur de la natalité and the Alliance nationale pour l'accroisement de la population. The other, established in 1930, was in support of the premarital exam, the major campaign of the French Eugenics Society in the late 1920s. This will be discussed in more detail in the next chapter.

CONCLUSION

The establishment and work of the National Social Hygiene Office hardly contradicts the assessment made by members of the French Eugenics Society that postwar sentiment was concerned with questions of human biology from the standpoint of both quantity and quality. Nor can the eugenics leaders be faulted for losing control of the social hygiene movement, especially once the national office was created. In addition to the movement's being too large and far removed from the leaders politically, there was another, larger development working against them: a transformation of the very notion of social hygiene. As the rigors and sacrifices of the war receded into the past, the emphasis of social hygiene shifted away from, in Duclaux's words, the "social viewpoint" of illness. With the return to normalcy came the tendency once again to view health and hygiene from the perspective of the individual, specific case. National campaigns might be waged, more because of their efficiency in reaching larger numbers of individuals than because of their view of the problems from the perspec-

tive of society or the human species as a whole. It is not coinciden-
tal that when the French Eugenics Society embarked on a new
campaign for a premarital examination law, the law could be presented as serving the interest of individual couples as well as the
larger eugenic goals of society.

6

The campaign for a premarital examination law

The campaign by the French Eugenics Society for a law requiring a physical examination before marriage was noteworthy in many respects. In the long run it produced the present French marriage law, which is the most obvious legacy of the eugenics movement's efforts to improve the population of France biologically. Although the present law requiring a blood test and tuberculosis x-ray is usually seen as a health measure, it was conceived and implemented in the name of eugenics and grew directly out of the legislation first proposed by Schreiber at the French Eugenics Society conference in 1920. Members of the society were central in proposing, lobbying, and keeping the idea of the premarital examination law before the French public between the wars. No other organization was as actively engaged in promoting the law.

In another sense, the premarital examination law was an important landmark in the history of the French eugenics movement because it represented the first major shift in emphasis of the society from positive to negative eugenics. Although critics argued with the law's effectiveness, there is no question that eugenicists saw the physical examination as part of a screening program whose ultimate purpose was to prevent procreation by the unfit. It is true that this point quickly became obscured (deliberately, one might argue, for political reasons) by related health diagnostic proposals aimed at detecting and treating certain diseases. But, as indicated by the history of the social hygiene movement in Chapter 5, ambiguity was typical of such measures. Moreover, as will be seen in Chapter 7, the advocacy of the premarital examination presaged a broader trend in French eugenics toward other negative measures that gained support in the 1930s.

The campaign for a premarital examination law was also very different from previous actions of French eugenicists in that it focused on legislation to accomplish its goals. Prior to the First World War, most members of the French Eugenics Society agreed with Léonce Manouvrier's modified redefinition of Galton's eugenics, which avoided the call for societal measures to achieve eugenic ends. They were satisfied to sit back in the ambiance of the Ecole de medécine, discussing various means of improving future generations, confident that the logic and value of their ideas would eventually filter out and persuade the public to follow them. At most, they invited politicians and social reformers to join them at meetings or to read the society's journal, content that the compelling logic of their arguments would carry the day. Although their postwar activities included a search for allies in the social hygiene movement, which itself had become increasingly involved in government activities, as late as 1925 French eugenicists had not followed the lead of their English and American counterparts in proposing specific legislative measures to achieve their eugenic goals. In other words, there was no French equivalent of the English Mental Deficiency Act of 1913 or the numerous American state laws on sterilization or the spectacular American immigration restriction legislation of 1921. Hence, Pinard's 1926 legislative proposal for a premarital examination law was probably most significant for bringing the tactics of French eugenics in line with the activities of eugenics movements in other parts of the world.

Like the parable of the half glass of water that can be seen as half empty or half full depending on one's perspective, the campaign by the French Eugenics Society for a premarital examination law was also indicative of its inability to implement a eugenics program as their counterparts in other countries had done. The proposal for legislation came late, in part because eugenicists were timid and apprehensive about public support. Moreover, once a law was proposed, there was much disagreement among eugenicists about its terms. In the atmosphere of political paralysis that characterized the Third Republic between the wars, little wonder that passage of the legislation was delayed until the Vichy regime created a new framework as well as a rationale for the measure.[1]

Contrary to the fears expressed by some eugenicists, there was nothing inherent in French society to prevent the idea of a premarital examination from receiving serious consideration. As mentioned in Chapter 2, the question of a premarital examination for eugenic purposes was widely discussed at the turn of the century, well before the American states began enacting laws requiring these examinations. In fact, as early as the Revolution of 1848, there had been a legislative proposal to prohibit marriages "by consumptives, the scrofulous [tubercular], syphilitics, and other sick people." It drew the attention of Lamartine, Thiers, and Arago, and in a foreshadowing of twentieth-century arguments, the measure was justified by analogy with the physical examination of recruits at the time of military conscription.[2]

Cazalis' 1900 book and proposals to the French Chamber, although not adopted, provoked an extensive debate in the French medical community. The Société de prophylaxie morale et sanitaire held several meetings on the subject from June through December 1903, and an issue of Cabanès' *Chronique médicale* that same year contained lengthy articles based on answers from prominent physicians and other leaders to the question, "Should marriage be regulated?"[3] Yet, French medical and health literature was slow to notice the new American laws regulating marriages. One reason was that, as always, the decentralization of the American political system left marriage regulation up to the individual states, making the new laws less noticeable than a national statute. In addition, it was not until 1909 that the state of Washington passed the first law making a medical certificate obligatory before marriage, and even then the law was soon revoked. Eventually, seven other American states passed similar laws but with differing requirements as to whether the future husband or wife or both were to be examined, and for what. Thus, most states tested for venereal disease and tuberculosis, North Carolina added a screening of "idiots, imbeciles and the insane," and North Dakota's law tested for "epileptics and inveterate alcoholics."[4] Thus the Americans, hardly offered a clear-cut example for the French Eugenics Society to follow in considering a premarital examination law before the First World War. It was only after the war that the idea reappeared in France, helped also by developments in the international eugenics movement.

The earliest postwar calls for a law requiring a premarital examination for eugenic purposes came from Charles Richet in his book, *Sélection humaine,* and Georges Schreiber in his talk before the conferences on the eugenic consequences of the war in the winter of 1920–21. Their reasons for the measure, however, were very different, and illustrate once again the diversity of opinion that existed in French eugenics. Richet's position was, typically, the more extreme. His book devoted a whole chapter to the subject of "Prohibition of marriage by the abnormal," and an example of the radical nature of his views is found in his conclusion.

It is very simple to require as authorization for marriage not the banal certificate of a complacent doctor but the decision of a control commission judging with even more severity than our military conscription boards. Excluded would be syphilitics, alcoholics, epileptics, the tubercular, the rachitic, those who have neither sufficient size nor muscular strength, those who would not be in condition to read, write or count. Rigorously excluded would be those with several criminal convictions, because it is completely useless to perpetuate families of criminals.[5]

Although he wrote the book before the war, Richet did not shy away from his convictions when the book was published in 1919. In fact, as mentioned in Chapter 5, the war had reinforced his opinion that the emphasis of eugenics had to be on improving the quality of the population, and Richet considered the premarital exam to be the most practical starting place. At a conference in 1921, Richet restated his position, including the analogy between the long-established physical examination required before entering the military and the proposed examination before marriage, and noting that "there is much less peril in introducing a feeble and incurable individual into a regiment than to permit this feeble, this incurable to have descendants." Moreover, Richet reminded his audience of a suggestion for an additional test before marriage that he had previously made only "half seriously," because he realized it had "no chance of being adopted."

It is to require before the authorization of marriage that each of the two young spouses swim across a large river, without any boat there to serve as a rescue. Too bad for the weak ones who would be carried off by the current![6]

Schreiber's proposal at the conference on the eugenic consequences of the war was much milder by comparison, even though he shared some of Richet's concerns about the negative consequences of the war. Commenting on the postwar emphasis that had been given to the question of depopulation, Schreiber pointed out that the war had left not only fewer males capable of reproducing but also, "by leaving men older, sick and suffering, by spreading certain illnesses especially venereal diseases, the war has left as survivors male reproducers of an incontestably inferior quality compared to peacetime." The result was that "without a doubt the war has effected a reverse selection for every belligerent country."[7]

Despite his gloomy general conclusion, Schreiber noted that there were some encouraging population statistics from wartime. For example, after it was realized that the extended conflict was having a disastrous effect on marriage and birth rates, the government instituted a rotating leave policy in the second year of the war. The success of the policy, Schreiber noted, was already reflected in the rise in the marriage rate from a low of 755 marriages in the IXth arrondissement of Paris in 1915 to 1,161 in 1917. Although the number of births lagged behind, by the first half of 1920 it was already showing a similar upward trend.[8] In fact, Schreiber went even further to claim that this wartime precedent of government concern and action in the area of marriage both justified and proved the need for a premarital physical examination law.

The benefits Schreiber predicted from the policy were much more limited than Richet's, and his approach was much more moderate. For example, on the question of whether examination results should be used to prohibit marriage, Schreiber admitted that "eugenics is not yet at the stage of furnishing a legal base in favor of such restrictions except in a very few number of cases." This meant that none of the illnesses usually mentioned in conjunction with the examination – cancer, tuberculosis, syphilis, mental illness, or alcoholism – would warrant the prohibition of marriage because, in Schreiber's words, "the laws of heredity that rule them can not yet be described with significant rigor to condemn certain subjects to mandatory celibacy."[9] This left only a few diseases about which enough was known to warrant such a drastic step, such as hemophilia or Huntington's disease. Although Schreiber was not proposing use of the examination as a general screening measure, he did wish to make it mandatory, at least as a first step. Accordingly, every future spouse would be required to have an examination before marriage by a doctor of choice who would indicate in writing "if he believed the patient to be suitable for marriage." It would be up to each individual, however, to act on the results, including whether to furnish them to the family of the intended.

This was clearly a moderate proposal, far less radical than Richet's and in keeping with the major thrust of French eugenics since its beginning. It is not surprising, therefore, that Schreiber's talk was included in the postwar conference sponsored by the French Eugenics Society. What is surprising – or rather, what illustrates again the willingness of French eugenicists to tolerate a variety of opinions – is that Richet's views were listened to as well. Richet, in fact, had become vice president of the French Eugenics Society at the first postwar meeting in 1920 – a testimony to his prestige as a Nobel laureate. Moreover, his 1921 talk was included with the papers from the 1920–21 conferences published by the French Eugenics Society in a volume entitled *Eugénique et séléction*. But toleration of opinion did not mean agreement with Richet's ideas, nor did it mean that the French Eugenics Society was ready to act even on Schreiber's call for a relatively moderate premarital examination law. It was to take four more years and further discussion of the idea in other quarters before the society took action.

Among the most important forums for these discussions were international eugenics meetings. With the growing interest in premarital examinations and the passage of laws in several countries, these meetings were natural places at which eugenicists could compare notes. As mentioned, the subject of eugenics and marriage regulations had been considered in Charles Davenport's paper at the First International Eugenics Congress in 1912 entitled "Marriage laws and customs."[10] After the war, the eugenics section of the International Institute of Anthropology held a conference in Liège at which Schreiber, Apert, and others heard a paper by the Czech Ladislaus Haskovec entitled "Matrimonial contract and public hygiene."[11] In the discussion that followed, it was decided that the premarital medical certificate should be one of the major questions studied at the next full congress of the IIA. In the meantime, each issue of *Eugénique* carried reports on the passage of premarital examination legislation throughout the world, including a Wisconsin law of 1914, a Norwegian law of 1919, and another in Denmark.[12]

As a result of these encouraging developments, Schreiber brought the matter up for discussion at two meetings of the French Eugenics Society in 1922. At the first meeting he essentially restated his earlier proposal for a mandatory examination without sanctions. Each spouse would be required only to furnish proof of having been seen by a doctor of choice.[13] The practical reasons for not proposing a stricter law became apparent in the discussion that took place at the next meeting of the society, for even this proposal was deemed too radical. Eugène Apert's reaction was typical. At first he expressed his sympathy with an idea he thought "useful," but he saw no possibility of formal intervention in the marriage process except "in cases where contagion was clearly feared." He argued that "what is needed first is the conquest of opinion." Lucien March, likewise, saw great merit in the proposal, especially in an age where "movement is facilitated by modern means of transport." By this he meant that "the ancestors of future spouses are often unknown. People marry without knowing one another."[14] Although he agreed that the premarital exam could help remedy the situation, March feared that passing a law requiring such an exam would be difficult. At best, he suggested, "it is appropriate to launch a campaign in order to demonstrate the advantages of it." Others at the meeting were no more encouraging, and emphasized the need first for "the preparation of public opinion by adequate publicity."

Appropriately, it was Pinard, the only deputy in attendance, who had the last word, offering both a review and summary of the status of the question. "We all desire to see healthy marriages," he began, and then noted that

the subject has previously been studied, in particular by Cazalis whose campaign at the Academy of Medicine produced few results. One can always propose a law, but a new law is difficult to get accepted. It is above all education that must be developed and the sense of responsibility that goes with it.[15]

Given Pinard's attitude, it was clear that Schreiber's proposal would not be acted upon by the society.

Over the next three years the question of the premarital examination continued to be a subject of discussion and study both inside and outside the French Eugenics Society. For example, in May 1923 an international congress of social hygiene was held in Paris, sponsored by the French government and presided over by Emile Roux, director of the Pasteur Institute. Among the papers presented were those on the premarital examination by Schreiber and by Henri Gougerot of the Ecole de médecine, who was a new member of the eugenics society. Haskovec also contributed a paper on the subject.[16] The following year, at the next meeting of the International Institute of Anthropology in Prague, one of the major questions designated for discussion was the premarital examination. Moreover, the location of the congress meant that Haskovec presided over the eugenics section of the meeting, and he proudly noted the work of Czech eugenicists since 1901 to secure modification of the marriage laws for eugenic purposes.[17]

Of even greater significance for French eugenicists at the Prague conference was the lengthy paper entitled "The marriage certificate and popularization of eugenic ideas," presented by the obstetrician and French Eugenics Society member Henri Vignes, that reported the results of a questionnaire sent to seventy-five people in France.[18] Although only one-third of those questioned responded, the study offers some proof that these questions were gaining a wider audience, because only three of those answering the questionnaire were eugenics society members. The respondents included six obstetricians and pediatricians, eight other doctors, three anthropologists, one biologist (Maurice Caullery), and three editors.[19] Opinions on the questions were mixed. Responses to some questions were almost equally divided, such as whether there was adequate scientific knowledge to make eugenic decisions; other responses, such as those on the utility of various types of premarital examinations (mandatory versus voluntary), elicited more fragmented responses. These ranged from complaints that measures were too harsh to opinions that they were too vague or mild to do any good.[20] Perhaps most noteworthy was that almost all responses were well-informed and revealed a familiarity with the subject, indicating that the premarital examination was hardly an obscure or new idea, at least to those who took the trouble to respond.

This is further demonstrated by an increasing number of articles on the premarital examination appearing in the general press as well as the medical press.[21] There is even evidence that the question had reached the political arena by 1925, when the council of the department of Seine-et-Oise passed a resolution "inviting the public and parliamentary powers to enact matrimonial legislation which will realize the wishes of modern science concerning public health and hygiene."[22] Similar resolutions were passed by the councils of the departments of Doubs and Côte d'or. Of further significance in the Seine-et-Oise resolution was the man behind it:

Louis Forest, publisher of *Le Matin* and a powerful force in the social hygiene movement, about whom more will be said later. In the meantime, Schreiber continued his own publicity campaign, including a radio broadcast on the premarital exam in September 1925.

Based on these developments, Schreiber felt confident enough to bring the subject up for discussion again at the French Eugenics Society meeting in December 1925. This time he was successful in securing the society's agreement to hold a series of public conferences at the Musée social the following spring. The Musée was a particularly appropriate site, for it had been a center of progressive social reform for three decades. Moreover, it was part of the social hygiene movement since the Alliance of Social Hygiene was founded there in 1904, and its president, Georges-Risler, was a member of the eugenics society.[23] Shortly thereafter, Lucien March agreed as French representative to the International Eugenics Federation to propose the premarital examination as the major subject for discussion at the next meeting of the federation to be held in Paris in July 1926.[24]

LEGISLATIVE CAMPAIGN

The conference on the premarital examination held at the Musée social in May and June 1926 was the beginning of the effort to pass the first eugenic legislation in French history. Although it took sixteen years, many study commissions, four revisions in the legislation, and ultimately a change in the government of France, a premarital examination law was decreed by the Vichy government in 1942 and retained by subsequent French governments. Despite the extraordinary circumstances under which the law was finally passed, the measure in force in France today is only slightly modified from the initial proposal that came from the 1926 French Eugenics Society conference. The fact that the current law is not seen as serving eugenic ends does not detract from the expressed intention of those proposing it in the 1920s and 1930s. The words of the 1942 decree made it quite clear that "for the first time a eugenics measure appears in French legislation."[25]

The outlines of the campaign for passage of a premarital examination law in France can be seen in the proposals and legislation that followed the 1926 eugenics society conference (Table 6.1).

Table 6.1. *Premarital examination legislation in France, 1926–45*

Date	Proposal
May–June 1926	French Eugenics Society conference
November 24, 1926	Pinard bill (Chamber of Deputies)
January 1927	Guérin bill (Chamber of Deputies)
December 1927	Duval-Arnould bill (Chamber of Deputies)
June 24, 1930	French Eugenics Society resolution
January 28, 1932	Justin Godart bill (Senate)
December 16, 1942	Vichy decree
July 29, 1943	Vichy decree (amendment)
November 2, 1945	Provisional government ordinance

Each new proposal or bill was consciously made as a modification or revision of the previous one, so that the lines of influence are clear and unbroken. Nonetheless, there were noteworthy disputes and changes as well as delays in the passage of the legislation that reveal a great deal about eugenic thought in French society between the wars.

The most important feature of the 1926 conference at the Musée social was that it was held at all, because it brought together for the first time since the turn of the century a group to examine the subject of the premarital examination in depth. Originally scheduled for two sessions in May, the conference elicited such a strong response that a third session was held in June. One reason for the interest was that Pinard, who presided over the conference, announced in his opening remarks that he not only supported passage of a premarital exam law, but also that he had drawn up a bill that he would introduce in the Chamber. The bill read as follows:

Every French [male] citizen wishing to marry or remarry can be entered in the civil registry only if he has a medical certificate dated from the day before, establishing that he has contracted no contagious disease.[26]

The questions raised by the provisions in Pinard's proposal were less important for the moment than the fact that he had changed his mind since the last discussion of the subject by the eugenics society.

Pinard's change of heart was news to everyone, including the

participants at the conference, who proceeded to deliver their prepared talks, which were generally more cautious in their approach
to the subject. For example, Schreiber's presentation, "The prenuptial medical examination in different countries," made clear his
long-standing view that the examination offered a more practical
way of "suppressing defectives and forbidding their reproduction"
than the sterilizations practiced in the United States and Switzerland that "our sentimentality finds too brutal."[27] Schreiber, however, chose to leave to others such controversial details as who
should be examined, by what doctors, for what illnesses or defects, and whether there should be sanctions against some marriages. Finally, after surveying the Scandinavian countries, Tur-
key, the United States, Belgium, Germany, Spain, Argentina, and
Austria, he concluded that France would probably not enact legislation until "the distant future." In the meantime, he could only
call for a propaganda campaign and an increase in the use of voluntary premarital consultations.[28]

Schreiber's experience in the early 1920s had made him by now
even more cautious than Pinard, but this was not the case with
some of the other speakers that followed him. For example, one
indication of the public awareness and acceptance of the premarital
examination was the talk by Louis Forest, editor of *Le matin* and
the member of the council of Seine-et-Oise who had earlier proposed and secured passage of a council vote recognizing the need
for an examination. To a nonscientist like Forest, the passage of
legislation did not depend on the technical provisions of the law
but on propaganda, pure and simple. His confidence in the prospects for achieving the goal was reflected in the analogy he made
at the end of his talk.

The French state spends enormous sums to improve lines of horses. Ask
yourself, after having taken so much trouble to improve the horse species, whether the hour has not arrived to do something to improve the
human species.[29]

Two other presentations at the first session of the conference —
Maurice Letulle's on tuberculosis and Louis Queyrat's on venereal
disease — strongly favored the examination, even calling for interdiction of marriage if the future spouses were found to be in particularly contagious stages of the diseases. But they conceived of
the examination more as a public health measure than a eugenic

measure, because they were both willing to allow the couple to be married after the illness had been cured. No mention was made of the potential inheritance of the disease. Georges Heuyer, the final speaker at the first session, did call for permanent screening of what he considered undesirable inherited traits such as delinquency and criminality through the prohibition of marriage. His only qualifications were that alcoholism and certain psychoses (manic depression, schizophrenia, and paranoia) required further study and should be judged on an individual basis until more was known.[30]

The next session of the conference included talks by Eugène Apert on the inheritance of family diseases and Georges Papillaut on the human unconscious. Both, however, placed more emphasis on recent technical developments in the fields than on assessments of how these developments affected the need for the premarital examination. Lucien March's talk was very different from the others because its purpose was to draw "general conclusions" from the conference. Although March was careful to note that all the previous speakers had unquestionably demonstrated the need for "judicious care of the health, physical and mental condition of those who wish to found a family," he also offered the first direct response to Pinard's opening proposal for a premarital examination law. It was a mixture of grudging support, guarded skepticism, and specific disagreements, foreshadowing some of the difficulties that French eugenicists would encounter in the following years during the campaign for passage of a law. For example, March reiterated his earlier support for such a campaign, but primarily because of its educational value.

Proposing a law will assure for our subject a wide publicity. It will indicate to all that it is an important, studied and desirable objective in the eyes of many well-intentioned people.

This was not exactly a resounding endorsement of Pinard's proposal, and March went on to make clear his objection to some of the specific language in the bill.

As to the text of this law – I hope our respected master and president, Professor Pinard, will be brought to this point of view – it seems to me that a mandatory medical examination would be a dangerous thing. For, if two lovers are legally forbidden to appear before a magistrate, is it not to be feared that they will go around him?[31]

Questions such as these continued in the discussion and general debate at the final session on June 11, and thus reveal an important new development at the conference – that it stimulated rather than settled disagreements about the premarital examination. Schreiber and Sicard de Plauzoles agreed with March that a proposal for a law was the best means of propaganda in favor of the examination, but others such as Queyrat were skeptical of any public or parliamentary acceptance. The situation in France was not like that "in Switzerland and other countries," he noted, where "anyone who spits on the ground must immediately pay a fine."[32] In fact, these differences produced no less than three other resolutions at the end of the conference on the premarital examination besides Pinard's, all of which were passed by those in attendance. One by March called for voluntary consultations to be publicized by the marriage registry; one by Queyrat went further by calling for a measure to require the registry to encourage the premarital medical examination as the form of consultation. Sicard de Plauzoles' resolution was in the nature of a compromise intended to reconcile all the parties as follows:

The assembly expresses the wish that a prenuptial medical certificate be made mandatory by law, and that in the meantime marriage registries distribute to people who come to register, advice regarding the necessity for a prenuptial medical exam.[33]

Pinard was unmoved by these warnings of disagreement among eugenicists, and in November 1926 he submitted his proposal, unchanged, to the Chamber of Deputies. In what followed, March and others were proven right because even though the proposal greatly increased public attention to the subject, passage was delayed for many years. A major reason for the delay, however, was the extensive debate among eugenicists themselves on what the precise nature of the law should be. In fact, as will be seen, this debate was to be a more important cause for delay than the anticipated objections from the general public.

DEBATE

The simplicity of Pinard's proposal both helped and hindered the prospects for its passage. The proposal was short, uncomplicated, and gave the appearance of being relatively easy to carry out. This

served the purpose of making it more palatable to the general public and natalists who might have opposed a highly complicated
premarital examination law. But the simplicity that made the proposal appealing to the public led to disagreements within the medical community, especially among those who favored the idea.
These specialists knew that certain features of the Pinard proposal
would have both explicit and implicit consequences that would
make implementation far more complicated. Despite these concerns and the debate that followed among eugenicists, in all the
revisions and subsequent proposals for legislation the essential
simplicity of the first Pinard proposal was retained.

Most of the issues that arose in the later debates can be seen in
the immediate responses to Pinard's submission of the bill to the
Chamber in November 1926. One was the question of who was
to be examined, which in the Pinard proposal was to be only the
future male spouse. To be fair to most eugenicists, Pinard was
unusual in calling for this provision, which reflected his very traditional view of male–female relations in marriage – "the woman
is impregnated when the man desires."[34] All subsequent legislative
proposals included provision for examinations of both future
spouses. Equally as idiosyncratic was Pinard's proposed timing of
the examination – the day before the certificate was to be presented to the authorities. Objections to this were not only practical, because it made no provisions for delays, but also medical,
especially from those who wished the examination to be a check
for venereal disease, which had a long incubation period. Critics
claimed that a day or even a week would not be long enough for
the most obvious symptoms to manifest themselves. Pinard's choice
of timing reflected his neo-Lamarckian view of influences on the
newborn. He was a firm believer that the condition of parents at
the instant of procreation was the most important environmental
influence on the offspring; and it followed logically that the closer
to this moment that the examination occurred, the better one would
be able to judge the fitness of the future parents. There is no record
of Pinard's openly calling for a procreation certificate (though this
is clearly what he intended the premarital exam to be), but he later
said that he almost included in his proposed legislation a provision
requiring a period of retreat and contemplation before the act of
procreation.[35]

The nature of the medical examination was left vague in Pinard's proposal, but this did not prompt as much debate as other questions. Although some critics raised questions about the qualifications of general practitioners to diagnose complex hereditary diseases, and the need for penalties against those who gave certificates after inadequate examinations or none at all, the language of subsequent proposals was, if anything, even more vague about the examination itself. Instead of Pinard's examination for "contagious diseases," these proposals spoke only of an "examination in view of marriage." Much more controversial, however, was whether or not presentation of the certificate as proof of examination should be mandatory, and to whom it should be shown. Most in the medical community who opposed a mandatory law were nonetheless in favor of the examination in principle. They simply feared that making it mandatory would jeopardize public acceptance. Like Schreiber and March, they thought that such a law would be seen as a restriction on marriage and hence would risk provoking opposition by natalists.

In contrast to these fears, the first major objection to Pinard's proposal in the Chamber came from a deputy who did not think the provisions were strong enough. In January 1927, Gustave Guérin proposed a different premarital examination law with important provisions far stronger than Pinard's. For example, he wanted the examination to be given to women as well as men, and foreigners as well as French citizens. Guérin also proposed an eight-day period within which the spouses were to be examined, and added that future spouses should be checked for "congenital malformations" as well as contagious illnesses. Finally, Guérin included a clause in his proposed legislation prescribing penalties for doctors found to have delivered false certificates and civil officers performing marriages without obtaining proof of the exams.[36]

Guérin's proposal was referred to the same Chamber subcommittee that was studying Pinard's. In the meantime, discussion of the premarital examination continued in many other forums. For example, articles appeared in medical as well as general-interest journals, and were both well-informed and surprisingly sympathetic to the idea, if not very optimistic about prospects for passage of a law. "In our country of liberty it is easier to overthrow the Bastille or ministers than established customs," noted Raoul Baudet in the *Annales politiques et littéraires*,[37] a remark reminiscent of Queyrat's at the 1926 eugenics conference. In addition, other organizations began studying the idea and lending it their support. In April the premarital examination received a boost when the Ligue des droits de l'homme made a mandatory examination law part of its "Declaration of the Rights of Children," whose goal was to ensure for the child the "right to a healthy life." This was largely the work of Just Sicard de Plauzoles, a eugenics society member who was also a member of the league's central administrative committee.[38] Later in the year the Pinard proposal was examined by the Conseil nationale de la natalité where, despite Pinard's membership, the proposed law was strongly attacked by Armand Siredey.[39]

It was more than a year – December 6, 1927, to be exact – before the chamber Committee on Hygiene made its report on the Pinard proposal. Paul Nicollet, a deputy from Lyons, presented a very long and detailed assessment of the proposed law. His presentation was undoubtedly colored by the fact that Nicollet himself was a doctor, with the greatest respect for Pinard. In fact, Nicollet described himself as "the student of a student of Pinard's" at the Ecole de médecine in Lyons.[40] In addition, he admitted that his twenty-five years of medical practice before entering the Chamber had long convinced him of "the necessity for such a law from the viewpoint of social hygiene and its exigencies." Nicollet's views are thus no small testimony to the influence of Pinard and the social hygiene movement in France at the time. Moreover, the experts whom he cited in his report were the by now familiar leaders of eugenics and social hygiene in the twenties – Schreiber, Queyrat, Richet, Jeanselme, and Paul Strauss, as well as members of the Lyons medical faculty such as Etienne Martin, Maurice Pehu, J. Rhenter, Eugène Villard, Joseph Nicolas, and Victor Augagneur (Nicollet's teacher). Virtually all agreed at least with the principle of the premarital examination, although some had general questions about its practicability (Nicolas) or specific suggestions for changes in who was to be examined and for what diseases (Rhenter, Richet).

Nicollet's report was addressed above all to fellow doctors; for he only briefly mentioned the possible objections of a nonmedical nature. Thus, he dismissed questions about civil liberties with the rejoinder that the examination would be no more an infringement on individual rights than the military draft or already existing laws requiring a minimum age for marriage. The additional inconvenience caused by the examination would be more than balanced by the general good it fostered. Nicollet was little disturbed by predictions of a rise in illegitimacy or prostitution that the law might produce. He expressed confidence that the good sense of his compatriots would make them see the need for the examination. Finally, to the potential objection of natalists that any barrier to marriage might have a negative effect on the birthrate, Nicollet responded with a quote from Cazalis that "of importance is not to produce many children but to produce them well." Moreover, Nicollet attempted to turn this criticism to his advantage by maintaining that

marriages will be easier to arrange because they will no longer entail the same uncertainty for the young women, families and relatives about the health of the future spouse. With a healthy marriage, there will certainly be a greater confidence of having children.[41]

Given Nicollet's views and the audience he was addressing, it is not surprising that a major portion of his report concerned the medical practicalities of implementing Pinard's proposal. For example, on the question of what constituted a "contagious disease," Nicollet advised the Chamber not "to enter into the 'jungle' of all the contagious or transmissible diseases," or the "controversies yet to be decided by renowned doctors," about syphilis, tuberculosis, or diabetes and their relationship to marriage.[42] Instead, Nicollet urged that it be left to the examining physician to detect conditions that might produce in a future offspring "a poor, defective being, sick, perhaps a monster and in any case a human misfit." To other questions, Nicollet's findings suggested far simpler answers. For example, to those concerned with the abilities of a general practitioner to diagnose complex hereditary diseases, he answered that patients could always be referred to specialists. Likewise, there was no need for penalties or provisions for lawsuits against those issuing incorrect certificates because the examination could never be 100 percent accurate, especially for diseases in incubation. Besides, Nicollet added, there is enough misfortune already when one of the social plagues strikes a marriage, without trying to determine blame where there is none.[43] Nicollet obviously identified more with his fellow doctors than with the spouse whose marital partner had passed a physical examination and later developed syphilis or tuberculosis.

The most attractive feature of Pinard's proposal, according to Nicollet, was its simplicity. And he pointed to this fact in the conclusion of his report in which he pleaded against those who would make revisions or additions. They would complicate matters, whereas passage of the law would only require

a simple certificate, clearly drafted without ambiguity, dated at most 24 hours before by any licensed practicing physician who has registered his diploma with the prefecture, freely chosen by the candidate for marriage, safeguarded by elementary precautions of sincerity.[44]

With this favorable report from committee, the stage seemed set for passage of the bill.

This was not to be the case. For immediately after Nicollet's report, a vote on Pinard's proposal was blocked by a counterproposal from another deputy. Once again the move came not from an opponent of the idea of the premarital examination but from a proponent, like Guérin, who wished to see a stronger law than Pinard's. This time it was Louis Duval-Arnould, whose proposal repeated Guérin's call for examination of both the future spouses and extended the time for the examination to within three days of presenting the certificate. Although Duval-Arnould dropped Guérin's clause concerning penalties against doctors and civil officers, he added a new clause that would require each spouse's signature as an indication of having seen the other's certificate. Thus, he hoped to calm the fears in the medical community about liability in the event of unforeseen problems developing after marriage, at the same time encouraging, without requiring, spouses to share the results by giving official notice that they had been examined. Stronger requirements might jeopardize the principle of doctor–patient confidentiality. Regardless of Duval-Arnould's obvious support for a premarital examination, this counterproposal meant that supporters were still divided. A vote was postponed, and it was to be more than four years before the matter was taken up again by the legislature.

It was obvious now that the reason for delay was the growing debate among eugenicists as to the exact provisions to be contained in a premarital examination law. This was glaringly evident in a eugenics society meeting held on May 16, 1928, at which Edouard Jeanselme, professor of cutaneous and syphilitic diseases at the Ecole de médecine, raised questions about Pinard's proposal

concerning timing, exclusion of women, the competence of doctors to do adequate screening, and the fact that results would not
necessarily be made known to the other party. Eugène Apert also
noted the criticisms raised earlier by Siredey as well as by Sicard
de Plauzoles' idea of basing the examination on the rights of the
unborn child. Schreiber was not concerned about the question of
medical competence. After all, he said, one could just as well ask,
"Is the military draft board competent? Yet the draft physical is a
useful institution."[45] Schreiber's preference now was modeled on
the existing law in Norway, which required an official declaration
by each spouse that they had been examined, one of the features
of Duval-Arnould's proposal. Jeanselme, however, wondered what
good such a law would do if only the fact of having been examined and not the results of the examination were reported to the
future spouse or government officials. Lucien March continued to
voice fears that a mandatory law was premature if public opinion
was not in favor, and Apert concluded the meeting with the observation that given the disagreements, no motion could be passed.
Instead, he noted agreement on only two points: "(1) the utility of
the premarital exam, and (2) the necessity for modifications so that
Professor Pinard's proposal be practicable."[46] Supporters of a premarital examination law were still a long way from resolving their
differences.

In the meantime, there were indications that March's fears about
public opinion may have been correct. The same month of the
eugenics society meeting (May 1928), the Medical Society of St.
Luc, St. Côme and St. Damen voted strong condemnation of Pinard's proposal on both medical and moral grounds. "Can one be
sure that a man who presents himself for an exam is not a syphilitic, and can one give him a certificate stating such in view of his
coming marriage?" asked Dr. Henri Martin, ex-intern of hospitals
at Pau. "Well, sirs, no and no!" he answered. The much acclaimed
Wasserman test was not sufficient because "given the current state
of knowledge, even negative reactions can hardly confirm healing,
let alone the absence of syphilis."[47] The moral objections Martin
raised included concerns that had been stated earlier about infringement on individual liberty and medical confidentiality, as
well as the observation that the only fair way to apply the law was
for both future spouses to be examined. This, Martin warned,
would mean an examination of the future bride that might raise

all sorts of delicate matters that doctors would want to avoid, such as the question of virginity.

More opposition to the examination law came in June 1928 when the prestigious Comité nationale d'études sociales et politiques considered the premarital examination at one of its monthly meetings. This semi-official group was created after the First World War to study and publish reports on a variety of domestic and international questions of the day. Experts on such subjects as war reparations, social hygiene, and the revolution in Russia would appear, present their views, and respond to questions from the group, and the proceedings of the meeting would be published shortly thereafter. The meeting on the premarital examination included all the sponsors of legislation before the Chamber (Pinard, Guérin, and Duval-Arnould) as well as Siredey, Jeanselme, Schreiber, Apert, and Edouard Jordan, a leading spokesman of the natalist and Catholic community. Not much new was presented at the meeting because participants essentially restated their previous positions, but one highlight was an exchange between Pinard and Siredey in which it was very clear that the questions first raised by Siredey at the Conseil de la natalité had not been resolved.[48] When the French Eugenics Society again considered the Pinard proposal at its May 1929 meeting, there was still no agreement on how the proposal should be modified. The society decided only that when the subject was discussed again in the Chamber, "an effort should be made to make known to legislators the conclusions which the Eugenics Society has reached."[49]

Despite this impasse, in the last half of 1929 and the first half of 1930, eugenicists were able to resolve their differences and reach agreement on the provisions for a premarital examination law. The first important new development responsible for this change was a lengthy report presented to the Nineteenth Congress of Legal Medicine held in Paris June 24–26, 1929, by Louis Verwaeck, director of the Belgian Penal Anthropology Service, and Jules LeClercq, professor of legal and social Medicine at the University of Lille. The proceedings of the congress ran to eighty pages and were cited in virtually all subsequent discussions of the exam as "the most complete and the most sensitive" study of the question.[50] The main body of the report was divided into three parts: an exhaustive list of the potential or actual objections raised to the idea, an assessment of current medical opinion on "pathological states constituting a temporary or definitive counterindication for marriage," and yet another survey of existing or proposed premarital examination legislation in France and other countries.[51]

The authors of the report shied away from endorsing any specific legislative proposal, but made clear their general support for the exam in their conclusion.

The medical exam before marriage appears to be a highly desirable eugenic measure, capable of making social life more healthy and realizing an effective prevention of degeneration and contamination which are sources of so much physical misery and moral disorder.[52]

As to the specific means of instituting it, they recommended only that both future spouses be examined, that professional confidentiality be respected, and that whatever the form of the attestation, it should be clear that only a "relative security" is assured by the examination, "which in no way implies a responsibility by the doctor" for the subsequent condition of those examined.

It was thus the thoroughness of the report rather than any new or specific conclusions that made it an important turning point in the campaign for the premarital examination. Indicative of this was a whole spate of articles it inspired on the subject.[53] In addition, a new element was added in June 1930 with the announcement that Alexandre Couvelaire, Pinard's son-in-law and successor at the Ecole de médecine and the Baudelocque Clinic, was opening a clinic to offer "the first prenuptial consultations in France for persons of both sexes who wish to be informed as to their state of health in view of marriage."[54]

The final step in reviving the premarital examination came June 24, 1930, when the French Eugenics Society unanimously adopted a proposal for an examination that included the following points:

1. The French Eugenics Society considers that the prenuptial medical examination is indispensable, and expresses the hope that a law make this examination mandatory.
2. It expresses the hope that from now on at the occasion of legal registration, notice be given to the interested parties emphasizing the fundamental importance of the prenuptial medical examination for future spouses and their descendants.
3. It desires that this examination should include the free choice of doctor.

4. It desires that this examination should result in the drawing up of a certificate establishing simply that *such and such doctor, at such and such date,* examined M. X or Mlle. Z, who declared that he [or she] had to be married at such a date.

This examination would thus serve neither as an authorization nor an interdiction of marriage, and the only sanctions envisaged would be against any marrying officer who performed a ceremony without requiring a certificate.[55] Later in 1930, the Propaganda Commission of the National Social Hygiene Office made passage of a premarital examination law one of the items on its list of national campaigns to be supported in the 1930–31 fiscal year.[56] The stage was now set for a new legislative initiative that was not long in coming. In January 1932, Justin Godart introduced a new proposal for a premarital examination law in the French Senate.[57]

CONCLUSION

The Godart proposal marked the beginning of a new phase in the campaign for a premarital examination law that is best understood as part of the broader discussion of eugenics in the 1930s in the next chapter. For now, it is worth noting that the history of the examination in the 1920s shows that Lucien March was both correct and incorrect in his predictions about what the results of the campaign would be. He was certainly correct that it would help publicize the premarital examination. This could be seen in the press and the medical community as well as in the national legislature. Another telling indication of how well established the idea had become was the number of medical theses devoted to the topic. Virtually every year after 1926 a medical thesis was written on the examination, with one by Laure Biardeau, published in 1931, becoming a standard work on the subject.[58]

March was proven incorrect, however, in his prediction that public opinion would be hostile to the examination. Opposition was isolated, or focused on specific features of its implementation. Some may have poked fun at Pinard's proposal, or used it as the basis for a subplot in plays, but no organized opposition developed against the premarital examination law. In fact, many eugenic leaders expressed genuine surprise at the amount of public support for the proposal. As Georges Schreiber admitted in 1928 in *Siècle médical,*

To be honest, we did not think that events would unfold with such a rapidity that has "accelerated" public opinion to the point of considering the premarital examination as a necessary, beneficent measure of preventative and eugenic medicine. We have been brought to the point of "restraining" the ardor of our deputies, who have suddenly become "more eugenic than the eugenicists themselves."[59]

This failure of the eugenicists to anticipate support was compounded by their own public disagreements about the specific terms of the law. The front-page headline of the article in *Siècle médical,* which quoted Schreiber, was hardly one to take advantage of the new-found backing for a premarital examination law. It read, " 'The law would be inapplicable,' Doctor Schreiber says," with the article describing the vice president of the French Eugenics Society as "an opponent of the mandatory premarital medical certificate, which confers on the doctor a right of veto."[60]

Lack of real opposition can be seen most clearly in the reactions of the two groups most likely to have opposed the law: natalists and the Catholic church. In each case, the premarital examination was met with indifference at worst, and at best with cautious support. For example, there was almost complete silence on the subject by the leading natalist journal. Only one article appeared mentioning the premarital examination in the journal of the Alliance nationale pour l'accroisement de la population française during the whole of the 1920s – a review of Marie-Thérèse Nisot's book on *La question eugénique,* which considered the premarital examination to be worthwhile.[61]

Catholic leaders paid closer attention to the proposals for a law requiring a premarital examination. In fact, Edouard Jordan's monthly *Pour la vie* carried coverage beginning with the eugenics society conferences at the Musée social in May and June of 1926. Jordan, who held the chair of medieval history at the Sorbonne, had close ties with both natalist and church groups, and he continued to monitor the progress of discussion about a premarital examination law to the end of the decade. As will be seen in the next chapter, he expressed an attitude of cautious support, which was typical of the attitudes of French church leaders toward eugenics in general until the papal encyclical of 1930. This shows that there was at least one benefit of the policy of moderation followed by the majority of French Eugenics Society members, who from the beginning of the organization sought to draw a distinction between themselves and their Anglo-Saxon counterparts. For the moment, then, the French eugenicists may have missed the opportunity for quick passage of the premarital examination law, but they had retained their image of moderation among the French public. Events in the 1930s were to change the situation dramatically.

French eugenics in the 1930s

It is clear by now that eugenics in France was hardly a static, un-changing movement. Even in the few decades since its formulation at the turn of the century, it was in an almost constant state of flux due to changes both in French society and the sciences upon which eugenics was based. Yet one can discern certain major turning points that help in understanding the broader development of the history of French eugenics. The First World War was one such turning point, and in many ways the 1930s was an equally profound if less abrupt juncture.

The most important reasons for the second turning point were undoubtedly the Depression and the rise to power of the Nazis in Germany. But also important for the history of eugenics was the proclamation of Pius XI's encyclical, *Casti conubii* [On Christian marriage] in December 1930, which specifically condemned eugenic practices. Although the effects of the Depression were ambiguous and complex, the actions of the Nazis in power and the results of the encyclical quickly sharpened the line of debate about eugenics in France, where definitions had always been fuzzy. For example, after the papal pronouncement, the full weight of the Catholic church was unmistakably opposed to eugenics, whereas the passage of Nazi eugenic laws beginning in 1933 put a eugenics program into effect for the first time on a national scale – for Europeans and the world to see. This chapter will examine the impact of these developments, which originated outside France, and it will also look at changes in the people and institutions within the country that made the nature of eugenics in the 1930s very different from previous years.

Studies of American and British eugenics have made the 1930s something of a controversial period, one side arguing that these years saw a decline in eugenics, and the other saying that developments only confirmed what eugenicists had maintained all along.[1] In France the 1930s saw a change in eugenics that can best be described as placing a greater emphasis on harsher, usually negative eugenic measures such as premarital examinations, immigration restriction, and birth control. Discussion even began about the use of sterilization. Although most of these ideas had surfaced in France earlier, with the exception of the premarital examination they had not been pursued or advocated in an organized fashion by the majority of French eugenicists. Instead, the prevailing opinion of those who were instrumental in founding the French Eugenics Society in 1912 was to improve the French population hereditarily by improving health and prenatal care. As mentioned, this approach to eugenics presumed a neo-Lamarckian inheritance of acquired characteristics and was fed by a strong fear of depopulation, very pronounced in France because it had been one of the earliest countries in the world to manifest a drop in its birthrate during the nineteenth century. The loss in the First World War of over one million men further heightened that fear; hence, in the 1920s the French Eugenics Society emphasized a program of fighting tuberculosis, alcoholism, and venereal disease by alliances with existing groups or by founding new ones. Thus, the society continued the prewar strategy of increasing both the quality *and* quantity of the French population.

The measures called for by eugenicists in the 1930s were in marked contrast to these activities. The most highly publicized measure was the proposal for a law requiring a physical examination before marriage. As shown in the last chapter, the campaign for a premarital examination had already begun in the 1920s, when Pinard introduced his bill in the Chamber to require an attestation of "no appreciable symptoms of contagious diseases" before a couple could register for marriage. Although the bill was delayed while eugenicists argued over the best way to clarify the vague language of Pinard's bill, it was revived again in the early 1930s by Justin Godart, a former health minister, who proposed new legislation in the Senate. Thereafter, the proposal was delayed only because it became entangled with the more general idea of a *carnet de santé*, championed by Louise Hervieu and others in the late 1930s, which proposed that a health card be maintained for everyone, from cradle to grave, to be presented at appropriate stages in one's life, including marriage. Support for this proposal was stimulated by the sympathetic response to the personal plight of Hervieu, a well-known painter and writer who suffered from syphilis contracted at childbirth. She dramatized her story in two novels, *Sangs* and *Crime,* which became bestsellers in the mid-1930s. Scientific and government support for Hervieu's campaign owed much to the same shift in opinion that the eugenicists had correctly gauged in proposing the premarital examination at the end of the 1920s.[2] A ministry of public health decree of June 2, 1939, made the health card mandatory, but defined it as "a strictly personal document which no one could require to be divulged." This restriction was removed in November 1942 by the Vichy regime in the same decree that established the mandatory premarital examination.[3]

Other eugenic measures that received increasing attention in the 1930s were immigration restriction and contraception. French eugenicists had first voiced their concerns about immigration in the 1920s when postwar political and economic dislocations brought a large influx of workers and refugees to France. Although some eugenic anti-immigration arguments were voiced by public health officials worried about the physical condition of those coming to France, it was not until the 1930s that a full-blown immigration restriction program was advocated, with eugenic warnings of biological decline from intermixing of incompatible races. An even more radical change in French eugenics in the 1930s was the call for more liberal laws on contraception. Implicit in this was a very different attitude toward the population question in France that went directly against the previous alliance between French eugenicists and natalists. A telling indication of how fundamental a change this represented in French eugenics was the first serious discussion of sterilization of the "unfit," a subject that had almost always been dismissed out of hand as being unacceptable to French mores.[4] It should not be concluded, however, that in the face of these developments, those supporting the milder eugenics of the 1920s simply faded away. In fact, they were strengthened in the late 1930s when French communists left finally entered the debate on eugenics, supporting a family and public health policy in the tradition of Pinard and the *puericulteurs.*

Before examining these changes in eugenic thought more closely, it is important to remember that there were also changes in personnel and organization that were independent of the major developments of the 1930s, yet also greatly influenced the nature of eugenics in France. For example, in the 1920s there was a change in generations of those active in French eugenics, with many of the founders of the French Eugenics Society either dying or retiring from active professional life. Louis Landouzy, the first vice president of the French Eugenics Society and dean of the faculty of medicine, died in 1917, as did Frédéric Houssay, another society officer. Edmond Perrier, director of the Museum of Natural History and the first president of the eugenics society, died in 1921, and Pinard who had already retired from the Ecole de médecine in 1914, ended his political career in 1928. The physiologist Charles Richet, a vice president of the eugenics society, retired from the medical faculty in 1925, and Lucien March, secretary-treasurer of the society, retired from the direction of the Statistique générale of France in the early 1920s. Although many in the new group rising to prominence in French eugenics – such as the pediatricians Eugène Apert and Georges Schreiber who became president and secretary respectively – shared the training and outlook of the founding generation, others such as the public health doctors René Martial and Just Sicard de Plauzoles, who began their careers at the turn of the century, had very different backgrounds and views of eugenics.

Related to this change in personnel was a change in the status of the French Eugenics Society itself during the 1920s that had important consequences in the following decade. As noted before, the society had close ties through its founders to the Ecole de médecine, where its regular meetings were held. There had also been sufficient membership in the organization to pay for the printing and distribution of its own journal. After 1926, however, this changed. With the cost of the journal exceeding income from membership subscriptions, a decision was made to publish the articles and minutes of the society in the journal of the Ecole d'anthropologie in Paris.[5] This was possible not only because of the participation of members of the Ecole in the eugenics society, but also because the Ecole helped establish an International Institute of Anthropology after the war that included a separate subdivision devoted to the study of eugenics. Local national committees had been formed in different countries, and in 1926 the eugenics society merged with the eugenics committee for France, most of whose members belonged to both organizations. The reconstituted committee, however, never met on a regular basis, and the result was that there was no institutional focus for eugenics other than the journal, *Revue anthropologique*.

This change did not bring an end to eugenic thought in France. On the contrary, as a result of the developments in the 1930s, there was an upsurge in writing and discussion of eugenic measures. Although the lack of organization hindered the practical implementation of a eugenics program, it did allow all sorts of people to enter the debate with new ideas.

One final organizational development in the 1920s that helps to explain the change in focus of the French Eugenics Society was the strategy of supporting or creating social hygiene organizations to combat such problems as venereal disease and tuberculosis. As shown in Chapter 5, the groups grew and expanded to meet these problems, but the immediate goal of relieving suffering replaced the long-range eugenic plans that the French Eugenics Society hoped to accomplish, and the society soon found itself without a program to champion. This loss of control of the social hygiene movement in the 1920s was one reason why the eugenics society undertook the campaign for a premarital examination in 1926. It therefore signaled the beginning of French eugenicists' search for new answers to the question of biological decline.

THE DEPRESSION AND THE POPULATION QUESTION

The internal evolution of the French eugenics movement indicates why there was general openness to new ideas and change, but it does not explain why certain ideas received more attention than others. It seems clear that the most important reason why the harsher negative eugenics program displaced the mild positive one in the 1930s was the coming of the Great Depression. Although for a short time France was spared its effects, by late 1931 the unemployment and economic decline that had been seen in other countries arrived in France. Whereas in England or America these developments undercut eugenic arguments that presumed that the conditions of lower, poorer classes were the result of biology – how could the ranks of the poor be multiplying faster than their birthrate?[6] – there was no such contradiction in French eugenics. One reason is, of course, that neo-Lamarckians presumed the opposite relationship between poverty and biology – that the lower classes were worse off biologically because they were poor, and not vice versa. An increase in their numbers only raised the fear of more rapid biological decline because of the effects of deteriorating environment.

The conclusions drawn by many French eugenicists from the Depression were therefore Malthusian – that is, the problems were the result of demography and economics. In words that would have made Malthus himself smile (albeit grimly), French eugenecists described a world with too many mouths to feed and too few resources. A new word entered the French eugenic vocabulary – "overpopulation." It was the cause not only of economic – and therefore, biological – woes, but of wars as well. Coincidentally, Europeans had a convenient example at hand beginning in 1931, when Japan invaded Manchuria. The image of the teeming "Asian masses" is an old one in Europe, but a book with that title written by Etienne Dennery on the eve of the Manchurian war expressed it in contemporary demographic language that was cited throughout the 1930s.[7] For example, Gaston Bouthoul's *Population dans le monde*, written in 1935, criticized the Japanese preoccupation with population in a manner that could just as easily have applied to the French natalists of the 1920s:

They are intoxicated with the dizziness of figures. "Tomorrow we will be one hundred million" is the theme of exaltation which is found in the Japanese newspapers. No matter that the difficulties and miseries will grow in proportion, the essential thing is that the numbers make them proud.

Bouthoul then repeated Dennery's observation about what such a growth of population brings.

To whoever has traversed these overpopulated countries, it is incontestable that overpopulation is a cause of their malaise, disorder and fundamental weakness. The abundance of the miserable, the unemployed, and those without skills makes a country anemic rather than reinforced. . . . The number of inhabitants does not necessarily increase the power of a country if it diminishes the output of each inhabitant.[8]

Bouthoul's own conclusion was an explicit attempt to view demographic questions in a more balanced light, and he warned that "those who maintain that the amelioration of humanity depends on the uninterrupted growth of the population are as far from the evidence as those who see restriction as the essential remedy of all past and present difficulties."[9]

This new view of the population question in France was possible in part because of new statistics from recent years that showed France's two rivals, England and Germany, with a steep drop in their birthrates. In fact, by 1932 the French rate of 17.3 births per 1,000 was actually higher than England's 15.3 and Germany's 15.1.[10] This general leveling off of the population in Europe was therefore doubly welcome to French observers concerned with France's relative position in an overcrowded world. The respected economist Charles Gide noted that "the density of the population in Europe appears to have attained almost the maximum compatible with its present-day resources." Some were even tempted to see France in a position of actual advantage because it had the lowest population density in Western and Central Europe, although others cautioned that "populations must be proportional to the resources and not just the surface of the territory."[11] Perhaps most telling of this change in perspective on the population question during the 1930s is the decline in the political influence of the natalists in the Chamber of Deputies. In the 1932 election, two-thirds of the natalists lost their seats, including their leader, Adolphe Landry.[12]

The 1930s also saw the appearance of authors who for the first time were critical of the technique of projecting long-range future population statistics from limited, short-term trends. This, of course, had been one of the standard techniques that accompanied the wave of fear about depopulation in France at the end of the nineteenth century. Bouthoul devoted a chapter to "demographic forecasting" in which he criticized such predictions as the common view in 1890 that Germany would have 100 million inhabitants by 1920, whereas France would have only 30 million.[13] In 1935, members of the Academy of Medicine heard a lecture entitled "On the pretended 'depopulation' in France." The premise of the author, Alexandre Roubakine, who had formerly been attached to the Hygiene Section of the League of Nations, was that natalists had erred in focusing their attention solely on birthrate, for although the rate in France and all of Europe was dropping, the mortality rate was dropping even faster. In fact, Roubakine prophetically noted,

If there is a decline in the birthrate in Europe, its population is, nevertheless, growing more rapidly than that of Asia. Moreover, since the habitable spaces are much more restricted in Europe than Asia, it is the expansion of the White race of Europe which presents the greatest danger for the world today.[14]

Such a dramatic change in perceptions of population growth had the obvious effect of softening attitudes toward contraception. By the mid-1930s, for example, new organizations such as the Association d'études sexologiques called for the repeal of the 1920 ban on the sale and advertisement of contraceptive devices, as did established organizations such as the Ligue des droits de l'homme. Standard medical reference works, such as the 1934 edition of the *Encyclopédie médico-chirurgicale,* justified the practice of birth control in cases of women "whose motherhood would be dangerous for themselves or for the future of the race, because of the inferior quality of the infants they would bring into the world." Although one of the reasons for this was a desire to diminish the estimated 500,000 yearly illegal abortions in France, the authors pointed to growing support for the concept of "motherhood by consent."[15] There were obvious eugenic implications in these new ideas of birth control and overpopulation that eugenicists sought to turn to their advantage. One of the most articulate and persistent advocates was Just Sicard de Plauzoles, president of the Ligue nationale française contre le péril vénérien, who became a leading spokesman for the revisionist eugenic view of the population problem in the 1930s.

SICARD DE PLAUZOLES

Sicard is a fascinating character who represents the new generation of French eugenicists coming into the movement in the 1920s and 1930s primarily from an interest and background in public health. Born in 1872 at Montpellier, Sicard's background was perhaps the most aristocratic of all eugenicists.[16] His family traced its origins back to a Raymond de Plauzoles, who was made a count in 1230 by the King of Aragon. In the 1700s, members of the family began pursuing medicine as a career, and no less than nine ancestors had been doctors by the time Just was born. His father, Henri Sicard, was a professor of medicine at Montpellier at the time. Shortly thereafter, he was named dean of the faculty of science and medicine at Lyons.

Sicard de Plauzoles attended medical school in Paris, where he studied with Pinard and Richet, but it was Landouzy who directed his work toward public health in general and tuberculosis in particular. After graduation he pursued his interest in "public medicine," as he called it, joined Fournier's Société de prophylaxie sanitaire et morale, and published books with such titles as *Tuberculose* (1900) and *Maternité et la défense nationale contre la dépopulation* (1909). Two other features of his later career were also evident in this prewar period – his membership in the Ligue des droits de l'homme in 1898, including election as a member of the Central Committee and vice president in 1911[17] – and his teaching of popular *cours libres* on social hygiene at the College libre des sciences sociales and the Sorbonne.

Despite the nature of his interests and contact with such leaders of eugenics as Pinard, Richet, and Landouzy, Sicard did not become associated with the French Eugenics Society until after the First World War. The manner of his affiliation then was as much the result of the society's postwar strategy of broadening contacts with social hygiene organizations (described in Chapter 5) as it was a change in Sicard's mind. In 1919, Sicard de Plauzoles began directing a tuberculosis clinic in Paris, and the following year he became the general secretary of the Commission des maladies vénériennes of the ministry of health. It was in this capacity and in search of support for a regular series of public talks on social hygiene that he joined the French Eugenics Society in May 1922. In December of that year the eugenics society created a Comité d'union contre le péril vénérien, which joined the Ligue national contre le péril vénérien headed by Sicard de Plauzoles. Twelve hundred francs were given to the league by the eugenics society, which at the same time agreed to cosponsor Sicard's *cours libres* (public lecture series) on social hygiene that had recently been approved by the Ecole de médecine.[18] Although Sicard de Plauzoles eventually became the head of the Société française de prophylaxie sanitaire et morale, and general secretary of the Conseil superieur d'hygiène sociale created by the ministry of health in 1938 (while retaining his other titles), it was this series of lectures given every year until 1941 that brought him the most notoriety and permitted Sicard the widest latitude in developing his eugenic ideas.

The *cours libres* began in 1922 and usually consisted of fifteen to twenty-five lectures, running from January through March. There had been some delay when the course was first proposed in 1920 because Léon Bernard, who occupied the chair of hygiene at the Ecole de médecine (which had to authorize the course), objected that it would duplicate instruction at the school. A compromise was worked out the following year whereby the lectures would be given instead at the Grand Amphitheater of the Sorbonne.[19]

This did not diminish the official sanction given to the course, as indicated from the attendance at the opening session each year by members of the French public health and medical establishment, including professors and deans of the Ecole de médecine, senators, deputies, and even ministers of health. Moreover, the list of other institutions acting as cosponsors of the lectures (besides the Ecole de médecine and the eugenics society) ranged from the ministry of labor and health to the Comité nationale de defense contre la tuberculose, the Ligue Franco-Anglo-Américaine contre le cancer, the Ligue nationale contre l'alcoolisme, and the Ligue d'hygiène mentale. When Bernard died in 1932, the *cours libres* moved to the Ecole de médecine, where Louis Tanon, the new occupant of the chair of hygiene, presided over the opening lecture that year and introduced Sicard de Plauzoles with the admission that the course had always belonged at the medical school.[20]

Sicard de Plauzoles' ideas on eugenics were implicit in his notion of social hygiene developed in the 1920s. In his lectures he always cited the work of Pinard and Richet, both of whom were obviously not opposed to having their names associated with his ideas, because they frequently attended and even spoke at opening sessions of the public hygiene course. From 1927 to 1932, Pinard attended all opening lectures except one; Richet attended in 1929, and ceremonially opened the series in 1930. By this time, Sicard's ideas were already reaching a wider audience thanks to publication of his book, *Principes d'hygiène*, which was based on the first five years of the courses and included a preface by Pinard.[21]

A key concept of the book that also reveals the influence of Taylorism on Sicard's generation of public and industrial hygiene was *"zootechnie humaine."* Sicard defined this as "the art of procreating, perfecting and utilizing man as a work-producing machine."[22] Eugenics' role in the process, he claimed, was to ensure that the best "human capital" would be produced, and social hygiene would help to ensure the best possible return on this invested capital. Continuing (one might say, belaboring) the economic metaphor, Sicard proposed the following equation:

$$P = n + p + i + a + e + r + m$$

where,

P *(prix de revient)* = cost of return
n *(naissance)* = cost of pregnancy and birth

p *(puericulture)* = cost of rearing
i *(instruction)* = cost of education
a *(apprentissage)* = cost of apprenticeship
e *(entretien)* = cost of upkeep
r *(retraite)* = cost of retirement
m *(maladie)* = cost of health

According to this formula, the value of an individual to society equaled the total productivity of that individual's life minus the total of these "maintenance" costs.[23] This balance-sheet view of humanity was not an original idea of Sicard de Plauzoles'. It was an example of a somewhat extreme extension of the positivist, Taylorist view of humanity found in the early French social hygienists such as Landouzy and Emile Duclaux. At the turn of the century, they dramatized the social costs of diseases such as tuberculosis by assuming a monetary value of human life – 25,000 francs was a commonly cited prewar figure – and multiplying it by the number of deaths caused by the disease.

Sicard de Plauzoles' attack on those who were content merely to count the number of births to determine the value of the population was first made in the opening session of his 1932 social hygiene course entitled "The future and the preservation of the race: Eugenics," with Justin Godart and Adolphe Pinard in attendance. He began with an admonition:

It is infantile to measure the vigor and future of a population by the number of births registered every year. What constitutes the value of a nation is the number of healthy adults in condition to work, produce and reproduce healthfully; . . . and what counts is less the number of births than their quality.[24]

Having stated the case for quality over quantity, Sicard then expressed alarm at the qualitative decline of the French population. This was happening, he insisted, because

the lower classes, the poorer classes, have a much higher birthrate than the upper, richer classes. . . . Misery, along with alcoholism, syphilis and tuberculosis, is a powerful factor of degeneration . . . and children of poorer classes compared to children of the richer classes show an inferiority of physical, intellectual and moral development . . . caused by fatigue and deprivation of the mother during gestation, by insufficient feeding in early years, by poor housing conditions and by working at an early age.[25]

Most important to Sicard was the fact that the inferiority did not disappear, because it was transmitted and increased from generation to generation.

Here was the greatest danger of all. For, assuming as Sicard did, that lower-class families had an average of five children while upper-class families had two, he was led to the arithmetic conclusion that in two generations the descendants of the lower half of the population would represent 85 percent of the people and in five generations, 99 percent. From this, Sicard predicted that

the increased swamping of superior classes of society by the lower classes will certainly result in the complete bankruptcy of the nation in gifted, capable and energetic individuals. It can not take long before the whole of the population is lowered to a level which today is that of the uncultured classes. . . . In summary, as the population grows in number, it diminishes in quality. It is the lower categories that are the most prolific: the defectives multiply; the elites disappear. The result is a progressive bastardization, a degeneration which is more and more pronounced. Anything that can reduce the proliferation of the lower classes, in any country, will be a benefit for humanity.[26]

The important point here is not Sicard's class prejudice nor the fanciful notions about differential birthrates that his fellow eugenicist Lucien March had done much to disprove in his prewar studies.[27] Rather, it is the fact that a serious program of class-based negative eugenics was being proposed that considered birth control, especially for the lower classes, to be the only solution to the decline of the species. The French government's efforts to encourage larger families was considered by Sicard to be a policy that "favors the multiplication of inferior classes and runs directly counter to natural selection and the progress of the species." Hence, he concluded that "birth control is justified as a means of artificial selection to prevent the evils that result from an unhealthy or exaggerated fertility."[28] In other words, Sicard was breaking from the long-held maxim of French eugenics that called for "quality and quantity."

There was at least one attempt in the 1930s to give this new approach an organizational base – the founding in 1931 of the Association d'études sexologiques, which included as members Sicard de Plauzoles and Justin Godart, as well as Victor Basch, the president of the Ligue des droits de l'homme, several deputies and senators, and a large number of doctors.[29] The chief organizer was

Edouard Toulouse, probably the best-known psychiatrist in France between the wars and head of the Ligue nationale française d'hygiène mentale.

Toulouse was similar to Sicard in that he represented another example of the broad interest in eugenics that existed in France separately from the organized eugenics society. Rather than coming from the public health field, Toulouse's background was in mental health. He was born in Marseilles in 1865 and came to Paris in 1889 to complete his medical studies.[30] After completing his medical degree in 1891 he wrote on a number of psychiatric topics then fashionable at the end of the century, such as melancholy, amnesia, and neuropathy. Toulouse gained prominence in psychiatry with a study of Emile Zola subtitled *Les rapports de la supériorité intellectuelle avec la neuropathie,*[31] and in 1897 he began editing the *Journal de psychiatrie*. Of even greater importance was his appointment in 1898 as médecin-chef at the Asile Villejuif, because it gave him an institutional base from which to launch his many projects.

The life work of Toulouse was mental illness – its causes, effects, and treatment. The most distinctive feature of his approach to the problem was the breadth of scope with which he viewed it, but there were disadvantages as well as advantages to this breadth of vision. To his credit, Toulouse saw the necessity of crossing disciplinary boundaries in order to examine the many influences on mental illness – psychological, physiological, and hereditary. In casting his net broadly to discover more about mental illness, however, Toulouse also drew in a variety of other ideas and theories current at the end of the century. These included innate criminality, sexology, and hereditary alcoholism, which were not only less useful but carried with them broad assumptions about social causes and effects that confused the problem of mental illness with many other issues.

This broad perspective, in turn, had a similar mixed impact on Toulouse's view of the cure for the problems. He saw the answer to mental illness in *prophylaxie mentale,* a vague term that recognized eugenics as the ultimate means of resolving the problem by eliminating the procreation of mental deficients. In the meantime he saw the necessity of identifying the mentally ill and treating them, if possible.[32] To his credit, Toulouse chose as his most important goal the provision of open and free treatment for the mentally ill, the Hôpital Henri Rousselle being the lasting legacy of his success.[33] On the other hand, he also supported extensive testing and screening of the population along the lines of the massive American IQ testing of army recruits for the First World War.[34] Toulouse saw broad advantages to such testing, not only in identifying those at the lower end of the scale, but also in selecting an elite and determining a proper place for those in between. Never one for understatement, Toulouse once proposed "that entry into every school and factory should be by way of a psychophysiological laboratory acting as an organ of selection and classification."[35]

Toulouse realized the importance of public relations, at least in the sense of informing the general public of the problems he saw and solutions he proposed for them. In fact, one reason for his success was the ability to mobilize political support for his projects. Before the turn of the century, he wrote columns for the newspaper *Le journal* and the *Revue bleue*. He also authored a series of "how-to" books for Hachette destined to reach the broad public.[36] After the war, he helped build support for his open psychiatric hospital by convincing the minister of hygiene to establish a Ligue d'hygiène mentale based on an American model described to him by a colleague who had visited the United States.[37] The result of all this activity was to make Toulouse's name virtually synonymous with psychiatry in France between the wars. One of his young interns later recalled that *"Eh, va donc chez Toulouse!"* became a common insult exchanged by taxi drivers.[38]

The Ligue d'hygiène mentale, like Sicard's anti-venereal league, was one of the postwar social hygiene organizations that paralleled the work of the French Eugenics Society. It followed closely and was a strong supporter of the campaign for a premarital examination. Partly because of the reduced activity of the Eugenics Society at the end of the 1920s, and partly in response to the new climate of opinion at the beginning of the 1930s, Toulouse created the Association d'études sexologiques in July 1931. According to its founding statutes, the new organization's goal was to examine and correct the many problems of the human race that resulted from the fact that

the procreation of children has literally been left to sentimental anarchy. And man, who early on was informed enough to seek the best return from domesticated animals whose strains he perfected and who came upon the idea of castration to make them more docile, appears little interested in his own offspring. So long as children are born from chance matings, many will be the carriers of defects requiring costly help and care, out of all proportion to the meager results obtained. Syphilis, insanity, and all morbid predispositions are given free rein.[39]

As mentioned, Toulouse was able to enlist several influential political as well as scientific leaders in the new association that backed many of the ideas that Sicard de Plauzoles had been writing about in the 1920s. For example, warning against "reverse selection," Victor Basch called for repeal of the 1920 law against birth control as the first order of business of the new association. Although Basch did not subscribe to all of the ideas of Sicard de Plauzoles, he did make clear that his reasons were based on eugenics, specifically citing Sicard's definition that eugenics

wants procreation to be no longer the result of blind passion and chance but, on the contrary, something of conscious will and reflection by healthy parents, vigorous in mind and body, wise and prudent, knowing the task they are undertaking, willing and able to carry it through to a good conclusion.[40]

Basch's support was significant because his Ligue des droits de l'homme was the most important civil liberties organization in France. It had been founded at the time of the Dreyfus affair, and was the rallying point of left intellectuals supporting Dreyfus after Zola's publication of *"J'accuse"* forced the affair into the public light.[41] After the First World War, the league increased its activities, not just in political matters but also in many social and health questions that were of interest to eugenicists. For example, the league took positions in favor of the premarital examination and opposed to the 1920 legislation against birth control, based on the right of the infant to a healthy life. The man behind both these league positions was Sicard de Plauzoles.[42]

Sicard had been a founding member of the league, and quickly moved into the inner circle of its directors. He became a member of its central committee in 1903 and a vice president from 1911 to 1919. In the 1920s, his renewed interest in social hygiene prompted him to bring before the league such matters as the mandatory declaration of tuberculosis and venereal disease (justified by the right of others to a healthy life), the mandatory declaration of pregnancy, the prohibition of work by expectant mothers just prior to giving birth (justified by the right of the infant to be born healthy), and mandatory breastfeeding in the first ten months of life (justified by the right of a child to its mother's milk). In fact, largely at

Sicard's instigation, the conflict between the child's rights and the mother's rights was brought to the attention of various committees of the league several times during the 1920s.[43]

In 1927, Sicard obtained the support of the league for the French Eugenics Society's proposed premarital examination law that would provide for the "protection of the child before procreation and during pregnancy." This was an extension of the concept of children's rights, which went back to the earliest days of the league and its concerns over the right of access to education.[44] The following year, Sicard brought up the matter of the legislation prohibiting publicity in favor of contraception, and secured passage of the following resolution by the league's central committee:

That the law of 31 July 1920 be revised; that all provisions contrary to the free expression of opinions be deleted; and that in particular paragraph 2 article 3 aimed at "publicity for birth control and against the birth rate" be deleted.[45]

In his article reporting the results of the central committee's decision, Sicard was not yet as strident in his criticism of the natalists as he would be six years later, but he did note that eugenics offered a middle position between the populationist doctrine of "go forth and multiply" and the Malthusian claim that increased population only brought "misery and suffering." Eugenics, he stated, concentrates "less on the number than on the quality of the products."[46]

After the creation of the Association d'études sexologiques, additional support for repealing the anti-Malthusian legislation came from Victor Basch who, in his capacity as president of the Ligue des droits de l'homme, made contraception "the question for October 1932" in the league's journal. He urged repeal of the Law of July 1920 and added a call for the creation of counseling centers.[47] In 1933 the league backed a bill introduced in the Chamber by the left urging amnesty for those guilty of breaking the 1920 law, and the following year the league formally protested the arrest and conviction of Jeanne Humbert for spreading neo-Malthusian propaganda.[48] In fact, the league was so outspoken on the issue that it had to publish a disclaimer in its journal in 1936, stating,

The league defends the rights of children . . . but it has not created any outside organizations to this effect, and it has no link with any group specializing in the defense of the rights of children.[49]

Evidently, Basch's and Sicard's participation in the Association d'études sexologiques did not constitute such a link.[50]

The ideas of Sicard de Plauzoles and others in the Association d'études sexologiques illustrate two of the most important effects of the Depression on eugenics and contraception questions in France during the 1930s. First, although the Depression did not create the birth control movement, it sufficiently changed the climate of opinion to provide an opportunity for those who favored the use of contraception as a negative eugenic measure to make their case. Second, the economic decline and rising unemployment undercut the natalist position that had dominated French eugenic thought for so long. An indication of how different the times were in the 1930s is the fact that the birth control question was only part of the Association d'études sexologiques' overall eugenics program, which soon went far beyond calling for repeal of the 1920 legislation against birth control. In February 1933 the association formally voted to support a six-point program that included a mandatory premarital examination and the creation of public clinics to give advice on contraception and perform sterilizations and abortions. The latter two could be voluntary, or performed for medical reasons such as those "in the public interest (physiological and mental hereditary defects, impulses of a criminal or sexual order) for which a list would be established according to the advice of competent medical societies."[51] The advocacy of such measures in the 1920s would have been unthinkable.

STERILIZATION

Of all the new developments in French eugenics during the 1930s, the one that was most directly tied to influences outside France was the use of sterilization. Here, however, it was the actions of the Americans and not, as is commonly believed, the Nazis that served as the inspiration for a discussion of the question. The event that sparked the discussion was the 1927 *Buck v. Bell* U.S. Supreme Court decision, which upheld the sterilization law of Virginia.[52] This was followed shortly by sterilization legislation in Sweden and the French-speaking Swiss canton of Vaud. All of these developments prompted a large number of talks and articles in France on the eugenic use of sterilization.[53]

The extent of this interest is indicative of the change in French eugenics starting in the late 1920s that opened up the movement to new ideas even before the changes brought about by the Depression. Only iconoclastic figures such as Charles Richet had seriously proposed sterilization before, but even he realized that it was unlikely to be accepted. As a result, in his 1919 book *Sélection humaine* he had called for the premarital examination as an expedient until public opinion changed.

Whereas previously the extensive California sterilization program was dismissed by French doctors as a manifestation of the American *"ouest adventureaux,"*[54] articles in French journals during the 1930s began examining the new American and Swiss legislation on sterilization seriously for the first time. Although they still contained abundant warnings of caution or skepticism, most of these articles included substantial descriptions of the new laws. Moreover, the authors almost invariably admitted explicitly or implicitly the legitimacy and scope of the problem sterilization proposed to resolve – elimination of, in the words of one author, "the refuse of life, the sickly such as tuberculars, incurable defects, the insane and also those socially dangerous because of nerves, alcoholism and especially the morally pathogenic such as criminals and socially demented."[55] Even those who thought sterilization was extreme endorsed the more moderate premarital examination as a means of achieving the same end.[56]

One of the earliest and most thorough examinations of the question was a 1930 article by Georges Schreiber, vice president of the French Eugenics Society.[57] His approach was to make sterilization more acceptable by first examining "therapeutic sterilization," before looking at the possibility of "eugenic, penal, economic or social" uses of the measure. The examples he chose from his experience as a pediatrician were intended to elicit sympathy for the women whose lives were threatened and in some cases even lost because of pregnancies they could not bring to term. For example, he spoke of

a woman who comes every week to my clinic. She has three young children and expects a fourth. The three babies have rickets, serious rickets. The father is an alcoholic, and the mother probably is too. At home, "there is misery!" says the visiting social nurse who follows them closely. They are piled into a small room, the father barely makes a living. This is a family in the worst possible condition. Yet the woman is pregnant again. Do you believe it would be desirable for this woman to bring into the world a fourth child?[58]

Having made his specific rhetorical point, Schreiber offered the following general conclusion about "therapeutic sterilization":

Uniquely from the practical point of view of daily consultation . . . there are cases where accumulated defects and misery make human sterilization legitimate.[59]

Schreiber was more cautious about what he called "penal and economic sterilization." For example, he cited Georges Heuyer's 1926 talk on the premarital examination, which identified the hereditary trait of "instinctive perversion" as the origin of criminality and delinquency, and suggested that sterilization would be justified to prevent its transmission.[60] On the other hand, Schreiber was critical of the 1909 California statute requiring castration for certain crimes, because it was too broad in its assumption of inherited criminal traits.[61] In the end, he concluded that the question should at least be studied further in France without "the false sentimentality which risks simply multiplying the number of miserable beings."

Early in 1932 there was a chance to sample a slightly broader cross-section of opinion when, as part of preparation for the Third International Eugenics Congress, the American eugenicist Chàrles Davenport sent a letter to the French Eugenics Society requesting "the opinion of the French public on questions of reducing the fertility of the 'socially inadequate,' " by means of sterilization and birth control. In response, Henri Vignes, a member of the Ecole d'anthropologie who had earlier surveyed opinion on the premarital examination, sent letters to twenty doctors and sociologists, half of whom replied.[62] This was hardly an exhaustive survey, but Vignes' limited results give some indication that French opinions on sterilization had changed since the 1920s. Whereas earlier mention of the subject in the French Eugenics Society had prompted immediate disclaimers, only a few of those surveyed in response to Davenport's letter condemned sterilization outright or saw no instances when it was justified. The view of most, which was shared by Schreiber and other observers of the day, was that sterilization provided another means, albeit extreme, to a laudable end – the prevention of procreation by undesirables.[63]

It was primarily the question of public acceptability that was most often cited by respondents as a reason for attempting other, less controversial measures to achieve the same ends. These included the premarital examination or Davenport's suggestion of agricultural work colonies segregated by sex to prevent procreation by the "socially inadequate." Significantly, the only respondent urging caution on the scientific grounds that not enough was known yet about human heredity to sanction sterilization measures was the one non-scientist Georges Inman, a novelist and lawyer.[64] The physicians, anthropologists, or psychologists who responded did not share this view.

The discussion of the sterilization question in France thus began well before the Nazis came to power in Germany. Hence, when the July 1933 Law for the Preservation of the [Aryan] Race was passed in Germany, the sterilization measures it contained were not significantly different from those called for in the February 1933 platform of the Association d'études sexologiques. The reaction in French journals, therefore, was simply to add the German law to the list of laws passed in the United States and Switzerland and under consideration in England and Scandinavia. The analysis of the Nazi legislation followed the general pattern: a detailed description of the laws and their rationale and application, with a short section listing support or objections, and occasionally one or two concluding paragraphs about the writer's moral qualms or skepticism about the accuracy of knowledge about heredity.[65]

Eventually, the Nazi measures did produce a divergence of views in France. For example, Georges d'Heucqueville, a doctor for the public insane asylums, was encouraged enough by the Germans to suggest sterilization for alcoholics who

(1) have already given birth to defective children, [and] (2) have already been hospitalized or committed at least two times, for example, in a state of alcoholic intoxication or simply demonstrate a permanent intellectual weakening by their incapacity to accomplish regular tasks.[66]

At the other end of the spectrum of opinion, a Dr. Lowenthal of the Academy of Medicine ridiculed the whole notion of sterilization on Lamarckian grounds that defects were acquired by action of the environment as well as through inheritance.[67] The one feature of the Nazi sterilization program that was immediately noted as being significantly different was the number of people involved. Even Georges Schreiber called "audacious" the fact that

16,000 sterilizations were reported in the first year after the enactment of the German law. Yet as late as 1939 an article in the *Concours médical* said of the German legislation, "These laws which appear at first sight to be an affront to individual liberty and consequently to the welfare of the citizen, have as their goal the rational pursuit of that welfare."[68]

On the whole, perhaps it would be most accurate to describe the response to the German sterilization program as muted. In part, as has been suggested, this was because it was seen as only one manifestation of sterilization programs that were already in effect in many other countries. Another reason for the muted criticism was that the measures were recognized as part of a wider program of population, eugenic, and race laws passed by the new Nazi regime. To be sure, some of these measures, such as the anti-Jewish race legislation, were strongly criticized in France, on both moral and scientific grounds. As will be seen, even right-wing French race theorists such as René Martial and the anthropologist Georges Montandon never agreed on the advantages of racial purity or even the possibility of achieving it. Other measures, however, were actually envied. For example, the decrees aimed at repopulation were lauded by the very natalist organizations in France who had come to oppose eugenics because of its new attachment to ideas of birth control. One 1934 article in the leading French natalist journal even reprinted a section of *Mein Kampf* describing how the state should encourage large families, and asked wistfully why no French prime minister spoke or acted like Hitler.[69] The communists, too, admitted the value of Hitler's program of making state loans to young couples setting up house.[70] The respected geneticist Lucien Cuénot, who had no love for the Germans since he lived through the First World War on the front lines at his university in Nancy, wrote admiringly in 1936 of the "great number of measures" passed by the Nazis – some eugenic, others "para-eugenic," and some repopulationist – that had as their goal the "practice of suppressing dysgenics" in the population. He concluded that as a result, Germany would be "in twenty years a power that could dare anything," and he warned with a not very subtle sarcasm that "France, headed toward ruin by its absence of a family policy, would make a very nice German colony."[71] Events would prove his time estimate conservative.

OPPOSITION TO EUGENICS

One final feature of eugenics in France in the 1930s was the appearance of organized opposition to it by the church and natalist organizations. Although the most striking fact about the opposition is how long it took to appear, there is ample evidence to indicate that some other rallying point of opposition would soon have developed even if there had been no papal encyclical in December 1930. The most likely catalyst would have been the attempt by some eugenicists to repeal the 1920 law against contraception, which certainly would have turned the natalist organizations against eugenics. Sicard de Plauzoles' complaint about "a system of assistance that favors the multiplication of inferior classes" was also a direct attack on the natalist campaigns for government financial assistance to large families that had been urged since the turn of the century. Hence, although the encyclical was directed against the increase in sterilization practices in the United States and the Anglican bishops who had endorsed contraception at the Lambeth conference,[72] most French churchmen and their allies in natalist organizations took it as a signal to end the equivocal position they had held on eugenics from its beginning. Yet the French church's position before 1930 can also be taken as a testimony to the effectiveness of the milder program of French eugenicists in securing allies in the 1920s and earlier. This is illustrated by the reaction of the church and natalist organizations to the campaign for a premarital examination law.

When the premarital examination was first proposed by the French Eugenics Society, some religious leaders were wary of how the procedure might be carried out. As mentioned in the last chapter, Edouard Jordan, a professor of medieval history at the Sorbonne who had been a prominent member of the natalist congresses and the Association of Christian Marriage, accepted the basic rationale for the measure proposed by the French Eugenics Society. In a 1926 article he pointed out that it would be "unreasonable to think only of numbers and not be concerned about the quality" of the population.[73] The premarital examination, Jordan agreed, appeared to offer a common ground for cooperation in that "everyone could agree that children should be born under the best of circumstances." He cautioned his fellow natalists, how-

ever, that "one can draw very different conclusions from eugenics, and according to the manner in which it is understood and
practiced, it could be a powerful ally or redoubtable adversary in
the campaigns that we will be pursuing." To illustrate what he
meant, Jordan described an institute in Hamburg named by Georges
Schreiber in his talk at the 1926 conference on the premarital examination. Although Schreiber said the institute provided marriage counseling when the couple underwent their physical examination, Jordan maintained that only about 10 percent of the
institute's work was with couples engaged to be married – the
other 90 percent came solely for contraceptive information. Jordan
also considered what was to be done with couples whose examinations revealed problems, and he saw an even greater difficulty
when Pinard announced his proposal for a law that would make
the premarital examination mandatory. Although Jordan stopped
short of opposing the examination, he noted that all along he had
presumed a voluntary examination. A mandatory certificate that
had to be presented to government authorities was to him "a rather
different hypothesis."

Despite these reservations, Jordan continued to participate in
the discussion about the Pinard proposal. He spoke at a conference
on the subject sponsored by the Comité national d'études sociales
et politiques. At the same time, church officials joined in offering
their ideas on eugenics in general and the premarital examination
in particular. As late as April 1930, René Brouillard, a Jesuit the-
ologian wrote, "In principle, Catholic morality does not condemn
all eugenic science."[74] Differences occurred, he said, when one
"passes into the realm of practice and forgets that man the animal
is not the total man."[75] Of the two most commonly mentioned
eugenic measures, he found sterilization "absolutely repugnant to
Catholic morality." On the regulation of marriage, however, he
had a more open attitude. A premarital physical examination seemed
a good idea to Brouillard in the overall practice of marriage counseling, but making it mandatory raised a question, because he felt
that negative results or not having a medical examination should
not be sufficient grounds for "a legal interdiction of marriage."[76]

Although Brouillard answered Jordan's question about a mandatory examination law negatively, he was not reluctant to discuss
eugenics or find a way to work with some of the ideas, and in this
respect he was typical of French church leaders. In fact, the next

month, May 1930, the Association du mariage chrétien held a national congress in Marseilles devoted entirely to "The church and eugenics." The attitude of most at the congress was summarized in a final address by Monsignor Dubourg, the Archbishop of Marseilles, who stated that

if the goal of the new science [of eugenics] is, as its name indicates, to assure good offspring, it can only inspire our sympathy and find in Christian morality an auxiliary, even a very precious guide, because we profess that if God commanded man to multiply, He did not wish him to multiply poorly.[77]

To be sure, the congress soundly condemned such eugenic practices as contraception, but Jordan in his preface to the published proceedings welcomed eugenics as "an invitation to reflect upon the responsibilities involved in procreation."[78] The words could not have been better chosen by Pinard himself. Jordan now even expressed support for an obligatory examination such as Duval-Arnould's, which contained provisions for the exchange of results by spouses.[79] This sentiment was echoed by Jean Arnould, former chief of gynecology at the Faculty of Medicine in Marseilles who spoke on the premarital examination to the "Church and Eugenics" congress. Arnould found the proposed mandatory examination law "morally, socially and eugenically" advantageous.[80]

Thus, on the eve of the papal encyclical, the French church still expressed a very open and cooperative attitude toward eugenics, based largely on an accommodation over the premarital examination. French Churchmen lauded the "discretion" of French eugenicists who distinguished their program from the much harsher "Anglo-Saxon eugenics" advocated in England and the United States.[81] Jordan himself summed up this position in an extraordinary work entitled "Eugenics and Morality" published in 1931 but written just before the December 1930 encyclical. It was clear to Jordan that the negative eugenic measures of the Americans and others – especially the sterilization laws and advocacy of contraception, which were being discussed more and more in Europe – were pushing eugenics in a different direction from the positive program that had been emphasized by the French Eugenics Society since its beginning. Jordan's book amounted to an extended plea to French eugenicists to return to their original track, to "continue their legitimate warnings against unfortunate births, and to

concentrate again on the improvement of the milieu, on the progress of medicine, on general hygiene, urban planning."[82]

Jordan was criticizing the Americans and British to be sure, but
his real targets were those French who were sympathetic to the
Anglo-Saxon ideas. The most complete statement of this position
(and the one most frequently cited by Jordan) was Charles Richet's
Sélection humaine, a book written before the First World War but
whose publication was delayed until 1919.[83] Despite Richet's importance in French science generally and eugenics in particular,
there could not have been a more inauspicious time for his dramatic negative eugenics program to have been proposed. The early
1920s was precisely when the positive program of social hygiene
reached its peak in an effort to recover from the serious loss of life
in the war. By 1930, however, conditions had changed, and it was
not surprising to see Richet's views revived by eugenicists such as
Sicard de Plauzoles.

The tone of Richet's book was now much more in tune with
the new conditions of the 1930s. The Depression had begun, and
many more readers were likely to be in sympathy with Richet's
observation that "the fact of nature is the crushing of the weak.
The fact of society is the protection of the weak. Thus, the social
state vitiates the grand law of selection which is essentially the
survival of the strong."[84] The various measures Richet described
as necessary to bring society in line with the laws of nature could
now be seen as frank, including segregation of the races and the
ending of care for the "mentally deficient." Earlier, Richet had
had to soften his call for the use of sterilization to prevent such
people from procreating, and recommended instead the practical
expedient of marriage regulation (such as the premarital examination) until such time as public sentiment found sterilization more
acceptable.[85] Now, public discussion of sterilization was quite
commonplace.

Jordan naturally found none of Richet's proposals acceptable,
even arguing against mandatory marriage restriction on pragmatic
as well as moral grounds. To those who suggested such restriction, he posed the question, "Which would be a better course of
action: forbid marriages by alcoholics or revoke the rights of dis-
tillers and limit the number of bars?"[86] Jordan juxtaposed the neo-
Lamarckian presumptions of the founders of French eugenics with
the existing mood of the times:

Take a poor family, because it is assumed by many eugenicists that a poor person is a degenerate. Raise the wages, find the family healthy lodging, family subsidies and try to raise the standard of living. Won't their health have a chance to be maintained and improved? But does a society which wants to do nothing effective against alcohol or degradation or slums or other social plagues, have the right to avenge itself, in a way, on the victims of its own inactions, and to have recourse to the contemptuous and harsh methods such as sterilization, on the pretext that it is simple and final?[87]

It is doubtful that Jordan hoped to dissuade proponents of such negative eugenic measures, but a more realistic hope may have been to plead with the Catholic church hierarchy to leave room for the positive eugenics that had been championed by the French. When *Casti connubi* was published, its contents clearly showed that Jordan had failed.

By most accounts, the encyclical was aimed at the Anglican bishops' endorsement of contraception at their Lambeth conference earlier in the year.[88] The church also took advantage of the occasion to condemn several other practices that were increasingly advocated in the name of eugenics. This included the American state sterilization laws that were passed and applied with greater frequency after the U.S. Supreme Court confirmed their constitutionality in 1927. Similar laws were under discussion or had been newly legislated in European countries as well. The encyclical directly condemned the attempts of eugenicists to sterilize "defectives" by legislation, because it would

deprive these of that natural faculty by medical action despite their unwillingness; and this they do not propose as an infliction of grave punishment under the authority of the state for a crime committed, nor to prevent future crimes by guilty persons, but against every right and good they wish the civil authority to abrogate to itself a power over a faculty which it never had and can never legitimately possess.[89]

The position of the church on sterilization was hardly surprising, and neither was the encyclical's condemnation of abortion on any grounds, "social or eugenic," even "medical and therapeutic," nor in the encyclical's words, "however much we may pity the mother whose health and even life is gravely imperiled in the performance of the duty allotted to her by nature." The encyclical went on, however, to condemn as well those who put eugenics before aims of a higher order, and by public authority wish to prevent from marrying all those whom, even though naturally fit for marriage, they consider, according to the norms and conjectures of their investigations would, through hereditary transmission, bring forth defective offspring.

Thus, the church also opposed the idea of a premarital examination – the very proposal that French Catholics had seen as a possible meeting ground for accommodation with the eugenicists. As if to remove any doubt, the Holy Office issued a supplemental decree on March 21, 1931, that "declared false and condemned the theory of eugenics, either positive or negative," and disapproved of the means it proposed, "to improve the human race, neglecting the natural, divine, or ecclesiastical laws which concern marriage or the rights of individuals."[90]

There was no mistaking the effect of the encyclical on French church and natalist organizations, who ended their equivocal position on eugenics. Writing shortly thereafter in the Jesuit review, *Etudes,* René Brouillard praised the encyclical and subsequent decree as being the catalyst for attacking the increased publicity given in recent years by the press to "eugenic views, even the most radical, without the most elementary reserve and with a sympathy that is out of place in [such a] publication of high moral principles as the [*Journal des*] *débats.*"[91] In his lengthy two-part article, Brouillard welcomed the papal condemnation of practices – abortion, birth control, sterilization, marriage restriction – that he noted were against church doctrine and too drastic to be justified by the uncertain scientific knowledge of genetics.[92]

At the end of the second part of the article, however, the author indicated that he was not willing to give up completely the idea of eugenics, at least the overall goal that it sought to achieve. Brouillard attempted to make the case for retaining a notion of eugenics that was different from what he called the "Anglo-Saxon, Galtonian" version. It is a remarkable testimony to the power and attraction of the idea of eugenics that even in the face of the new church edicts, Brouillard still sought to define a "Catholic eugenics – a eugenics of life" – as opposed to the "eugenics of death" preached in the United States and England.[93] Reading between the lines of the encyclical and emphasizing what was not condemned rather than what was, Brouillard spelled out what he hoped the new eugenics would be:

Sanctification of marriage and the duties of spouses; attention to morality and health at the time of conception and birth; action by the state, associations and the church against public immorality, social diseases, alcoholism, slums, etc. to develop the economic well-being, general hygiene, puericulture, healthy dwellings, the prosperity of families . . . , all of which would constitute a moral, family, social and Christian eugenics.[94]

Thus, Brouillard continued to hope for a version of eugenics in France completely purged of the harsher negative elements with which it had so long coexisted.

In hindsight, the overall effect of the encyclical was more to quell support for eugenics by the French church in the 1930s than to stimulate strong or vocal opposition. Catholic publications and conferences ceased their consideration of eugenics that had proliferated in 1929 and 1930, shifting their attention instead to the depopulation problem and the dangers of neo-Malthusian activity.[95] As late as 1937, however, Edouard Jordan's sympathies with eugenics were still evident in an article for *Etudes* entitled "Natalité dirigée," which warned:

There exists if not a caste then at least a class, often very prolific, in which the worst physical and moral defects are transmitted from generation to generation through the effects of heredity or by the persistence of the same deplorable living conditions. They are costly to society, for whom their numerous offspring are too often a burden and not an asset. The fact is that no one of good sense would maintain that all births are equal.[96]

Jordan stopped short of endorsing eugenic measures as a remedy, despite the terms he used to describe the problem. His rather weak excuse was that in the United States and England, "they preach neo-Malthusianism by invoking eugenic arguments; but inversely, many are undoubtedly happy to find in eugenics a decent and special pretext to recommend neo-Malthusianism."[97] Jordan's only suggestion was that a natalist policy needed a complementary "social" policy.

The major reason for the break between French Catholics and eugenicists in the 1930s, therefore, was the question of contraception. The situation was aggravated by individuals such as Sicard de Plauzoles and organizations such as the Association d'études sexologiques who continued to express their views and even de-

clare themselves more openly in support of such measures condemned by the church. Soon the major natalist organizations joined
with the church in the attack. For example, in January 1931, Fernand Boverat of the Alliance nationale contre la dépopulation wrote
the first attack on eugenics in the organization's journal. This article was in striking contrast to a 1928 review of the first volume
of Marie-Thérèse Nisot's *La question eugénique dans divers pays,* which
was called by the natalist journal, "an indispensable repository for
all those . . . interested in the future of the race."[98] When the Association d'études sexologiques adopted its program in 1933 calling for a mandatory premarital examination and the creation of
public clinics to give advice on contraception and perform sterilizations and abortions, the reaction of the natalists was equally as
vigorous in opposition. This was particularly necessary, Boverat
noted, because it was proposed by a serious group that, "contains
among its officers and members a large number of distinguished
personalities belonging especially to the medical world."[99]

The opposition obviously did not silence or overwhelm these
proponents of the harsher eugenics of the 1930s. It is clear, however, that the effect of the papal encyclical and other opposition
was at least to destroy the old coalition of groups that had joined
together before the war to found a French eugenics movement.
One other effect of the timing was that this organized opposition
had already developed before the Nazis came to power and began
carrying out their eugenics program in 1933. Hence, the new German laws were not seen as something radically new or different in
principle. Only after the measures were in effect for some time
was their scale seen to imply something new. The overall result
was to dampen criticism, because the lines in the dispute had already been drawn before the German laws were passed. Although
this resulted in the existence of ready-made criticism of the laws
as soon as they were passed, the opposition was not focused specifically on the German practices, nor did it possess the immediacy
and vigor that might have been the case had the opposition been
organized directly in response to the Nazis.

THE LEFT AND EUGENICS

Criticism of eugenics by the church and natalists in the 1930s did
not spell the end to the movement in France. As mentioned, ad-

vocates of the harsher eugenics measures continued to voice their opinion and mobilize new bases of support. In fact, shortly after the change in church and natalist positions, another powerful group proclaimed a family and public health policy that was very close to the long-held moderate eugenic position that Brouillard and Jordan had hoped to retain. The irony is that the group was the political left, and the fact that some form of eugenic policy was being advocated across the political spectrum from extreme right to left shows how widely the idea of eugenics was employed by the end of the 1930s.

The new position of the left in France was not comparable to developments in other European countries where distinct "left-wing" programs had developed from the earliest days of eugenics. The closest had been Paul Robin's grass-roots working-class neo-Malthusian "Regeneration" league at the turn of the century. Although it contained many eugenic elements, Robin's movement was soon caught in a bitter debate on the question of birth control.[100] Robin, therefore, did not have the opportunity to develop a broader program, and few other socialist or labor leaders supported him, even on the issue of contraception. Left-wing policy on the broader eugenic-related questions of the prewar years was most notable by its absence. With the exception of occasional debates on issues such as alcoholism, there was little mention of health, let alone contraception, social hygiene, or eugenics in socialist publications. The postwar years removed these questions even further from the focus of attention of the left as it became engrossed in the communist/socialist doctrinal split prompted by the Bolshevik Revolution in Russia. In addition, the 1920 legislation against contraceptive propaganda had the effect of ending for a time this aspect of the question in all public legislative debate.[101]

The first mention of any eugenic or related topic in the publications of the Communist Party came in the early 1930s – exactly when other voices were being raised over the previously taboo questions of contraception and sterilization. In this case it was the subject of abortion, which was discussed in two articles in the *Cahiers du bolchevisme* in 1931 and 1932. As might be expected, the articles were highly critical of the "repressive" French laws, which the author of the first article claimed not only failed to prevent abortions, but also had the effect of making it possible for only the wives of the bourgeoisie to pay the high price for safe, clan-

destine abortions by doctors and midwives. Women of the working class had to resort to other, more dangerous methods. As the
author, Tilly Abeau, succinctly put it, "Done by people without
medical instruction, with crude instruments, under conditions of
miserable hygiene, these operations present very grave dangers
and result . . . in a very high proportion of death and injuries."[102]
Not surprisingly, Abeau contrasted the French situation with that
in the Soviet Union, where abortion was legal and accessible in
clinics, making the death and injury rate almost negligible. It is
significant that Abeau also made special note of the fact that the
Soviet population continued to grow at a rate of over 2 million
inhabitants yearly; hence, she was aware of the wider natalist
issue.

This article was clearly an exception, with no references to previous positions on the issues having been taken by the French
communists or socialists. The next year, another article called for
legalization of abortion, but none of the articles gave any indication of the sweeping legislative proposal to be introduced in 1933
by the communist deputies of the Chamber.

The proposal, entitled "Law for the protection of maternity and
childhood," was prompted, according to its authors, "by the economic crisis which has struck the capitalist world," leaving 50
million workers unemployed, not to mention the hundreds of
millions in the Far East and India.[103] Among the effects of this
desperate situation in other countries was a more relaxed attitude
toward the use of contraception, but according to the authors of
the legislation, the French bourgeoisie in its short-sighted approach to the problem of birthrate had retained the law of 1920,
the result being an increase in the number of clandestine abortions.
The communist deputies called for a sweeping revision of existing
laws and the introduction of new legislation to resolve the complex problems of maternity and childhood. For example, they
proposed the creation of offices to coordinate existing programs
for pregnant women and new mothers. They also wanted to expand the number of refuges for expectant mothers and provide
day nurseries for new mothers, if other programs would not allow
them to stay home with newborns. The most controversial features of the proposed legislation, however, were the final two sections, which called for revocation of the Law of July 31, 1920 that
had outlawed publicity about contraception, and for a complete

revision of the statutes on abortion. Legal abortions would be permitted when the health of the pregnant woman was endangered and "for eugenic reasons when necessary to prevent the procreation of defects or insanity."[104]

The communist deputies admitted that the bill had "no chance to be supported let alone adopted by the majority of the Chamber," despite the fact that it complied "with the suggestions and current evidence of eugenics, medical and surgical sciences," not to mention "the interest of all human society."[105] As communists, they reasoned that the existing situation suited capitalist interests.

The presence of hundreds of thousands of unemployed, the presence of an army of momentarily non-productive reserve workers constitutes for [the capitalists] an argument and a pretext for lowering salaries and thus augmenting their profits.[106]

The communist predictions proved to be correct, and for two years the matter lay dormant. Then, in November 1935, a series of articles appeared in *L'Humanité* and the *Cahiers du bolchevisme* that introduced a full-scale family policy retaining many of the features of the 1933 bill, and significantly dropping others. The policy was similar to the natalist position of the French Eugenics Society, the program that Brouillard had hoped the Catholic church would support after the 1930 encyclical. The first indications of this policy shift came in a speech by Maurice Thorez, head of the French Communist Party, on October 7, 1935. It was clearly part of a larger change in strategy by the communists prompted by the rise of the Nazis in Germany and the growth of right-wing movements in France and the rest of Europe. The result was a call for cooperation between left and center groups that culminated in the electoral victory of the Popular Front coalition in 1936.

In order to succeed, the communists had first to broaden their appeal to the French voting public. The theme of Thorez's 1935 speech could not have been broader in appeal, touching on motherhood, children, and country.

The working class does not want a weak France, with a degenerate people. It wants a hard-working and powerful France. What can be done to achieve it? We want to institute immediately a policy of effective protection for the mother and child.[107]

Thorez also sought to refute one of the common notions about the cause of the declining birthrate in France.

The sterile and degenerate bourgeois say, and have their journalists write, that the wives of workers and peasants, the whole of the people of France, do not want children. It is not true. . . . What is true is that they are afraid of the father unemployed, of the mother without work, of not being able to meet the needs of the family. . . . They are afraid of not being able to give birth to children in full health, robust and intelligent instead of being the misfortunes who will only know a life of misery.[108]

The following month, a series of articles appeared in the Communist Party newspaper *L'Humanité,* written by its editor, former deputy Paul Vaillant-Couturier, entitled, "Au secours de la famille." His opening article revealed the more moderate position, which described the problem of the family in political terms. The right, he pointed out, accused the left of "destroying, degrading and sterilizing" the family, while the left accused the right of being "repopulators" for military or religious reasons. Vaillant-Couturier deliberately chose to occupy the middle ground, but significantly his front-page article stated the issue in eugenic terms:

How to make motherhood a social function of the highest order – by combating misery, low salaries, unemployment, prostitution, slums, clandestine abortions, social diseases, alcoholism, infantile mortality – because upon it depends the continuity and improvement of the species.[109]

The next day, Vaillant-Couturier further defined his position by citing Sicard de Plauzoles as one who wished to resolve these problems by limiting births, and Fernand Boverat, a leading natalist, as an advocate of exactly the opposite course. The article ridiculed Boverat for representing "the interests of the directing oligarchies . . . which want to produce men above all for purposes of war," and Sicard for his "scientific preoccupation with the question of human breeding which unfortunately sinks to a Malthusian confusion of the facts."[110]

Before Vaillant-Couturier could elaborate on his own position, however, he was flooded with hundreds of letters from readers (if the editor can be believed), which he made the subject of what became virtually a daily column on the front page of the newspaper for the next six weeks.[111] These were exactly the kind of personal stories of ordinary working people that *L'Humanité* prided itself on reporting – men and women wanting to marry and have families but not being able to afford it. The letters were also used to help define the new moderate position of the party. For example, they stressed the value of marriage and the family – which contradicted many of the radical notions attributed to the left, such as the portrayal of marriage as a bourgeois institution of slavery for women. In two articles on November 22 and 24, 1935, entitled "Lenin talks on love" and "Lenin and the family," Vaillant-Couturier quoted the rather prudish father of the Russian Revolution as follows: "Neither monk nor Don Juan – sport, gymnastics, swimming, exercise, all sorts of physical exercise and varied moral interests . . . are better for youth than endless discussions on sexual questions."[112]

Most of the articles were directed toward the natalists in order to demonstrate that the working class desired larger families but simply could not afford them. A November 30 article was dedicated "especially to Boverat and the directors of the Alliance nationale contre la dépopulation," with quotes from letters and pictures of slums printed on the front page. Another article on December 8 entitled "Law and money versus motherhood" complained of inadequate subventions for mothers and families who were evicted from apartments for having too many children. An article on December 21 featured a picture of the recent winner of the Cognacq-Jay Prize, given yearly to exemplary large families in France, but which the article called "an exception without social value that serves to mask the failure of society with regard to the family." The communists had obviously found a way of beating the bourgeoisie with its own stick of natalism. The clear and unmistakable message of these articles was that the working class wanted to marry and have families. The problem was the capitalists, who would not hire them or pay them enough money to live decently.[113]

When Vaillant-Couturier finally got around to his long-delayed article entitled "Remedies," which described the Communist Party answers to these problems, he placed great emphasis on the features of the 1933 legislative proposal calling for support of motherhood and children, but made only passing reference to its call for revoking the statutes against birth control and abortion.[114] Yet the essentially eugenic viewpoint remained. As Vaillant-Couturier noted in the beginning of the article, "The guiding principle of our proposition resides *in the recognition of motherhood as a social function.*"[115]

The importance of the revised program to the communists can be seen in another bill introduced in the 1936 Chamber, sponsored by the now much larger communist delegation that had been elected in the Popular Front campaign. Gone were the references to legalizing abortion; gone also was the call to revoke the 1920 law against contraception. What remained was a bill for "effective protection of maternity and childhood" that hardly anyone could oppose. It included the call for creation of a national office of the mother and child to coordinate all existing legislation on their behalf, passage of new legislation that would "protect mothers effectively before, during and after pregnancy," encourage breastfeeding, and protect all children through three years of age.[116]

The Popular Front was not in power long enough to enact this legislation, but the issues remained a part of the Communist Party program in the years that followed. Speeches by Thorez and articles in the *Cahiers du bolchevisme* covered subjects that could just as easily have been found in earlier issues of *Eugénique:* "Depopulation and childhood misery," which cited Pinard, Richet, and even Fernand Boverat, or "The battle against slums," on the effect of poor living conditions on the birthrate.[117] At the end of January 1936, Thorez warned that "the population decreases instead of growing. If this unsettling phenomenon continues or grows, it will be a catastrophe for our country. In a few decades we will be a nation of the elderly, a weak, diminished people on the road to extinction."[118] In other articles, Georges Levy, a communist deputy who had been trained as a physician, reviewed the history of the public health movement in France since 1902, covering in turn the problems of slums, alcoholism, tuberculosis, and syphilis. Although Levy's stated purpose was to show "the human inequality in sickness and death" resulting in rates in the poorer quarters of Paris that were double those of the rich quarters, his language and descriptions were clearly drawn from twenty years of social hygiene and eugenic writing. For example, Levy made much of the concept of "human capital" that Sicard de Plauzoles had used in order to justify increased expenditure on health measures.

One forgets too often that the expenses for the protection of public health are excellent investments, because in the future they prevent the degeneration of the race, sickness and death; and they decrease expenses for hospitalization, insane asylums, welfare, prisons and lost work days."[119] Levy also had little doubt that "there is heredo-alcoholism like heredo-syphilis," which he proved by citing statistics claiming that half the crimes in France resulted from alcoholism.[120] In sum, most of the positive, neo-Lamarckian eugenic position developed in the first three decades of the twentieth century is evident in Levy's program, without the negative measures designed to eliminate the undesirables.

The communists' "policy of protection of the family and childhood" was not a program of some fascist league, but a demonstration, in the party's own words, of a "preoccupation with this important problem, both in the parliamentary field as well as the courts." Thorez gave special attention to the question at a November 21, 1938, meeting of the Central Committee of the Communist Party by making "protection of the family and childhood" one of the points of the party's ten-point program.[121] Although this program did not support a mandatory premarital exam, it did call for "prenatal consultation." In fact, it is a testimony to how far the left had moved on these questions that virtually every other point of Pinard's puericulture was included – from "surveillance of pregnant women," including "a longer rest period before and after pregnancy," to encouragement of breast-feeding.[122] It goes without saying that included also was support of most legislation proposed by natalists for bonuses, subventions, and tax breaks to encourage large families. Thorez even echoed one of the natalists' favorite proposals calling for "the advantages accorded to large families to be paid for by taxes on the unmarried and households without children."[123]

What would cause such a dramatic change in policy by the left, aside from a genuine response to the sympathetic chord evidently struck by the *L'Humanité* articles? Natalists were openly skeptical when they first heard of their new-found allies, although Boverat admitted that the new policy, "whatever its faults denotes serious concern for the population problem." He also noted the fact that the left had at least put it in the form of a legislative proposal, which was more than could be said of many natalists, whose longtime support was "warm but vague in principle."[124]

In the context of the mid-1930s and the preparations for the creation of the Popular Front, it is not surprising that such a policy was embraced. For example, in April 1936 Thorez attempted to make peace with the Catholic church in his famous *"main tendue"* speech – the communists' "outstretched hand" to Catholics and the members of fascist youth leagues during the mid-1930s as part of the party's campaign against its right-wing foes. Peace was also extended to the Ligue des droits de l'homme, which the party had opposed since 1922.[125]

The new position on family and health thus fit in well with this new policy. It challenged no important part of the programs advocated by the left, and to those who feared that the party was abandoning its revolutionary mission, Thorez replied simply, "We do not want to take power in a diminished, amputated country. We want to take power with a strong people, a healthy and numerous people."[126] If legalizing abortion had to be dropped, this was no major revision because the issue had only been briefly taken up in previous years. Moreover, Thorez was very conscious of the potential political danger of the position.

We do not wish to repeat on this precise matter the tragic error of our comrades in the German party. For some time they had made abortion one of the essential articles of their program. This article caused them extreme harm. The Nazis went out in the countryside and among the workers and said, "here are men who wish to weaken our country, to the advantage of foreigners."[127]

The left certainly had no qualms about government intervention in the private sphere. More important, the family policy could take advantage of the broad appeal of natalist, social hygiene, and eugenic ideas that had been developing in France since 1900. In first announcing the change in policy, Thorez complained that "the fascists pretend to be guardians of the family tradition and say 'the communists want to destroy the family.' " His family program was consciously designed as a response, which he admitted "is a veritable turning point in our policy on this question, but it is also the path toward the masses of our country."[128]

The concluding paragraph of a 1939 article in the *Cahiers du bolchevisme* on family policy read as follows:

What higher goal [is there] to achieve for our party, if its militants set themselves to the task with their habitual ardor; to realize the great work of national renovation, the effective protection of the family and child-hood to which are attached at the same time the recovery and future of our country.[129]

These words could just as easily have introduced the new family policy of the Vichy regime one year later.

The communists' family program deliberately picked up eugenic ideas as part of remaking its image of respectability during the era of the Popular Front.[130] In addition to what this says about the broad applicability of ideas concerning biological regeneration, the fact that they were adopted by a wide range of political movements meant that the eugenics question in France was similar to that in other countries by the end of the 1930s. A full range of eugenic proposals was openly advocated – from the most moderate, positive support of motherhood to the most extreme calls for the use of sterilization. Despite the efforts of leaders of the French Eugenics Society to carve out a compromise position based on the idea of a "Latin eugenics" complete with an international congress in Paris in 1937,[131] the old alliance of population regenerators could not be put back together. This is not surprising, given the polarization of political and ideological views in France at the time. The Third Republic, which had been founded and thrived on the spirit of compromise, survived until the end of the decade, but only in the face of many new and more radical ideas. These ideas will be spelled out more clearly in the next chapters, which look specifically at the questions of race and immigration in French eugenics.

8

Eugenics, race, and blood

In the 1930s, new eugenic arguments for improving the French race gained prominence. Although proponents of the milder, positive eugenics attempted to rally support from a diminishing base, the most significant trend of the decade was the growth of a more strident, negative eugenics. The issues and developments that prompted the change have been discussed in the last chapter: the economic decline of the Great Depression, the large number of immigrants in France, the rise of the Nazis to power in Germany, and the papal encyclical of 1930. This chapter examines one important feature of the new French eugenics: its racism.

The racist eugenics of the 1930s was only in part a return to the older tradition of Gobineau and Vacher de Lapouge. Like the earlier eugenics, it was also based on new anthropological definitions of race, but with different scientific underpinnings. Whereas older definitions had relied on certain cultural characteristics and specific physical features of skin color, hair texture, and the size or shape of the skull to distinguish races, new discoveries in the twentieth century of human blood groups and their distribution patterns among populations offered a seemingly more clear-cut and "scientific" basis for defining races. Although the theoretical explanation offered by blood groups was elegantly simple, the notions of "blood" and "race" were so fraught with historical and psychological implications that the result was confusion and misapplication of the new discoveries in ways that the first medical and anthropological researchers would never have thought possible.[1] This change can best be appreciated by examining the development of racial thought among French eugenicists in the first four decades of the twentieth century.

RACISM AND FRENCH EUGENICS BEFORE THE 1930S

Of all the early eugenics writers, Georges Vacher de Lapouge placed by far the most emphasis on race. It was literally the basis of his eugenic determination of "superior" elements of the population to be conserved. And although Lapouge was almost completely ostracized from the French scientific community after 1900 – he remained at provincial libraries for the rest of his life and published almost exclusively in foreign journals – his standing in other countries was quite high. No less a figure than Kaiser Wilhem II is supposed to have remarked, "The French possess only one great man, Vacher de Lapouge, and they ignore him." The statement, however, may say as much about the Kaiser as it does about Vacher de Lapouge's esteem in Germany.[2]

When Lucien March and Lucien Cuénot went to the Second International Eugenics Congress in New York after the First World War as official representatives of the French Eugenics Society, they found that the Americans had also invited Vacher de Lapouge to address the congress. Likewise, Margaret Sanger invited him to speak at the Sixth International Birth Control Congress in New York in 1925.[3] For his part, Vacher de Lapouge returned the favor for one of his American hosts by arranging the translation and writing a preface for the 1926 French edition of Madison Grant's *The passing of a great race*. More will be said of this American connection later.

Although Vacher de Lapouge's influence in France paled by comparison with his foreign reputation, one can hardly say that French racism was dead at the turn of the century. If anything, the 1890s and the Dreyfus affair witnessed the most violent and widespread anti-Semitism France had seen in modern times. Not only did the affair become a *cause célèbre* for nascent anti-Jewish publications such as Drumont's *La libre parole* and the Catholic church's *La croix*, which reached hundreds of thousands of French readers, it also was the inspiration for the establishment of more formal organizations such as the Action Française, which became centers of continuing racist thought.[4]

Another facet to French racism that was often overshadowed by anti-Semitism was the belief that Asian and African peoples were biologically inferior to Europeans.[5] Although this sentiment went against the much-lauded French assimilationist colonial theory that French culture rather than Frenchmen's physical attributes was what made the French superior to others, the expansion of French colonial rule in Africa and Southeast Asia at the end of the nineteenth century brought French government officials and intellectuals face to face with the practical aspects of assimilationist theory.[6] The real test was whether or not the new colonial subjects would be treated as equals or potential equals of Frenchmen in such matters as schooling and political rights. They were not, and because this ran counter to the long-held assimilationist tradition, it is telling proof of how deeply racism was rooted in French perceptions of outsiders. Moreover, it is relatively easy to demonstrate that the perceptions were reinforced by scientific scholarly thought at the time, most notably among French anthropologists.

The presumed inferiority of Africans and Asians was so deeply ingrained that it was taken for granted by most anthropologists and other thinkers of the day. No lengthy arguments were seen as necessary to prove the existence of a racial hierarchy; instead, anthropologists concentrated most of their attention on measuring physical features and classifying the peoples of the world according to these measurements. The work of Paul Broca, founder of modern French anthropology, illustrates this clearly. Although he is recognized now for pioneering studies in mapping the brain, and his organizational achievements in creating the separate discipline of anthropology in France, Broca's chief concern in physical anthropology was a study of differences between humans.[7]

Broca's subjects for comparison were not individuals but groups, and his most frequent categories for comparison were sex and race. In all of the studies one can find a continuing presumption of a hierarchical relationship between the groups. As a recent study of Broca points out, "Conclusions came first and Broca's conclusions were the shared assumptions of most successful white males during his time – themselves on top by the good fortune of nature, and women, blacks and poor people below."[8] With males assumed to be superior to females, and Europeans superior to Africans, the question that remained was to find the physical attribute that could be measured and correlated to the hierarchy already taken for granted. Broca's answer was the rather simplistic notion that skull volume as a measure of brain size was the best indicator of intelligence, hence superiority. Not surprisingly, his conclusions fit his presumption:

In general, the brain is larger in mature adults than in the elderly, in men than women, in eminent men than in men of mediocre talent, in superior races than in inferior races. . . . Other things being equal, there is a remarkable relationship between the development of intelligence and the volume of the brain.[9]

In a telling remark made during a debate about methodology with a colleague Broca himself admitted what came first in his thinking. "The superiority of Europeans compared with the African Negroes, American Indians, Australians and the Negroes of Oceania, is sufficiently certain to serve as a point of departure for the comparison of brains."[10] As anomalies arose, Broca's theory became more complex, eventually involving the number of folds of the brain and its position relative to the spinal column, but the presumption of inferiority and superiority always preceded the "proof."

The point here is not that Broca was a racist but rather that what we call "racism" – a presumed hierarchy of peoples based on biology – was normal among anthropologists, not just in France but throughout Europe and America in the nineteenth century.[11] Like Broca, they were also white, male, and of European ancestry, and they did not question their superiority to females, non-whites and non-Europeans, though they may have disagreed about the reasons for it and whether it was a permanent situation. Given this intellectual climate of racism, it is not surprising that French eugenicists shared these racist presumptions long before the 1930s. They may have paid less attention to racial hierarchy than eugenicists in other countries, but this is explained by the French preoccupation with more pressing problems such as depopulation. Also, they did not see an immediate biological threat, as in the United States, from blacks or Asians. In fact, some French neo-Lamarckians even argued that new immigrants could be biologically as well as culturally assimilated, according to a law they called "the dominance of the autochthonous," whereby offspring of parents of mixed ancestry showed greater resemblance to the parent in whose home country they resided.[12] This view was exceptional, and usually when French eugenicists considered other races it was with a presumption of inferiority, as did anthropologists and most other thinkers of the day. Enough examples of nonassimilation existed, moreover, for most French eugenicists to be openly fearful of a biological decline that might come from the influx of inferior peoples and interbreeding with them.

An excellent example of the continuity of racism – from Vacher de Lapouge's writings before the turn of the century to the French racists of the 1930s – was Charles Richet's *Sélection humaine*. As mentioned in Chapter 4, this work, written before the First World War but published in 1919, was frequently cited both by eugenicists and opponents not only as a clear and complete general statement of French eugenic thought, but also as a guide for eugenic ideas on race.[13] This was because Richet's book attached a great deal of importance to racial questions. When other French eugenicists were outdoing themselves in calling for measures to repopulate France, Richet began his chapter "The inferior races" with the following dictum: "Above all, one must avoid all mixture of superior races with inferior human races."[14] Realizing where this statement placed him in traditional French debates about equality versus inequality, or assimilation versus nonassimilation, Richet was typically blunt in describing the assumptions behind his rule.

I do not comprehend how by aberration one can equate a negro with a white. When I read works which talk of the unity of the human race, I wonder if I am daydreaming. Whether of single or multiple origin, it does not matter. The fact is that today in 1912 they are different, as different as a curved line differs from a straight one, as a crayfish differs from a lobster, and the sun from the moon. Whether I am crucified, whipped or made to suffer the most varied or clever tortures, I will never admit that the negro, with his curly hair, thick lips, receding facial angle, long arms and black skin is identical to a white with blond hair, blue eyes and pink skin.[15]

Nor was Richet merely describing differences; he was equally pointing out that his main purpose "concerns less the difference between whites and blacks – this cannot be denied – than the superiority of whites over blacks." From this conclusion, Richet went on to call for the prohibition of marriage between whites and non-whites as an essential prerequisite to other efforts at arresting degeneration from other debilitating causes within European society.[16]

As with Broca, the point is not simply to add Richet to the list of French racists, but rather to show that he was typical. Nor was Richet terribly imaginative in his proof of superiority, which was little more than a citing of the number of books written, scientific discoveries made, and art created as measures of what he called "intelligence."[17] Today, the simplicity of his ethnocentrism is almost pathetic, although one must give him credit as least for attempting to prove white superiority, unlike Broca, who did not even see the need. Moreover, Richet's delineation of the races was not particularly novel; if anything, it was even more superficial than the proof of intellectual superiority. "I am content with a very simple division," Richet said, "essentially true, though it may not be scholarly. Blacks, yellows, whites. Blacks are in Africa, yellows occupy Asia, the whites are in Europe and America."[18] To Richet's credit, however, his analysis had the effect of minimizing differences between groups in his white race, such as the Caucasians and Semites. As he put it, "Between these two races, from the standpoint of intelligence, I do not believe it possible to establish a preeminence. Even though my admiration for Arab or Jewish civilization is mediocre, I would not have the temerity to pretend that the Semitic races are inferior to Caucasian races."[19] This was faint praise, indeed, but praise nonetheless.

Richet's delineation of the races was almost a caricature of anthropological thought of the day, especially compared with Broca's and others' elaborate physical body measurements and their breakdown of groups in subcategories. But its most fundamental feature – the presumed racial hierarchy – was typical. Richet's book had been written in prewar days, and his concern resulted from France's and other European powers' having established vast colonial empires in Africa and Asia.[20] In fact, his stated goal was to avoid a repetition of race mixing as had occurred in South America. Richet preferred instead to see the colonization of Africa follow the example of the racially segregated United States. Such views did not inspire much of a following in the prewar heyday of assimilation. But as with the delayed appreciation of Richet's other negative eugenics, his views on race also received later approbation by French eugenicists when the possibility of race mixing became more real in France with increased immigration after the First World War.

As will be seen in the next chapter, the influx of immigrants to France in the 1920s was spurred by several developments: the revolutions and disruption in Eastern Europe, the establishment of U.S. immigration quotas, and the labor shortage in France that was heightened by a fear of depopulation from war losses.[21] All combined to bring unprecedented numbers of foreigners into the country, in the face of which the "law of autochthonous predominance" offered little comfort. The first discussion of the problem by the French Eugenics Society was at a December 1922 meeting at which general secretary Georges Schreiber raised the question of controlling immigration because, in his words, "there are eugenically undesirable elements among those who flock daily toward us."[22] He did not specify the nature of the elements, but Eugène Apert, vice president of the society, responded to Schreiber's remarks with a list of foreigners he could identify coming in large numbers, including Italians, Poles, and North African Arabs. In addition, he noted that there were regiments of Vietnamese Senegalese soldiers garrisoned in the south of France, where "mulattos are beginning to appear."

A second, extended discussion of the problem occurred at a meeting of the eugenics society in May 1923, when it was announced that an organization had been formed to monitor the placement of younger immigrants, aged thirteen to sixteen, with families in rural France. The Comité des enfants immigrés was created as part of the effort to recruit manpower from outside France to relieve the shortage of labor after the war. Youngsters placed with farm families, it was thought, could help meet the need for agricultural labor and be more easily assimilated into French society. Given the age of the children, special precautions would have to be taken for their protection, but this might also provide a mechanism to control selection of these workers. Schreiber, who along with Apert had been named to the committee because of his work on childhood diseases, reported to the French Eugenics Society in its May meeting that the screening of the young immigrants could be done from a eugenic standpoint in two ways: individually, according to moral and physical fitness, as well as by what he called a "séléction des races."[23] To illustrate the need for the latter criterion, Schreiber warned of women being brought to France from Martinique to relieve the shortage of domestic help. His anti-black bias was similar to that in Apert's remark about mulattos being seen near garrisons of Senegalese soldiers. But this time, comments from Georges Papillaut, vice president of the Société d'anthropologie, elicited an even clearer indication of racial hierarchy. Such a ranking of races was necessary, he noted, because "the productive white races can be considered capable of furnishing to France good elements of immigration." In other words, Southern and Eastern Europeans should not be excluded by a general ban on immigrants.

By the end of 1923 the question of immigration had become so important to the French Eugenics Society that it was the subject of the next two major addresses at its meetings: one by Apert on "The problem of races and immigration in France," the other by Lucien March on "Immigration and the birthrate." Apert's talk, drawing on his experience with the Comité des enfants immigrés, began by reassuring the society that the peoples coming to France mostly fell within Papillaut's definition of "production races." As a precautionary measure, however, Apert reported that he had suggested that the committee ban "the introduction of children of the black or yellow races." His justification was based specifically on Richet's ideas as stated in *Séléction humaine*.[24]

On the positive side, Apert indicated that the danger from either the West Indian domestics described by Schreiber or the African and Vietnamese regiments stationed in France was minimal so far, but only because their numbers were so small. Of greater significance in the talk was the fact that for the first time he made distinctions between the peoples making up the "white" immigrants to France. These he grouped into categories of people closely related to the French – such as the Belgians, Spanish, and Italians – and more distant white populations such as Arabo-Berbers and Balkan and other "diverse Slavic peoples." Apert avoided open condemnation of the rapidly increasing Polish immigration, but he mentioned the findings of a recent medical thesis on the effects of race mixing on the character of descendents, in which the author found a higher incidence of "moral, mental, and pathological defects" among the offspring of French-Russian, French-German, and Anglo-Greek marriages. Apert's conclusion was that immigrants from the more distant white races were in need of close scrutiny, because they formed a middle rank in the hierarchy between the black and Asian immigrants, who should be banned, and the Belgians, Italians, and Spanish,[25] who should be welcomed openly.

In the lively discussion following Apert's talk, there was little questioning of his categories. Papillaut, if anything, urged stricter controls, quoting an Arab proverb that "God created man and the devil made the half-breed." Schreiber argued against being too severe in judging the middle category of immigrants, but heartily agreed that "the collective introduction of subjects from the black or yellow race should be prohibited." March's talk at the next meeting of the eugenics society was essentially in agreement with Apert, although naturally it concentrated more on the effects of immigration on birthrate. Discussion afterward produced some comments about Latin peoples being more prone to assimilation into French society than Slavic peoples, but most attention was focused on the need for the government to control immigration policy rather than allowing employers or labor organizations to determine policy in piecemeal fashion.[26]

It is clear from these discussions that racism continued among French eugenicists well past the First World War, insofar as the races of the world were seen in a biological hierarchy. Nor was this unusual, given the views on race of most French thinkers of the day, including anthropologists. If there was a common thread linking their perceptions of differences between the French and others, it was perhaps the sense that the degree of difference was proportional to the geographical distance of the country of origin from France. Beyond that, however, there was little agreement about whether the differences were sufficient to warrant the exclusion of certain groups from France, or even about basic questions of what constituted a race. Richet had glossed over the latter problem by completely minimizing differences among whites, but he was the exception. Other French eugenicists who considered Eastern Europeans different enough to warrant closer scrutiny reflected traditional views of anthropologists, but even they were finding it increasingly difficult to draw these racial lines. In fact, by the 1920s so many questions had arisen that they threatened to undermine the whole system of racial classification that French and other physical anthropologists had helped to create in the last third of the nineteenth century. The new methods that evolved to answer these questions in the 1920s and 1930s had important consequences for French eugenicists as well as for race theory in general.

FROM THE CEPHALIC TO THE BIOCHEMICAL INDEX

The system of racial classification that Broca helped establish as the basis for the rest of physical anthropologists in the world emphasized two essential features: precision of measurement and comparison of data. Broca was not the first to measure human anatomy for these purposes or to make comparisons between human groups based on physical appearance. But it was the care and precision of measurement and the exhaustive manner in which he compared his data that gave rise to the claim that French physical anthropology was a scientific approach to discovering the differences between human groups. This included standardized procedures and the use of new instruments to improve the accuracy and comparability of measurements. For example, several body parts were singled out as standards for comparison. Typically this was done according to size and shape, such as the volume of the brain, which Broca thought to be crucial to intelligence and therefore evolutionary development, or the facial angle (the slope of a line from forehead to jaw), a steeper angle indicating a higher stage of evolution.

By far the most commonly used of these measurements was the cephalic index – the relationship of the width of the skull to its length. It was first proposed by the Swedish anthropologist Anders Retzius in the 1840s as a way of distinguishing between the so-called dolichocephalic ("long-headed") blond Aryan peoples of northern Europe and the inferior brachycephalic ("broad-headed") darker peoples of the south and east. Broca had questioned some of the simplistic claims of this craniological theory. For one thing, the majority of Frenchmen, including Broca, were brachycephalic; in addition, he was much more interested in the volume of the skull than its shape, because he considered it to be a better measure of brain size, hence intelligence. Other Frenchmen, such as Vacher de Lapouge, made the cephalic index the cornerstone of the division of races in Europe. Moreover, when Léonce Manouvrier challenged Lapouge's theories at the end of the nineteenth century, it was not on the skull-based definitions of race but rather on the characteristics Lapouge attributed to them, especially psychological ones. The cephalic index was easily understood, and soon became the most widely adopted means for the classification and comparison of races.[27]

Despite the widespread acceptance and use of craniometry and other measures in physical anthropology, by the 1920s there were many who saw the need for a new way to classify the races. For example, serious questions had been raised about anthropometry by the dean of American anthropologists, Franz Boas, who found in his famous 1911 study of immigrants that there were significant differences in the cephalic indexes of foreign and American-born Jews and Italians living in America. This led Boas to the conclusion that "the head form, which has always been considered one of the most stable and permanent characteristics of human races, undergoes far-reaching changes due to the transfer of the people from European to American soil."[28]

These studies were nothing new to the French who had long considered such changes as confirmation of the Lamarckian link between environment and heredity.[29] Other, more fundamental questions were raised about anthropometric methods by French researchers, among them Alfred Binet, the French psychologist who is best known for his formulation of what came to be known as IQ testing. Binet claimed that he was led to develop his aptitude measurements only after failing to achieve acceptable results using Broca's procedures for measuring intelligence from skull size. In 1900, after three years of work using these methods in French schools, Binet concluded,

I was persuaded that I had attacked an intractable problem. The measures had required traveling and tiring procedures of all sorts; and they ended with the discouraging conclusion that there was often not a milimeter of difference between the cephalic measures of intelligent and less intelligent students. The idea of measuring intelligence by measuring heads seemed ridiculous.[30]

Paul Rivet is another example of a famous French anthropologist trained in the old anthropometric method who questioned the use of the cephalic index to classify races, let alone to determine intelligence. Part of the problem, he pointed out, was the result of proponents' promising too much from their methods. Writing in 1930, Rivet recalled the earlier claims of those using Broca's so-called metric method.

One had the illusion then that the metric method was going to allow the classification of human races with an absolute rigor, to grasp the differences and establish relationships that the eye could discover only with difficulty and uncertainty. Moreover, it was thought that the study of such and such an isolated relationship (cephalic index, nasal index, orbital index, etc.) would furnish the essential characteristic of each human type. These hopes, it must be admitted, have in large measure been in vain. No matter which feature is considered, nor the rigor with which it is measured, its significance remains uncertain.[31]

As proof, Rivet cited a whole series of measurements made by him and others showing the wide variation of indexes for individuals within specific ethnic groups. He pointed out that

if a table is made of averages calculated for the different populations, classifying them in ascending order, it is clear that ethnic groups which are morphologically very different, lie close together. One finds, for example, the same average nasal index for ancient Pompeians and California Indians of Santa Rosa (46.6), for Ainus and the Japanese (50.7); the same cephalic index for Great Russians and Andaman Islanders (80.6), for Tyroleans and natives of Tonga (84.2); the same height for Turks in the Balkans and the Banda [of West Africa] (166 centimeters).[32]

It is, therefore, fitting that Rivet had welcomed and even helped arrange for the publication of an article after the First World War in the French journal *Anthropologie* by Ludwik and Hannah Hirszfeld entitled "The application of serological methods to the problem of races."[33] The article proposed a revolutionary new way for anthropologists to define race.

As mentioned before, differences in visible features of anatomy were the most common way to distinguish between human groups – the color of hair and skin, the shape and size of face and bones. The Hirszfelds' work was revolutionary because it measured something new – blood group, a chemical property of the red cells and serum in human blood. In 1900, Karl Landsteiner, an Austrian physician, had found that if blood samples of two human subjects were mixed, they sometimes clumped together, or agglutinated. Systematic research showed that a constant property in any individual's blood always produced agglutination with the blood of some individuals but not of others. Soon the outlines of the ABO blood system were discovered, with its four blood types – A, B, O, and AB – whose existence could be determined by whether and when the blood clumps together with the other types.[34]

The most immediate application of the blood group discoveries was in the practice of blood transfusion. With larger numbers of individuals tested, Ludwig Hirszfeld, then an assistant to Emil von Dungern in Heidelberg, discovered in 1910 that blood groups were inherited according to the Mendelian laws of heredity. This suggested several new avenues of research, but the outbreak of war in 1914 interrupted the plans. The research for the Hirszfelds' 1919 article was conducted while they were with the Serbian army medical corps on the Allies' eastern front in Greece. The Germans had pinned down a sizeable number of Allied troops around Salonika after they had been evacuated from the disastrous Gallipoli campaign. The troops came from England and France and their Eastern European allies, and from their colonies in Africa and Asia. Because there was very little military activity – they could not advance for military reasons nor withdraw for political ones – this setting proved to be an ideal laboratory in which to test whether blood types could serve as an indicator of race. Hirszfeld and his wife Hanna, who was also a physician, did blood tests on several hundred individuals from each of nineteen different ethnic groups, ranging from English, French, Greek, and Bulgarian to Senegalese, Indian, Malagasy, and Vietnamese. In all, over 8,000 tests were made.

The Hirszfelds could not have expected each nationality to have possessed only one blood type. Landsteiner's and others' research had already shown all groups to be present among the subjects of all their studies. What differed was the frequency. Hoping to determine how extensive these variations could be, the Hirszfelds found not only a wide range but a startling pattern to the proportion of blood types found in a given nationality. Simply put, the percentage of individuals with type A blood (so named originally because it was the one found most frequently by Landsteiner among the Austrian co-workers he tested) was significantly lower among Asians and Africans (27–38%) than among Europeans (42–48%). Even more striking was the higher percentage of type B blood among non-Europeans. Whereas only 7.2% of the English tested were type B, 29.2% of Senegalese, 28.4% of Vietnamese, and 41.2% of Indians from the Asian subcontinent were found to have type B blood.[35]

The Hirszfelds plotted their results on a double bar graph and found almost a straight-line increase in the percentage of type B blood for each nationality, with a somewhat more irregular decline in the percentage of type A (Table 8.1).

The most striking correlation they found was between the pat-

Table 8.1. *Results of Hirszfelds' 1919 research*

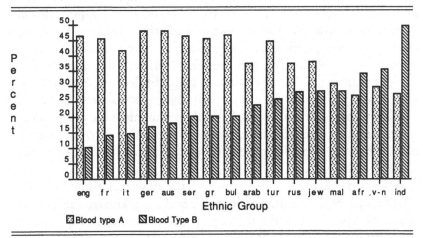

Source: Ludwig and Hanna Hirszfeld, "Essai d'application des méthodes sérologiques au problème des races," *Anthropologie,* 29 (1919).

tern of frequency of blood type and the geographical origins of the people tested. As the Hirszfelds put it,

It is remarkable that the distribution of A and B corresponds exactly to the geographical situation. The closer one is to central and western Europe, the more one finds A and the less of B. The closer one is to Africa and Asia, especially India, the less one finds A and the more of B.[36]

To quantify results for comparison, the Hirszfelds used a simple ratio of type A to type B blood for each of the peoples tested, and called it a biochemical index of races. This assigned Europeans the highest index (4.6 to 2.5), Asians and Africans the lowest (less than 1), thus preserving a hierarchy, whether intentional or not. Moreover, the Hirszfelds went on to suggest an explanation for their results – the independent origin of type A and B blood from two primeval races: one in India, the other in north or central Europe. In sum, the Hirszfelds' study suggested a new basis for distinguishing between human subpopulations.

APPLICATIONS OF THE NEW DEFINITION OF RACE

Given the problems that had arisen in classifying races according to traditional anthropometric means, it is not surprising that the

Hirszfelds' discovery was welcomed by physical anthropologists, not just in France but elsewhere in Europe and America. In fact, the study of troops on the Greek front helped set in motion a flood of new field work on the blood types of ethnic groups. By 1926, studies on fifty peoples had been made, ranging from the native American populations of the Western United States and Canada to the continent of Europe, Russia, the Middle East, South Asia, China, and Japan. By the early 1930s, over 1,000 articles had been published, based on almost half a million individual tests. The most recent definitive compilation, by Mourant et al. in 1976, reported that 15 million people had been tested for the ABO blood system alone.[37]

A second reason for the spread of the new technique was the relative ease of determining blood types. Using known samples of A and B type blood and a microscope, a researcher could quickly and definitively identify the blood being tested as one of the four types of the ABO system. Moreover, techniques for preserving and transporting blood had been developed almost as quickly as the new discoveries were made, thanks to advances in citration and refrigeration during the First World War, permitting testing in the most remote areas.[38] Was it not difficult to obtain the blood samples? Compared with the difficulty of keeping subjects still for the elaborate craniometeric measurements, drawing a few drops of blood from a finger was easy. A third reason for the welcome researchers gave to the Hirszfelds' new approach was its apparently more scientific and exact results. The process involved chemistry rather than linear measurement, and an individual could have only one of four blood types in the ABO system rather than the infinite number of lengths, shapes, and volumes obtained from anthropometric measurement. Hence, determination of blood type seemed to offer a welcome change from the somewhat arbitrary divisions that had been made between brachycephalics and dolichocephalics, not to mention the overlapping middle group of mesocephalics, which had to be created when no clear-cut dividing line emerged between long and round heads.

Despite what has just been said, it would be wrong to think that the Hirszfelds' idea was copied everywhere with the same thoroughness and speed. For one thing, there were differences in the availability of subjects to study as well as in the importance attached to the question of races. Poland, where Ludwig Hirszfeld set up a new research facility, became an important study center, but so too did Rumania, Hungary, and other central and eastern European countries whose new boundaries established by the First World War peace settlements cut across many ethnic groups. For example, one of the first anthropological blood group studies published after the Hirszfelds' 1919 article was by Frigyes Verzar and Oskar Weszeczky and showed differences in the blood-type distribution of Hungarians, gypsies, and descendants of German colonists living in Hungary. Likewise, in 1924 Sabin Manuila and Georges Popoviciu published studies on the differences in the blood-type distribution of the Rumanian and Hungarian populations living in the newly annexed Transylvania region of Rumania.[39] Studies in Germany focused on the increased incidence of type B as one moved east in the country, and on attempts to correlate the blood types with the older measures of race, such as hair color and head shape. Extensive blood group studies were also conducted in the Soviet Union during the flowering of biological research in the 1920s.[40] The United States, with its native American population in the West, its black population in the South, and its immigrant population in the eastern cities, was another society in which racial differentiation was important. Hence, there were numerous American researchers who were concerned with the anthropology of blood groups. Likewise, the far-flung reaches of the British Empire offered both the possibility and apparent need for such work.[41]

In France, despite the influx of immigrants after the First World War and the acquisition of new Asian and African colonies, anthropological blood group research was not done as quickly or on a comparable scale with that in other countries. For example, an analysis of the three major anthropological journals published in France (*Anthropologie, Revue anthropologique,* and *Bulletin de la société d'anthropologie*) shows that after the appearance of the Hirszfelds' article in 1919, the next article in any of the French journals presenting original research did not appear until 1925, when Popoviciu presented his findings on the frequency of blood types among Rumanians and Hungarians living in Transylvania.[42] The first article on the population of France appeared in 1929 in *Revue anthropologique,* the journal of the Ecole d'anthropologie. The first similar article in *Anthropologie* after the Hirszfelds' did not appear until 1936, although an article by a Dutch researcher on populations in the East Indies had appeared two years earlier. The *Bulletin de la société d'anthropologie* did not publish a single article of original research on blood groups until after the Second World War started – a 1941 article on the populations of French Indochina based on research done just before the outbreak of war.[43]

Despite the delays and some questions raised about the claims of the proponents, in these countries, as in France, the new work was seen as valuable. Henri Vallois, for example, wrote an article in *Anthropologie* in 1929 entitled "Preuves anatomiques de l'origine monophyletique de l'homme," which drew on all standard measurements of physical anthropology to make the case for a common human descent, and two full pages were devoted to the new blood group discoveries.[44] Although it took some time for the study of blood groups to make an impact, it was part of the mainstream of physical anthropology in most countries by the end of the 1920s.

Generally the reason for the delay in the publication of blood group studies in journals of anthropology was that doctors were the primary researchers, and they tended to publish in medical journals, even though the results might be primarily of anthropological importance. For example, the French journal in which the findings of blood group research were most frequently published was *Comptes rendus de la société de biologie* which, contrary to its name, published works in medicine.[45] It was in this journal, for example, that Hirszfeld and his students published most of the results of their work in Poland during the interwar years. Naturally, most French researchers working on blood group research also published their findings in the journal – as for example, Paul Michon in Nancy, working on problems in transfusion, or E. Balgaires and Louis Christiaens, who began working in the 1930s at the Institute of Legal and Social Medicine in Lille. More relevant to the question of blood and race was the fact that Nicholas Kossovitch, who dominated research in France on the anthropology of blood groups between the wars, published his findings most frequently and earliest in *Comptes rendus,* beginning in 1925.[46] Only in 1927 did a new, specialized journal, *Sang,* under the direction of Pierre-Emile Weil, appear in France devoted entirely to studies in the new field of serology.

Another reason for the delay in the blood-group discoveries' influencing physical anthropology was that the new research re-

quired a new kind of training and background. Physical anthropologists had traditionally been trained in medicine, in general
physiology or comparative anatomy rather than the microbiol-
ogy, biochemistry, and serology that were necessary in the new
blood-group research. Although France possessed one of the most
respected research facilities for this work, the Pasteur Institute,
blood research there was oriented more toward practical problems
of diseases in the blood rather than basic blood physiology, which
was being studied in Germany or Vienna.[47] As a result, in France
after the First World War very few individuals were engaged in
blood group research that could be applied to physical anthropology. Proof of this is the fact that Kossovitch, who was the first in
France to conduct research comparable to Hirszfeld's, was not
trained in France but rather by Hirszfeld himself in Salonika during the war.[48] When Kossovitch, a native Serb, went to Paris after
the war he obtained a position at the Pasteur Institute working
with Raymond Dujarric de la Rivière. Only after establishing
himself there did Kossovitch make contact with French anthropologists and eventually secure a joint appointment at the Ecole
d'anthropologie in 1931.

Kossovitch was by far the most frequent author on the anthropology of blood groups in French anthropological journals, beginning with his 1929 article on blood group distribution among the
French and continuing with articles based on his work in Morocco
during the 1930s.[49] An even clearer indication of Kossovitch's
dominance, and the corresponding lack of French-trained serologists working on the anthropology of blood groups, can be found
in *Comptes rendus,* which was much more likely to be the journal
in which research on all aspects of blood groups was published. A
survey of articles published in the journal between the wars shows
that most French blood researchers, such as Michon in Nancy and
others in Paris, worked on problems of transfusion, the correlation of blood groups, and the incidence of tuberculosis and cancer,
whereas Kossovitch and Dujarric de la Rivière at the Pasteur Institute dominated the work published on the anthropology of blood
groups. The first two articles on the subject by a French researcher
were by Kossovitch in 1925 on the blood groups of Czech soldiers
garrisoned in Salonika during the war. This was followed in 1927
by a study of Armenian emigres in Paris. In 1929 and 1930, Kossovitch published the results of his work on the French population

in general and Alsatians in particular, and also published the first results of his work in Morocco during the 1930s in *Comptes rendus*.[50] Of course, Kossovitch was not the only one in France doing such work, but a 1929 study of the blood groups of inhabitants of French Equatorial Africa was sponsored and supplied with test serum by Kossovitch and Dujarric de la Rivière at the Pasteur Institute, as was a 1933 study of Eskimos and a 1936 study of West Africans.[51] In fact, it was only after 1937 that the results of more than occasional studies appeared independent of Kossovitch in *Comptes rendus*. This reflected the work of a second generation of researchers, such as Balgaires and Christiaens in the north of France, Farinaud in Indochina, and others in Madagascar and West Africa.[52]

The pattern of this research also suggests another reason for the delay in blood group research among French anthropologists besides lack of trained personnel – lack of available subjects to study. France's indigenous population did not have the diversity of peoples immediately close at hand for the study of blood groups. Compare the French situation with the United States, for example, or the new Eastern European countries, where subjects for research along these lines were easier to find and the results were charged with potentially important political ramifications. By contrast, Kossovitch's first studies were of displaced peoples who happened to be accessible – Czech soldiers and Armenian immigrants. After his studies on the French, Kossovitch had to go to Morocco for his first field work among populations significantly different from the French. An opportunity to use the large number of other immigrants to France in the 1920s was missed, and it was not until the 1930s that the climate of opinion turned sharply against them, making the determination of differences between immigrants and the rest of the French population an important matter of public concern. It also was not until the 1930s that France was well enough established in its more remote African and Asian colonies to do blood-group research comparable to the work the British could do immediately in Australia, the Middle East, and China, or the Americans in their large eastern cities, in the South, or among the Indians in the Far West.

As will be seen in the next chapter, the way blood group studies entered French anthropology had consequences beyond the simple delay in moving away from anthropometry as a basis for studying

human populations. In some countries where more extensive research was done by several different investigators on the blood
group distribution among diverse populations – the United States,
and later England – problems began to arise in trying to fit the
results to the pattern suggested by Hirszfeld in his biochemical
index. In fact, the difficulties soon resembled those that had arisen
from skull measurements. Although there was only a limited
number of possible types in a given blood system, almost all na-
tionalities were found to possess all blood groups. As a result,
Hirszfeld's biochemical index was just as much an average of percentages as the old cephalic index. Moreover, the biochemical indexes were found to vary considerably, arranging themselves on
a continuum not unlike the craniometric indexes. Finally, as additional studies were done, the same problem arose that had plagued
anthropometric classifications of race – peoples with very different historical background and physical features had precisely the
same distribution of blood groups in their populations. For example, the Cantonese of China were identical serologically (at least
as far as the distribution of ABO types) to the Katangese of the
Congo and the Kazans of Russia. Likewise, the inhabitants of
Greenland matched the aboriginal population of Australia.[53]

For some anthropologists, these problems called into question
not just the concept of serological indexes but the very notion of
race.[54] Although the Nazis' wild claims and heinous policies were
most important in provoking public reaction to racism, the scientific rejection of the concept had independent roots in these earlier shortcomings of anthopometry and seroanthropology. This
was still not widely apparent even in the late 1930s. Among French
anthropologists, for example, the only group that was studied
enough to raise these questions was Jews, whose biochemical indexes were found to vary significantly depending on the geographical location of the population studied. In fact, since the beginning of the scientific racist studies in the last third of the
nineteenth century, confusion and disagreement had existed even
among Jewish scholars on the question of whether there was a
Jewish "race."[55] Because this controversy was closely tied to the
immigration of Jews to France in the 1930s, it will be examined in
more detail in the next chapter. Suffice it to say that the questions
raised by serological studies of Jews did not automatically lead to
the conclusion that the whole concept of race should be aban-

doned. Some maintained that Jews were not a distinct race but a religious group that usually intermarried with the local populace; others claimed that Jews were a race, but the biochemical index was not an accurate measure of race. In France, as in most other countries, there had not been enough serological studies of different populations by the end of the 1930s to warrant the latter conclusion. Instead, most anthropologists took the results as proof that Jews were not a distinct biological race.[56]

Such fine distinctions were not, however, made by most the violently racist anti-Semites of the 1930s, who were quick to pick up the new ideas on blood groups and race for use in their diatribes. As will be seen in the next chapter, these racists had welcomed Hirszfeld's original use of the biochemical (or racial) index, with its hierarchical scale of northern and western European populations at the top and central Asians at the bottom, because it served the same pseudoscientific purposes that the cephalic index had served for Aryan racists at the end of the nineteenth century. Even Hirszfeld eventually recognized the misapplication of his theory, especially by the Germans. Writing in 1938, Hirszfeld, who was born Jewish and later converted to Catholicism, wrote,

I wish to separate myself from those who attach the blood groups to the mystique of race. We have created the notion of serological race as an analogy to that of biological race. . . . The actual distribution of groups on the earth reflects the crossing of races and constitutes further proof that humanity presents a mosaic of races.[57]

It was not just in Germany that racists used the new blood group discoveries to support their claims. Kossovitch, having been trained by Hirszfeld, used the biochemical index in all of his blood group research. Each new study dutifully calculated the index of the particular ethnic group and fit the number into the hierarchy established by Hirszfeld in 1919. Because Kossovitch had almost a complete monopoly in France on research and writing about the anthropology of blood groups in the 1920s and the early 1930s, there was no questioning of the biochemical index by French researchers as there had been in the United States. As a result, when French immigration theorists such as René Martial wished to find a more rational basis for selecting and controlling the influx of people into France, they turned to Kossovitch's work with its use of the biochemical index as proof that the influx of blood from the

East would lower the racial index of France by bringing in more group B blood; and the index for France, they said, was already lower than the English or German thanks to race and blood mixing in the past.

In the long run, the discovery and application of new knowledge about blood groups to the study of physical anthropology was of crucial significance in moving the discipline away from comparative anatomy toward the study of gene frequencies among different populations. Blood groups were quite simply the earliest recognized and most easily tested traits that are genetically inherited.[58] In the meantime, however, many unwarranted generalizations were drawn from incomplete data and untested hypotheses. Among them was the biochemical index as a definition of racial difference. In France, because of the particular way blood group research was introduced, these notions fed and supported the racist thought that was part of the occupation and Vichy regimes. Nowhere was this more apparent than in the race theories that eugenicists and others applied to the question of immigration to France in the 1930s.

9

Race and immigration

In February 1940, Eugène Apert published an article in the journal *Pédiatrie* entitled "Eugenics in France," which was one of the last of his writings to appear before his death in April of that year.[1] It was a timely moment to reflect on eugenics in France, because the course of events was about to alter its nature dramatically. Apert was certainly qualified to assess the work of French eugenicists. He attended the First Eugenics Congress in London in 1912, was one of the founders of the French Eugenics Society later that year, and had been an officer in the society from the start – first as general secretary, then vice president, and finally president, beginning in 1934.

In describing the major accomplishments of French eugenics, Apert listed three as being most important: the campaign in favor of a mandatory premarital examination, work on arresting the population decline, and the monitoring of foreign immigration to France. Previous chapters have shown the great deal of attention paid to the first two of these accomplishments, as well as some of the concerns about immigration expressed by members of the French Eugenics Society in the 1920s. For eugenicists to be concerned with the question of immigration was not unusual. In the United States, for example, they made it a major issue after the First World War, and lobbied successfully for the Immigration Act of 1924, which put quotas on the so-called inferior populations of southern and eastern Europe.[2] The prominence of the immigration question in Apert's article on French eugenics, however, is surprising because immigration, by comparison with depopulation or the campaign for a premarital examination law, had been an issue of recent and sporadic importance for the society during the 1920s. Why then did Apert include immigration along with the other matters? The answer is the growing importance that the question had assumed by the end of the 1930s and the growing influence of the eugenic view of immigration in France.

Apert's list of eugenicists actively working on the immigration question included René Martial; in fact, his work is mentioned even before that of Schreiber or Apert himself. A major figure in French public health who had long specialized in questions of immigration, Martial only became associated with eugenics in the 1930s, when his views on immigration changed as a result of the new ideas of race described in the last chapter. This chapter will focus on that change as part of an examination of broader French reactions to immigration during the interwar period. It will show how changing conditions combined with the new blood-group race theory to produce a very strong anti-immigrant position with explicit eugenic underpinnings. Hence, it provides a striking example of the increased emphasis in French eugenic thought during the 1930s on the more strident, negative measures.

Martial's life and work covered the whole span of the Third Republic.[3] He was born in Paris in 1873 when the National Assembly was drafting the provisional constitution to replace Louis Napoleon's Second Empire. He began his medical studies under Mathias Duval in 1892, the year of the Panama Canal scandal, and received his medical degree in 1900 in the midst of the Dreyfus affair. His career actually outlasted the Third Republic, extending not only through the Vichy era but into the Fourth Republic, and his last book was published in 1955 when he was 82.

Martial's professional career in public health began with an appointment in 1902 at Leredde's clinic treating venereal disease, but of note at this early stage of his career was an interest in Taylorism and industrial hygiene. Hence, like Sicard de Plauzoles, Martial is another example of a physician inspired by ideas of health "efficiency" who later turned to eugenics as a means of achieving that goal.[4] At the time, however, Martial's work led him in another direction. The new Public Health Law of 1902 had created many opportunities for those working in the health field, and in 1909 he became the first director of the Bureau of Hygiene in Douai near the Belgian frontier.[5] This meant that one of his major concerns was now the large number of foreign workers in coal mines and other industries of the region. Martial often mentioned in later years how he had seen, while in Douai, trainloads of Eastern Europeans arriving to work in local zinc factories, with little or no attention given to their legal papers, let alone their health or physical condition. His main concern, however, was with more typical health matters, such as the problems of tuberculosis and alcoholism.[6] In addition, Martial's early work showed two characteristics that would continue through his later career – a flair for reaching the general public by means of talks and exhibitions he gave at the city hall, and maintenance of his status with professional colleagues through correspondence and publishing articles for journals.[7]

The First World War interrupted Martial's work in the north, when he was mobilized as an army health adviser and sent to Montpellier. These health advisers were given the task of monitoring the health of military and related personnel in camps as well as workers in war industries. As a result, Martial learned a great deal about the health consequences of mobilizing a large part of the French population previously isolated from many diseases, as well as problems stemming from the influx of soldiers and workers from French colonies in Africa and Asia. For example, he was in charge of organizing the health services for a camp at Castres that employed 6,000 Vietnamese workers. Another of his responsibilities was the creation of health checkpoints for immigrants from Spain in the department of Pyrenées Orientales.[8]

After a brief tour as director of hygiene for the department of Aisne in 1919–20, Martial learned firsthand about the health problems of non-French peoples when he spent three years in Morocco as director of health services in the city of Fez. He returned to France in 1923 to become director of the Bureau of Hygiene in the Paris suburb of Alfortville, but he continued his firsthand observations of the homelands of immigrants to France with trips to Poland in 1927 and Czechoslovakia in 1931, as well as an extraordinary voyage aboard a tramp steamer carrying immigrants from Eastern Europe to Brazil and Argentina. This trip also gave him a chance to study Argentina's immigration system and compare its policies with those of France.[9]

Because he continued to publish the results of his work in major medical journals, Martial was well respected as an expert on questions of immigration. For his work in the war he was made a Chevalier de la légion d'honneur in 1920. He was also elected a member of the Academy of Medicine, and in 1929 he began teach-

Table 9.1. *Foreigners residing in France 1876–1968 (selected years)*

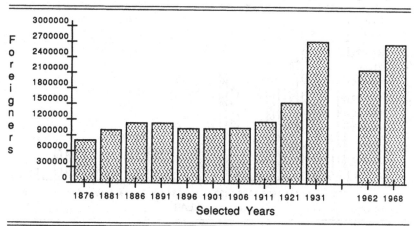

Source: Gary S. Cross, *Immigrant workers in industrial France* (Philadelphia: Temple University Press, 1983), pp. 21, 169; Gary P. Freeman, *Immigrant labor and racial conflict in industrial societies* (Princeton: Princeton University Press, 1979), p. 23.

ing a course on immigration at the Institut d'hygiène of the Ecole de médecine. In 1930, Louis Tanon, editor of *Revue médicale française*, called Martial the best authority in France on the question of immigration and health.[10]

RESPONSE TO FRENCH IMMIGRATION IN THE 1920S

During the 1920s, questions about immigration became more and more prominent in French political and health circles.[11] Although the tradition of immigration to France had a long prewar history, especially from countries such as Belgium, Italy, and Poland, it was the increased number of immigrants after the war that attracted the public's attention. As Table 9.1 shows, there was a significant but stable number of foreigners residing in France from the late nineteenth century up to the outbreak of the First World War. The sharp increase in immigrants during the 1920s brought the number of foreigners in the country by the following decade to about the figure for present-day France. The 1920s thus marks the most important watershed in immigration to France in the past 100 years.

Table 9.2. *Official foreign immigrant entries to France, 1920–52*

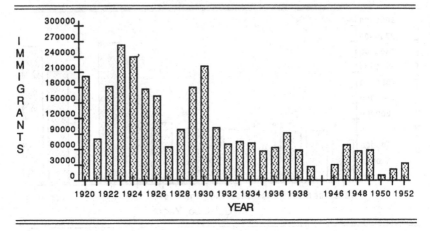

Source: Gary S. Cross, *Immigrant workers in industrial France* (Philadelphia: Temple University Press, 1983), pp. 60, 195; Gary P. Freeman, *Immigrant labor and racial conflict in industrial societies* (Princeton: Princeton University Press, 1979), p. 22.

France was not alone in receiving large numbers of people driven out by political and economic upheaval in Central and Eastern Europe after the First World War. And the shortage of French workers to rebuild the country added to the influx. Moreover, the migration of peoples from French colonies in North Africa continued after the war, and the situation was further aggravated when the United States began drastically restricting immigration in 1921, eliminating the country that in prewar years had been the world's largest recipient of immigrants. All of these developments increased immigration to France fourfold after the war. By 1931, a full 11 percent of the workforce was foreigners; some individual sectors – mining, metallurgy, and construction – had as many as 30–40 percent of immigrant workers![12] More specifically, figures for the number of official immigrants to France in the 1920s (Table 9.2) show between 150,000 and 250,000 entries per year for all but three years, before the Great Depression of the 1930s alleviated the demand for foreign labor. The post-Second World War era never reached even the 50,000 mark.

This dramatic influx of foreigners produced a strong reaction in France, such as that of the members of the French Eugenics Society described in the last chapter. Marital's writings on immigration during this period are therefore worth noting, not only because of the authority and respect he commanded on the subject, but also because on the whole and in marked constrast to many of his colleagues, he demonstrated a very tolerant attitude toward the foreigners. For example, a riot in 1924 involving North African workers prompted a popular and even legislative outcry against foreign immigration. No less than three bills were introduced in the Chamber to restrict immigration by the end of the year.[13] In response to these and other outbursts, Martial, just home from Morocco, wrote numerous articles expressing a particular annoyance with use of the label "undesirable" to describe the foreign workers because, as he said, it "ignores the present-day economic necessities and applies this epithet too quickly to a workforce which is absolutely indispensable and which we ourselves have called here."[14]

Martial tried to show in his writings that not all foreign immigrants were alike, offering as an example the different health problems that existed among immigrants from different countries. Using his own experience in the war, Martial described the Spanish as being prone to smallpox, Moroccans to typhus, Asians and North Africans to malaria, and Indochinese to internal parasites. Then there were the more obvious cultural differences. Martial admitted that the North Africans involved in the 1924 riots had been "brutally ignorant of our contemporary customs." But rather than blaming the foreigners alone for the problems, he also accused the employers and industrialists who recruited them in their home countries, only to

throw them on the streets of the cities without any precautions, left to themselves, living in infested boarding houses, indulging in alcohol, deprived of all moral guidance, the butt of jokes, only knowing their factories, bars and slums, seeing only bad examples.[15]

Martial's solution called for nothing less than having the companies provide housing, food, and religious guidance appropriate to the Moslem way of life. This was, in effect, an attempt to help create the conditions similar to those Martial had observed in the north of France, where Poles maintained their own churches, newspapers, and even banks in the mining region around Lille.

These ideas were all the more remarkable by comparison with

the views of others looking at the immigration question at the time. Members of the French Eugenics Society, it will be remembered, were quite clearly opposed to all immigration of Asians and Africans to France, and were only conditionally willing to accept immigrants from selected European countries. Martial also demonstrated a more tolerant attitude toward foreign immigration than many of his colleagues in the French medical community. Although their primary concern had usually been adequate medical screening of individual immigrants, many doctors grew increasingly concerned in the mid-1920s about the possible cumulative health and biological effects of the large-scale migrations to France. For example, the Société de médicine publique made immigration the chief topic of consideration for its Thirteenth Annual Congress, held at the Pasteur Institute in October 1926. In the keynote report by Georges Dequidt of the ministry of the interior and Georges Forestier, a departmental health inspector, the authors introduced their findings by describing these population movements as nothing less than "the advanced indices of the twilight of our Western Civilization and the decline of the white race." Their reasons could not have been expressed in more explicit biological terms. "The best representatives of this race restrain their birthrate and favor the swarm of inferior, undesirable types who eliminate them by biological competition."[16]

The eugenic character of these statements was no accident, for the authors specifically cited in the introduction to their report one of the leaders of American eugenics, Madison Grant, whose book *The passing of the great race* had been translated into French only a few months earlier.[17] Dequidt and Forestier quoted most extensively, however, from the fourteen-page preface to the book written by Georges Vacher de Lapouge, whose words were quoted to the members of the Société de médicine:

Do not forget that the first waves of Orientals and Slavs that are breaking on France presage the invading flood which threatens to submerge that which is left of our civilization and the health of our race. We have allowed certain of our provinces to become Macedonianized [a name taken from the salad of mixed vegetables but also a play on the immigrants' eastern European origins]. It is time to react.

As evidence of these dangers, Dequidt and Forestier cited several studies of French hospitals and jails that showed large numbers of foreigners in these institutions, higher as a percentage than their proportion of the population as a whole.[18] Such studies were very widely quoted in France at the time. Even an organization like the Ligue des droits de l'homme, which generally opposed immigration restriction because it was too easily used against political refugees, called the situation "from a health point of view an incontestable peril." According to a report of the League's central committee, 20 percent of the hospital beds in Paris were occupied by foreigners.[19]

This is only one example of the xenophobic hysteria of the time that often used statistics uncritically to illustrate general conclusions that were out of touch with logic. For example, the League's central committee members should have realized that employers would hardly be interested in recruiting unhealthy individuals in Eastern Europe for work in the mines and factories of France. Evidence from Polish historians today, for example, describes a "rigorous" screening process in the mining valleys of Poland, not just from a health standpoint, but from a political one as well.[20] In addition, pregnant women were routinely eliminated, and altogether in a typical year (1924), 12 percent of applicants were refused permission to leave the country.

Such information would not matter, of course, to those who viewed the foreigners as an "invading flood" or peril. Nor did Dequidt and Forestier offer much hope for the assimilation of immigrants, at least as indicated by other quotes they used from the Lapouge preface in their report to the 1926 public health congress.

The prince can no more make a Frenchman from a Greek or a Moroccan than he can bleach the skin of a negro, make round the eyes of a Chinaman or change a woman into a man. . . . The nation is a biological ensemble, a material thing not a juridical fiction, something which is apparently forgotten by economists, statisticians and jurists who confuse the qualities of a Frenchman with the rights that are attached to him.[21]

This use of Lapouge's work is telling both of the climate of opinion at the time and of the fact that the "anthroposociologist" was again an influence on the French scene. His reappearance in the 1920s is noteworthy for two reasons. First, Lapouge is usually thought of – and he did much to foster the idea himself – as an outcast, rejected by his compatriots after the turn of the century, better appreciated by the Germans, and only rediscovered posthumously in the late 1930s and early 1940s by the racist supporters of the Vichy regime.[22] Instead, we see him unabashedly cited in the mid-1920s with no apologies, by very well established and well respected members of the French public health community. One can only conclude that it was Lapouge's own self-imposed exile rather than the unpopularity of his ideas that had kept him from the French public. The xenophobic, racist eugenics he preached struck quite a sympathetic chord, as indicated in Dequidt and Forestier's report.

What then prompted the end of Lapouge's exile? Here is the second noteworthy reason for his reappearance in the 1920s – he was assisted by the work of American eugenicists who helped give wider circulation to his ideas in the United States and then returned the ideas to France. This began when Madison Grant wrote to Lapouge after the appearance of his (Grant's) book, *The passing of the great race,* in 1916 to see if Lapouge would translate it into French. Because of the war, however, the two men did not make contact until 1919.[23] At that time, Lapouge declined the request, in part because of his own earlier difficulty in publicizing similar views, but his sympathy with Grant's ideas and the high esteem in which the Americans held him prompted a long and frequent correspondence that reached the top leadership of the American eugenics movement. Among those with whom Grant shared Lapouge's letters were Henry Fairfield Osborn, professor of Zoology at Columbia University and president of the American Museum of Natural History; Charles Davenport; and, most significantly, Albert Johnson, chairman of the U.S. House Immigration and Naturalization Committee, who was the chief sponsor of the Immigration Act of 1924.[24] Davenport was so impressed with Lapouge's letters that he reprinted several in the *Eugenical news,* which he published as director of the Cold Spring Harbor eugenics research station.[25]

As mentioned in the last chapter, Lapouge was invited to the Second International Eugenics Congress in New York in 1921 and returned again in 1925 for Margaret Sanger's International Birth Control Congress. He was impressed by both the eugenic leaders he met in the United States and the country itself, although his perceptions were based on rather sketchy evidence. On his arrival at New York for the eugenics congress, he noted in his diary, "I am happy. In the streets of New York there are no dogs, no priests,

no cafes, no urinoirs." When he returned to France, Lapouge agreed
to help Grant find a translator and a publisher, and even offered to
write a preface for the book. Of these tasks, finding a publisher
was the most difficult. Both Masson and Flammarion declined. It
took the intervention of fellow American eugenicist Lothrop
Stoddard, who wrote to Payot, which had earlier published his
Rising tide of color. Even then, Payot only accepted Grant's book
after he had paid a $1,000 subsidy.[26]

Given these problems and Lapouge's pessimism about French
opinion, Grant naturally expected the book to receive a "stormy
reception." Yet the clippings and reviews Lapouge sent him at the
end of 1926 struck Grant as being "very satisfactory, much more
so than those I obtained in England."[27] The following year he
wrote, "I am delighted to know that my book, thanks to your
great influence, has received such favorable reviews"; and Grant
even went on to suggest that Lapouge

do for France what Gunther did for Germany and Lundborg has done
for Sweden, by writing a book with illustrations on the racial transfor-
mations now going on in France. It would be a great service to France
and to the better elements everywhere.[28]

Lapouge never wrote the book, but judging from the response to
the Grant book, it was not for lack of a receptive climate of opinion. The anti-immigration reaction had apparently done its work.

As we shall see, the book Grant had called for was eventually
written by René Martial, but in the mid-1920s Martial was still
very far from the biological view of immigration that would prompt
him to write it. Instead he emphasized differences in the immigrants' cultural traits and the failure of the French to accommodate
them as the explanation for the problems that had prevented assimilation. It was not that Martial ignored the health dangers, but
he saw them as being easily remedied by measures such as the
United States had taken in screening individual immigrants at their
point of entry into the country.[29] Much more fundamental to him
was the question of assimilation. In an article published at the time
of the 1926 health congress where Dequidt and Forestier reintro-
duced Lapouge, Martial reiterated his call in previous writings for
such measures as *"foyers musulmans,"* where

the poor "sidis" unfortunately set loose in our European life by ignorant
industrialists unconscious of what they have created, can remake for

themselves if not a true home, at least a common meeting place for moral comfort, something for which they have so great and intense a need.[30]

The following year, an economic recession brought on by the devaluation of the franc raised even more questions about large-scale immigration, and prompted the French government to take certain actions that seemed to agree with Martial's position. In February 1927 the ministry of interior required that a medical certificate be presented by all new immigrants entering France, and to help speed the process of assimilation, the first changes since 1893 were made in the naturalization laws to cut the residence requirement of immigrants for citizenship from thirteen to three years.[31] The latter measure was, however, at least as much inspired by pressure from natalist groups interested in promoting the growth of the French population as it was by those wishing to mitigate problems arising from immigration. Moreover, the French industrialists who recruited most of the foreign workers could easily take care of the health certificates, thus preventing a large government commitment to screening of immigrants on the model of Ellis Island.

As Table 9.2 shows, even without serious health screening, the economic downturn dramatically reduced the demand for foreign workers in 1927. This only underscored Martial's overall complaint about French immigration – that short-sighted government and industrial decisions left control of immigration to the unpredictable shifts and changes in the economy. The rational, long-term policy that Martial developed in the next few years was negative and racist because it was eugenically based on a biological view of immigration that differed greatly from his earlier, tolerant views. His working model was partly based on the U.S. policy of quotas begun in the 1924 legislation whereby an absolute ceiling of 150,000 immigrants a year was to be divided in proportion to the size of each ethnic group already in the population of the United States, according to the 1890 census.[32] Martial's major departure was that he did not accept totally the American "country of origin" basis for quotas. In fact, except for the exclusion of Asians, he evolved completely different criteria for selection.

The first formal expression of Martial's new line of thinking was his 1928 proposal for a policy of "interracial grafting."[33] The notion of grafting, borrowed from arboriculture, likened immi-

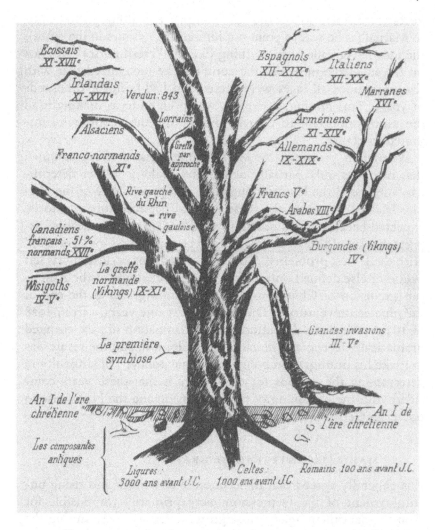

Figure 9.1   Martial's "Interracial grafting." [Source: René Martial, *Notre race et ses aïeux* (Paris: Secretariat général de la jeunesse, 1943)]

gration to the taking of a cutting from one tree or plant and embedding it in the trunk or branch of another (Figure 9.1). It was a seductive metaphor that incorporated Martial's previous concern with assimilation (the ability of the graft to take hold), but it also placed a great deal more emphasis on the *selection* of the graft than just a simple concern for its health. Race now was seen as an important consideration in the selection process, although to be fair to Martial (as he was to point out himself many times in the 1930s), the idea never called for anything like the "racial purity" of Nazi or Aryan ideologues. On the contrary, he recognized that with few exceptions all races were mixed and had been for thousands of years. This mixing, however, was pointed to as making it all the more important to control and choose the people who migrated to France.

When first proposed by Martial, interracial grafting assumed that race was only partially defined by biology. Other determinants included the history, language, and psychology of the people. Martial's concern for these cultural determinants was to be expected because of his previous emphasis on the "malleable" aspects that would allow immigrants to be assimilated, or "grafted," with the fewest problems. A biological basis for exclusion was left vague or else defined only by the extreme example of the American exclusion of Chinese and Japanese immigrants at the end of the nineteenth century.[34] During the next five years – from 1928 to 1933 – Martial's definition and determination of race changed dramatically to become much more biological, and the result was to make his immigration policy a eugenic policy. The difficulty in determining the reasons for the change is that these years coincided with the beginning of the Depression and the Nazis' rise to power in Germany.

MARTIAL'S INTERRACIAL GRAFTING

It is generally agreed that the economic downturn and rising unemployment of the Depression were primarily responsible for arousing sentiment against foreign workers in France during the 1930s. Even though as early as June 1930 there were still complaints of worker *shortages* in French mining and metallurgical industries – the Depression arrived somewhat later – by the end of that year organized labor was demanding restrictions on foreign workers. Bills to this effect were introduced in the National Assembly, and in early 1932 some mildly restrictive measures were passed into law.[35] It would be wrong, however, to say that the economic decline alone prompted the anti-immigrant views or shaped their expression. We have already seen that there was a strong xenophobic current in France during the 1920s that was reinforced by the economic problems of the following decade. This prompted even the leading natalists to set limits on those who might be welcome in France to offset the country's demographic decline. "France could not without harm open its borders to all immigrants," said Fernand Boverat, secretary general of the Alliance nationale contre la dépopulation in 1935. "Like every other nation of Europe and America, she has a primordial interest in not allowing coloreds [hommes de couleur] to establish themselves here."[36]

Martial's ideas on selection of immigrants also began to develop well before the Depression began. Moreover, there had always been Frenchmen who saw immigration as more than an economic matter. Although he had earlier pointed out the economic benefits that foreign workers brought, Martial usually sought to dissociate himself from the strict economic view of immigration, because he saw it as too short-sighted and subject to the whims of a changing economy. In fact, one of Martial's distinctions in the 1920s was that he took a long-range view of immigration, a perspective he was to hold in the 1930s even as his views on race became more pronounced.

Martial's views in the 1920s lend some credence to his own contention that the new ideas on immigration resulted not from economic or political developments in the thirties but from the new discoveries about human blood groups, especially Hirszfeld's biochemical index of race. The appeal of the index to someone like Martial, who was concerned with controlling immigration, is easily shown. Here was a seemingly scientific way of selecting the specimens for interracial grafting. The closer the biochemical index of the graftee's race to that of the host population, Martial reasoned, the better the chance that the graft would "take" – that is, the more likely the immigrant would be assimilated. The indexes calculated in the 1920s also seemed to fit Martial's analysis of the French historical experience with immigrants, most of whom (Belgians, Italians, Germans, Spanish, Dutch) had an index close to the French index of 3.2. This also meant that the index would justify exclusion of peoples to the east with lower indexes. Martial also used it, however, to explain why the English never migrated or assimilated into the French nation. Their index was too high (4.4) to be compatible with that of the French.[37] In other words, higher was not always better, at least to someone in France.

A more important effect of Martial's use of the biochemical index was his claim that he had a scientific approach to immigration. In blood groups he saw the same apparent advantages that physical anthropologists had seen over older definitions of race based on skull shapes and sizes. This also meant that Martial became a champion of Mendelian inheritance, because one of the earliest discoveries about the blood groups was that they did not change during an individual's life, and were inherited according to Mendel's laws. Thus, because Martial accepted the blood group research, he was an early proponent of Mendelism in France.[38] In fact, by the late 1930s, when anti-fascist critics attacked Martial's immigration policy, they often criticized his assumptions about Mendelian inheritance. For example, one 1939 book maintained that differences in soil, vegetation, and food changed inherited characteristics, including blood groups.[39] Thus, in France there was the ironic situation that rather than the "best" scientific theory being used to attack eugenic thought, it was used to support it.

This scientific plausibility also explains why so eminent an anthropologist as Paul Rivet hesitated to attack Martial's ideas. Still mindful of his experience with those who made great claims from measuring skull shape, Rivet cautioned that it was "premature" to draw ethnological conclusions from the blood group studies, especially if one wanted to "utilize them for selection as one does with livestock." He did, however, acknowledge their value in determining racial ancestry, and in the climate of the 1930s this lent credence to Martial's other assertions.[40]

Martial was very persistent in claiming a scientific basis for his ideas. This, and the simplicity of the theory (reminiscent of the one-gene one-trait controversy in the United States), helps explain the wide appeal of Martial's writings. Consider the following 1935 article for the general readership of the *Mercure de France:*

We have today two elements which permit us to understand and guide the phenomenon of immigration in a scientific manner and to add the exact procedures of racial selection to psychological ones, all of which permits us to arrive at a durable and high quality interracial grafting. What I am saying applies, moreover, to other countries in need of immigration besides France. This means that it is no longer necessary to leave immigration to empirical chance. . . . The scientific elements that we possess are on the one hand the hereditary laws of Mendel, and on the other the recently acquired ideas about blood groups.[41]

Despite these claims, Martial was hardly rigorous in his application of the biochemical index. He could not have been, because as noted in the last chapter, serologists soon discovered that the index did not always coincide with obvious physical and cultural differences between population groups.[42] For example, the Polish biochemical index of 1.2 was much lower than the French, yet Martial's historical analysis found a long-standing flow of immigration and assimilation of Poles into France. If this ran contrary to the biochemical index, the explanation was cultural or, as Martial called it, psychological:

They are authentic Slavs, but Slavs profoundly and radically modified from a psychic point of view by intensive Latinization since the year 1000. Psychologically they have undergone the same impregnation by Roman Latinization. Psychology intervenes here with history. The trilogy operates fully. Psychology and history compensate for the weakness of the index.[43]

Martial's experience with Polish workers in the north of France, along with his study trip to Poland in 1927, obviously left their mark on him. He even authored a travelogue volume complete with illustrations entitled *The Poland of yesterday and today* when he returned from his visit.[44] There are, however, indications that the biochemical index had at least made Martial somewhat wary of long-term problems with Polish immigration. As he put it,

Franco-Polish marriages produce very good results; but one must recognize that even when grandparents and parents have been absorbed into the French milieu, occasionally one sees several grandchildren revert back to the Slavic – return to Poland – like the Indochinese half-breed reverts unfailingly to the Yellow.[45]

Like French eugenicists of the 1920s, Martial was not convinced of the law of autochthonous predominance.

Martial was thus willing to overlook the difference in biochemical index in order to condone Polish immigration. At the same time he ignored a similarity in the index when cautioning against an influx of Jews. In this case, studies of biochemical index showed that some Jewish populations were very close to the French. As mentioned earlier, most serologists and anthropologists had found that the distribution of blood groups among Jews usually mirrored the distribution in the populace where they lived. For ex-

ample, in 1932 the most experienced blood-group anthropologist
in France, Kossovitch, wrote an article in *Revue anthropologique*
reviewing all blood group research on Jews as well as his own new
data from field work in Morocco. It showed that the biochemical
index of Berlin Jews was similar to that of the German population,
the Jews of Russia had a similar pattern of blood group distribution to the Russians, and Moroccan Jews showed a similar pattern
to the Arabs. From this, Kossovitch concluded that "there exist
Jewish communities of different races, and the tie that binds Jewish society is only religious. It is the common religion that has
produced certain characteristic traits, certain customs, which they
have in common."[46]

Martial did not accept this finding, even by such an authority as
Kossovitch, nor was he willing to accept the most obvious conclusion that the biochemical index suggested allowing Jews into France
from regions with a high biochemical index. (Kossovitch cited
figures of 2.7 and 2.6 for Dutch and German Jews.) Instead, Martial invoked nonbiological elements to justify taking great care in
scrutinizing all Jewish immigrants. Once again he argued that
"psychology" influenced the biological findings of Jewish blood
groups, but this time he used the opposite position from the Polish
example.

These biological facts must be examined with care and comparison to
psychological ones, because the most important result of cross-breeding
resides in the psychological value of the half-breed, in his capacity to be
incorporated into the environmental, ethnic and national psychology.
Not that physical qualities are to be rejected, but the one does not exclude the other.[47]

This may sound reasonable enough at first sight, but when Martial
gave examples of the psychological differences that Jews exhib-
ited, it was clear that his was far from a dispassionate, scientific
analysis. For example, he mentioned the "grand artistic sense" of
Jews, though they lacked a sensitivity to the beauties of nature. In
addition, he cited the "nervousness and nomadism" that prevented Jews from "staying long in the same occupations or identifying with one country."[48] In saying that the Poles were similar
to the French and that the Jews were not, or that their ability to
be assimilated was different, Martial ignored the biochemical index. In fact, he was repeating some of the oldest anti-Jewish prej-

udices. Much like Broca's method mentioned in the last chapter, Martial began with assumptions about similarities or differences between peoples, then sought "scientific" evidence to support them.

It would be wrong, however, to see only anti-Semitism in this aspect of Martial's ideas. It was also typical of his general lack of rigor in following the scientific method he preached. This failure is most apparent in Martial's attempts at original research on race and blood groups – which were unproductive at best, and outright prevarications at worst. For example, one of his goals was to correlate the blood group distribution for a given people with the old cephalic index of head shape that physical anthropologists of the late nineteenth century had employed to determine race. In order to achieve the desired results, however, Martial had to reverse the correspondence of A and B blood with long or round-shaped heads, depending on the group under study. And when no correlation was found, he invented a term called the "index of parallelism," which was little more than a measure of how far the skull and blood indexes for a given people deviated from each other. Martial then tried to claim support from the fact that they both came out exactly the same, whereas in reality it simply indicated that the skull index was as far from the blood index as the blood index was from the skull,[49] a refutation of correlation.

Even worse was Martial's comparison of the results of race mixing (i.e., children produced by racial intermarriage) with blood transfusion between people of different blood types. His specific warning was that intermarriage could produce hemolytic shock – the physiological reaction that occurs when blood of one type is transfused to someone with another type. The implication was that mixing of races with different biochemical indices would produce similar results, which was not only meaningless because the indices were only averages, but also patently false because everyday experience showed that the offspring of parents with different blood types would simply have a blood type determined by Mendelian inheritance. There was no literal mixing of blood.[50]

As seen in the last chapter, one of the fundamental problems with the concept of biochemical index was that it only represented an average of blood type distribution among individuals in a given population. Martial's response to such criticisms, however, was the observation that the frequency of type B was the most important variable in determining a high or low index, because the original Hirszfeld formula for the index was I = (A + AB)/(B + AB). So that for immigrants coming to France from the East, Martial's oft-quoted advice was the following simple rule: "Keep the O's and the A's, eliminate the B's, only keep the AB's if the psychological and health examination is favorable"[51] (Figure 9.2).

It is clear how the biochemical index fit into Martial's ideas on immigration and race. One final word might be said, however, on the timing of the change in his thinking, before looking at the influence of his ideas during the remainder of the 1920s. Martial first mentioned the blood groups in February and March of 1933.[52] In other words, the timing is suspiciously close to the Nazi takeover in Germany, and far removed from the first appearance of the biochemical index in scientific literature more than a dozen years earlier. Martial said nothing in his writings, however, to indicate inspiration from across the Rhine, and he consciously tried to distinguish his ideas from the Nazi goal of racial purity. Moreover, as noted in the last chapter, French scientific journals generally published blood-group studies later than elsewhere in Europe and the United States (with the exception of *Comptes rendus de la société de biologie*). Hence, the most logical explanation for the timing of Martial's new ideas on race was his belated discovery of the new medical findings on blood groups.

THE 1930S

Regardless of the immediate inspiration, Martial's new theory of interracial grafting was particularly well timed and placed for the debate on immigration in France during the 1930s. His writings on the subject continued to be prodigious, with over a dozen articles and several books appearing by 1940. Now, however, his audience was much wider than the French medical community. Articles appeared with more frequency in general-interest periodicals such as *Mercure de France* as well as related scientific journals such as *Hygiène mentale*. By the end of the decade Martial was in great demand as a lecturer at such places as the Institut d'hygiène and the Ecole d'anthropologie. He also gave a series of *cours libres* at the Sorbonne on the "anthropobiology of races," beginning in the academic year 1938–39.[53]

Such popularity indicates the appeal of Martial's views to many different groups. For example, although he continued to disclaim

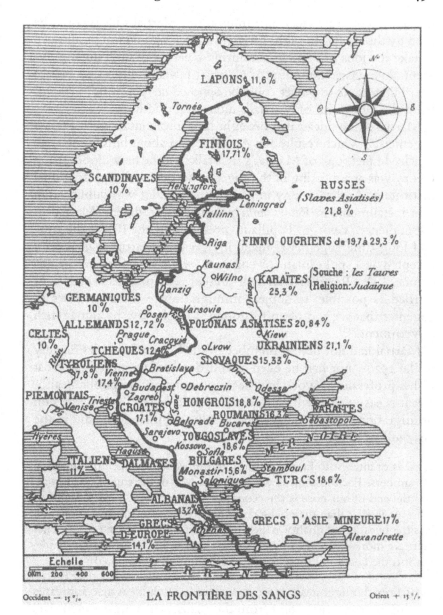

Figure 9.2 "Frontier of blood" (defined by the frequency of
type B blood in a given population, with the "frontier" delim-
iting a frequency more than 15% east of the line and less than
15% west of the line). [Source: René Martial, *Notre race et ses
aïeux* (Paris: Secretariat général de la jeunesse, 1943)]

the strict economic view of immigration, Martial's ideas could be used by those who thought foreign workers should not be allowed to take the jobs of Frenchmen during a period of high unemployment. Likewise, the influx of German Jewish refugees to France after Hitler came to power could be opposed on "scientific" grounds from the viewpoint of Martial's interracial grafting.

Martial's new ideas also brought him into contact with French eugenicists, which resulted in Apert's claim about him in the 1940 article. In fact, one of Martial's first talks on the new blood group theory was at a meeting of the eugenics section of the international Institute of Anthropology in March 1933, and it was published in two installments in *Revue anthropologique*. Introducing Martial to the audience, Georges Papillaut, president of the IIA at the time and long-time eugenicist, made it clear that Martial was already accepted as a spokesman for eugenics, when he informed the audience, "Dr. René Martial will present a plan to us which is as learned as possible: to subject immigration to the strict laws of eugenics that are too often forgotten, I might say, by our French government."[54]

Martial had not been a member of the French Eugenics Society in the 1920s, nor had he even attended any of its meetings. Most of his professional work had been in medicine and public health. Yet it is easy to see why eugenicists found Martial's new ideas on immigration so welcome, when he phrased them as he did in the 1933 talk at the IIA:

What is of interest to France in immigration is not so much the question of numbers. For those of us who see farther than the end of our nose – and the end of our nose is the economic point of view – for those of us who see farther than material gain, who envisage the future of our race, it is the question of quality which must intercede in the first place. That there are more or fewer foreigners who come, is not of great importance, but it is the quality of these foreigners that must be examined.[55]

That French eugenicists were receptive to such ideas also indicates the difference in viewpoint from the 1920s, when most eugenicists were careful to balance a concern with both the quality and quantity of the French population. Martial's concern was only with quality.

The audiences of these new organizations and publications that Martial now reached indicate his broader appeal as a result of the increased interest in questions of immigration, race, and biology. Several of his writings, for example, appeared in *Revue anthropologique*, which since the 1920s had published the minutes and articles of the French Eugenics Society. Beginning in 1935, Martial was listed as lecturer for the Ecole d'anthropologie, which published the journal. That same year, Martial addressed another congress of the International Institute of Anthropology in Brussels on the subject of the correlation of cephalic and blood group indexes. Martial even delivered a paper at the 1937 meeting of the Latin Eugenics Congress in Paris, although his ideas were not entirely in accord with the rest of those in attendance.[56]

With his emphasis on racial selection, Martial found himself identifying with one of the older traditions of French eugenics – that of Vacher de Lapouge. In his 1934 book, *La race française,* Martial praised the work of Lapouge, but this paled in comparison to the admiration Martial expressed after Lapouge's death in 1936. Martial's tribute in *Mercure de France* called Vacher de Lapouge "one of the greatest anthropologists of the times," whose most original scientific insight was his foreknowledge of blood groups. This was based on Vacher de Lapouge's reference to blood and skull shape correlation, a subject dear to Martial's heart. Vacher de Lapouge, like most nineteenth-century racists, spoke a lot about blood and its importance as an indicator (or even determinant) of inheritance. What Martial found most striking was references to dolichocephalic, brachycephalic, and mixed bloods.[57] Looking back, it seems that Martial was making much out of a relatively minor reference by Lapouge to blood in the nineteenth-century sense of ancestry, but from the broader standpoint of ideas about race and hierarchy, it is appropriate that Martial saw himself in the tradition of Vacher de Lapouge. It was no accident that Martial called his course at the Sorbonne, "Anthropobiology of races," a conscious identification with Lapouge's "anthroposociology."

It is difficult to assess how much influence one man could have on discussions about immigration in the 1930s, but in the case of Martial the task is made easier by the new use of blood-group studies he introduced into popular notions of racial definition. One testimony to his influence is how quickly his ideas were attacked by those who disagreed with him. Among the earliest and most consistent of these were French Jewish and other anti-fascist organizations. In particular, the idea of barring all those with group

B blood from France as expressed in *La race française* came under severe attack. One journal, *La terre retrouvée,* an organ of the Zionist Keren Kayemeth l'Israel, carried a review of Martial's *Race française* by Horace Goldie of the Pasteur Institute that was so critical of Martial, his methods, and his motives that Martial filed a lawsuit against the editors for defamation of character.[58] This was no minor incident. Not only was it reported in the French dailies – the headlines of *Paris Soir* for May 26, 1936, read, "A great racial trial in Paris" – but *La terre retrouvée* secured Paul Reynaud as its defense attorney. Eventually the suit was settled out of court, with Martial dropping charges in exchange for the journal's printing his rebuttal and its own apology for having suggested that Martial had been an anti-Dreyfusard.[59]

Another group opposed to Martial's ideas was the publishers of *Races et racisme.* This anti-racist journal was founded in January 1937 with the goal of studying the new racial doctrines, which "risk sowing division inside countries and menace gravely the peace of the world." Although the attention of the founders of the journal was clearly on Nazi Germany, contributors to *Race et racisme* also made direct and indirect references to Martial's ideas. For example, Julius Brutzkus, a recent emigré doctor from Lithuania by way of Germany, wrote an article in 1938 on blood groups among Jews, showing how the biochemical index varied according to the population among whom the Jews lived. Echoing Kossovitch's earlier work, Brutzkus concluded,

Contrary to established public opinion, the Jews of different countries do not represent a homogenous race, but are the result of cross-breeding of different populations. . . . Serological examination of blood confirms completely the absence of homogeneity in the racial composition of the Jewish people, united only by religion and historical tradition.[60]

Brutzkus even claimed that the Jews of Berlin were "purer Europeans than the German Berliners whose index was slightly reduced because of a considerable mixing with Slavs who until the twelfth century populated the entire country beyond the Elbe."[61] The well-known author Georges Lakhovsky gave much wider circulation to Brutzkus' findings in his 1939 book *La civilisation et la folie raciste,* attacking Martial's ideas, particularly his analogy between blood transfusions and race mixing.[62] That same year the biologist Jean Rostand attempted to minimize the import of Martial's ideas, labeling them a petty little racism (*"petit racisme ano-din"*), although he admitted that the ideas were currently receiving a noisy propaganda (*"une propagande tapageuse"*).[63]

The opponents of Martial were not very effective in blunting his influence. Despite their protests and criticisms, the interracial grafting view of immigration was very widely accepted in the France of the 1930s. The articles and publications of Martial and his lectures at the Sorbonne have already been mentioned. But the concept of interracial grafting was also picked up and repeated by more popular, general-interest writers who reached far wider audiences. This included the United States, where Joseph Spengler summarized Martial's immigration policies in his 1936 book, *France faces depopulation*. In fact, Spengler predicted that Martial's program would "probably be recognized in the form of governmental action," although the fear of depopulation made it unlikely that the quality of immigrants would receive as much attention as Martial desired.[64]

An even better example closer to home of the influence of the wider audience reached by Martial's views was the remarkable series of articles by Raymond Millet appearing in *Le Temps* in 1937 entitled, "Visites aux étrangers de France." The fact that the most influential newspaper in France carried a seven-part series on immigrants is yet another testimony to the importance of the immigration question in France a year before the events of Kristallnacht and developments in the Spanish Civil War increased the public's concern by adding even more refugees from Germany and Spain to the list of foreigners in France.[65] As a result of the interest in immigration, Millet published a book in 1938 entitled *Trois millions d'étrangers en France*, which also included selections from the lively exchange of letters that the original articles sparked. Much of the book was a background description of foreign immigration to France and issues raised by the large number of foreigners in residence – their role in professions, the "Jewish problem," and the question of naturalization. But in the last two chapters of the book devoted to the future of immigration, Martial's ideas were central. In fact, to answer the most crucial questions, "whom to pick and according to which criteria," Millet went first to Martial. Hence, the interracial grafting thesis dominated the conclusion of the book. To be sure, Millet attempted to remain neutral by quoting from Martial's critics, including Brutzkus, but this did not diminish the centrality of Martial's ideas to the debate on immigration at the end of the 1930s. On the contrary, it only underscored their importance, whether one agreed with them or not.[66]

When one turns to the out-and-out French racists and fascists, it is impossible to say that Martial was solely responsible for their anti-republican and anti-Jewish ideas. They were hardly the types to be persuaded by debates in scientific or even popular journals. Martial's interracial grafting did, however, offer a legitimacy and respectability for them that was part of what Michael Marrus and Robert Paxton have called "enlarging the scope of the thinkable" in the late 1930s.[67] It was a process whereby credence was given to ideas that in other times most likely would have been summarily dismissed as products of the lunatic fringe. Hence, a racist pamphlet by Jean-Marie Baron, *La grande découverte: Les juifs et le sang B*, published in 1938 by the Centre de documentation et de propagande, triumphantly cited "Dr. Martial and his allocutions to the Academy of Medicine," along with the work of Mendel, Kossovitch, and Landsteiner (not realizing that he was Jewish) to support its racial interpretation of history. People, the author stated, with blood of "groups A and O, whose properties can be different, have a common share of rectitude, morality, altruism and courage which allows them to live together," whereas B blood "is the source of all social ills."[68] In other words, one-gene one-trait had been replaced by one-blood one-trait.

Although the conclusions of this pamphlet might be considered an extreme view by a fringe publication, *Mercure de France* in the same year carried an article entitled "Races et groupements sanguins," which illustrates the effect of the extreme conclusion. After stating flatly that "there are four different blood groups in the world which coincide absolutely with the ethnic characteristics of the principal races" (note that the concept of a biochemical average was already gone), the author then identified these groups as "A and AB in the Aryan race, B among Orientals, Jews and Negroes; and absence of A or B among Indians and Eskimos." As an example of ethnic, blood, and racial characteristics coinciding, he offered this: "One can predict without great fear of error that a child of group B will be more apt at retail trade than bearing arms."[69] Although this conclusion was less openly hostile than Baron's, it went a long way toward granting scientific legitimacy to old shibboleths that previously would have been dismissed as racist diatribes.

The stereotypes of the Jew as merchant and the Aryan as warrior were now not only presented as scientifically proven but as moderate conclusions as well. Similar ideas were expressed in publications ranging from the establishment pages of *Le temps* to Jacques Doriot's *Liberté*.[70] And when anthropologists such as Georges Montandon criticized the idea current in the late 1930s of revoking French citizenship for Jews or all individuals of group B blood, his reason – "it would be like burning the house to cook an omelette" – still accepted the fact that individuals with group B blood presented a problem. He agreed that an omelette was to be cooked; the only disagreement was how.[71]

These last two chapters have shown both continuities and differences in racial eugenic thought in France from the turn of the century to 1940. There is no question that racism was deeply engrained in France throughout the whole period, but its theoretical basis changed, just as it did in other countries. Likewise, attempts to apply this racial theory to achieve eugenic purposes, especially in immigration policy, also changed as the theory of race changed. Other influences – political and economic – were important and perhaps overriding, but French eugenics of the late 1930s cannot be fully understood without appreciating the shift in underlying thought including, at last, an acceptance of Mendelian heredity.

In the end, however, the Third Republic survived the 1930s without enacting the immigration restriction or any of the other eugenic proposals that were made during the decade. It took the military defeat in 1940 and the creation of the new Vichy regime to accomplish that. Nonetheless, these changes after 1940 were not imports; the ideas supporting them came from French sources, hence they represent yet another continuity. It is time, therefore, to consider some of the specific results of four decades of eugenic thought in France once changes in government made possible the establishment of legislation based on these new biological ideas.

10

Vichy and eugenics

The split in French eugenic thought that widened in the 1930s was typical of much in French society on the eve of the Second World War. In the initial months of the conflict, these divisions were temporarily masked until the disastrous failure of the French armed forces in the spring of 1940. The military defeat and formal political changes of June 1940 had dramatic consequences for French eugenics, as it did for the rest of life in France. It was now possible for the racist, anti-immigrant proponents of harsh, negative eugenics to install themselves comfortably in Paris and attempt to implement their ideas not simply unfettered by the lethargy of the Third Republic, but encouraged by the Nazi occupiers. The neo-Lamarckian, natalist eugenicists who had favored a program of positive measures to improve the overall hereditary health of the populace also saw the delays and restrictions of the Third Republic give way to the new Vichy regime, which proclaimed the family as one of the three pillars of society. This setting even permitted the implementation of proposals that were the result of more idiosyncratic eugenic thought, such as that of Alexis Carrel, whose Fondation pour l'étude des problèmes humaines was chartered in 1941.

This chapter will examine these developments during the complex years of 1940 to 1944. It is not a definitive analysis of all racial and eugenic aspects of the Vichy era. Rather it considers the period to be a transition. In some ways, the Vichy years were the culmination of many long-building ideas and proposals for the biological regeneration of France; in other ways, Vichy laid the groundwork for new or revised ideas that carried into the postwar years. As Chapter 11 will show, one thing the period did not represent was an end to eugenic thought in France.

PARIS AND THE FRENCH RACISTS

When Eugène Apert summarized the progress of eugenics in his article of February 1940 for *Revue anthropologique*, he may have been anticipating that the war would bring changes. It was impossible, however, for him to have foreseen the startling turn of events on the battlefield in the following months, which brought the defeat of France and the complete collapse of the Third Republic. The French Eugenics Society, such as it remained in 1940, was particularly ill-prepared to survive in the new environment. With Apert's death in April 1940, the society lost both a well-respected leader and its ties to the French medical community, which had provided support for eugenics from the start. This left the Ecole d'anthropologie and its *Revue anthropologique* as the only institutional supports for meetings and publications of the society.

Henri Briand, who remained as the most active leader of the society, was a member of the Ecole d'anthropologie, but the status of the Ecole itself was greatly changed with the arrival of the Germans in Paris. The director of the Ecole, the nationalist ex-deputy Louis Marin, had run afoul of the Nazis at international anthropology meetings in the late 1930s, and when the Germans began closing in on Paris, he made arrangements to disband the Ecole d'anthropologie and its museum. Its collection of skulls dating back to Broca was given to the Musée de l'Homme, and the school's library was sent to the Sorbonne, but Marin's orders to suspend courses and the publication of *Revue anthropologique* were never carried out. The result was that they temporarily fell into the hands of Georges Montandon, a professor at the Ecole who became one of the leading raciologues of occupied Paris.[1]

For a short time, Briand and his colleague Henri Vignes published a few articles on such subjects as alcoholism and "physical education as a safeguard of the race," the latter praising the new Vichy laws requiring physical education and sports in the schools.[2] The influence of the German occupiers was evident immediately. For example, a course in "Eugenic laws of the Third Reich" was given at the Ecole d'anthropologie in 1940–41. And, as mentioned in Chapter 1, Otmar von Verscheuer and Eugen Fischer spoke at the Institut allemand in 1941 on German racial legislation.[3] Briand's report on the Fischer talk in *Revue anthropologique* appeared in the last issue of the publication, in which he concluded, "We note that

Prof. Fischer had the courtesy to make his speech in French, in a manner of great purity of expression."

Despite the presence of the Germans, their role as instigators of racial ideas should not be overemphasized. In fact, the appearance of German eugenicists and race theorists was as much a reflection as it was a cause of the increased attention paid to race by the French after the fall of the Third Republic. As shown earlier, the French could draw on their own race theorists and practitioners, such as Vacher de Lapouge and René Martial, whose ideas on race and immigration were debated widely during the 1930s. Martial, Montandon, and others found new and larger audiences during the Vichy era, as the French anti-racist opposition was quashed and new institutions were created for race study and propaganda.

The most important of these institutions was the Commissariat général aux questions juives (CGQJ), created in March 1941 at the suggestion of Theodor Dannecker, head of the SS branch for Jewish Affairs in Paris.[4] Although it served as a funnel for German money and influence, the CGQJ was actually created, staffed, and largely funded by Vichy legislation to operate throughout all of France. Moreover, it was no small office – its funding began at 30 million francs in 1942 and rose to 40 million the next year.[5] One indication of the abundance of Frenchmen with the credentials to serve as its directors can be found in internal German documents containing lists of potential collaborators such as Darquier de Pellepoix, Claude Vacher de Lapouge, Georges Batault, Fernand Céline, and Georges Montandon – names drawn simply from lists of individuals with prewar reputations as raciologues. Xavier Vallat, who eventually was named the first head of the CGQJ, is reported to have said to Dannecker during a heated discussion, "I have been an anti-Semite far longer than you," reminding the 29-year-old SS officer, "What's more, I am old enough to be your father."[6] These were merely the best-known of French racists. Others who eventually found employment with the CGQJ included opportunists such as Gérard Mauger, a former student of Montandon's who helped him edit a new journal begun independently of the CGQJ entitled *Ethnie française* (Figure 10.1), and Charles Laville, who became editor of *Question juive,* the official journal of the CGQJ.

Ethnie française grew primarily out of Montandon's own peculiar background and ideas on race. He was born in Switzerland and spent time in Russia after the revolution, where he met his

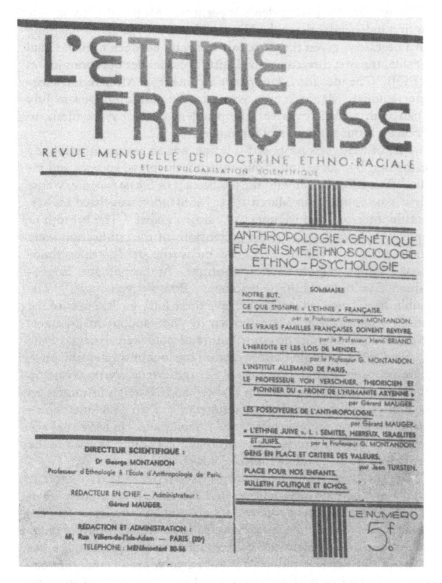

Figure 10.1 Cover of the first issue of *Ethnie française*.

wife. While a professor at the Ecole d'anthropologie in the 1930s, he developed a concept of human subgroups that he called *"ethnie,"* a category that differed from traditional concepts of race because it included linguistic and cultural as well as physiological determinants.[7] These credentials permitted Montandon to operate at first independently of the Nazis, although it was also something of a necessity, given the personal animosity between him and Paul Sezille, the first director of the Insitut d'études des questions juives (IEQJ).[8] The idea for *Ethnie française* came from Montandon's former student, Mauger, who wrote to the anthropologist in July 1940 with a plan to solve "the problem posed by the influx to France of four million [sic] foreigners."[9]

Part of Mauger's proposed solution was an ambitious publicity campaign by "an action group utilizing the press, speech, and radio." The effort began with the publication of *Ethnie française,* whose first issue appeared in March 1941. Montandon was listed as "scientific director" and Mauger as "editor-in chief." The breadth of approach as well as scientific pretensions of the publication were indicated in its subtitle, "Revue mensuelle de doctrine ethno-raciale et de vulgarisation scientifique. Anthropologie. Eugénisme. Génétique. Ethno-sociologie. Ethno-psychologie." The publication failed, in fact, to achieve these lofty goals. Most of the articles, for example, were written by Montandon and Mauger. Nonetheless, among the contributors of note were Briand of the Ecole d'anthropologie, who wrote on the low birthrates of French families, and immigration expert Georges Mauco, who wrote on the "Demographic situation n France" and "Foreign immigration in France and the problem of refugees."[10] Two of Montandon's articles were on blood groups and *"l'ethnie juive."* In May 1943 the journal ceased publication after Montandon became director of the reorganized IEQJ and its journal *La question juive.*

The IEQJ was set up by Dannecker in May of 1941, two months after the Vichy government created the CGQJ, apparently in an effort to exercise more direct German control over Jews. Its personnel was entirely French, coming from a marginal group of thugs and opportunists headed by Paul Sezille, a street fighter in the last years of the Third Republic.[11] Within a year, even Dannecker became exasperated with the group, and it was in an effort to make the IEQJ more respectable that Montandon was named director in March 1943. Up to that time, the most notorious of its ventures had been the exposition "The Jews and France," which toured the country in late 1941 and 1942 and was so wild in its accusations that it provoked protests from French non-Jews.[12] A more sustained publicity effort by the IEQJ was the publication of *La Ques-*

tion juive, a self-proclaimed, "monthly review of the institute," which began in March 1942 with Charles Laville as its editor. Much of its copy consisted of press reviews and news of anti-Jewish agencies in France, but articles by Laville also made a strong effort to demonstrate the scientific basis of racism, often citing the work of René Martial.[13]

Martial's influence in this period now went far beyond the influence of those on the German payroll in Paris. His writings were published by well-established French houses, and reached audiences even larger than in the prewar period. *Les métis,* published by Flammarion, was a summary of his pre-1940 writings, with special emphasis on the negative results of race mixing. *Français, qui es-tu?* was a more popular tome published by *Mercure de France* that Martial prefaced with these words.

Who are you? You know your parents and grandparents, but not your ancestors. You ignore everything about your geneology and your race. You have been told that race does not exist, that a negro or a Jew are as good as a Breton; that you can marry any woman. You have lost the instinct to preserve the race.[14]

Martial even wrote a children's primer entitled *Notre race et ses aïeux,* published by the Secretariat de la jeunesse in 1943.

In December 1942, an Institut d'anthroposociologie was created by the CGQJ, headed by Claude Vacher de Lapouge, son of the organization's founding spirit, and Martial was included among its directors. The stated purpose of the institute was to reach "exclusively scientific and specialized circles." Although the organization was dissolved just a few months later during the reorganization of the CGQJ, its inspiration was a clear attempt to raise the tone of discussion above the petty squabbles of racists, while giving greater legitimacy to the whole of the CGQJ.[15] Eugenics was to provide the overarching theoretical framework, as indicated in the official statement of purpose.

The responsibility of this institute concerning racial questions will be extended to breeding and agriculture. To insure a clean break with the past, the institute will admit no one among its ranks who was concerned with raciology before the war.[16]

The eugenic justifications of anti-Semitism could also be found in the most widely diffused propaganda efforts of the CGQJ –

radio broadcasts. This went beyond the work of the blatant German propaganda of Radio-Paris, which went on the air shortly after the occupation of the capital.[17] In the fall of 1942 the French government's Radiodiffusion Nationale began a series of ten-minute programs every Monday, Wednesday, and Friday evenings on "the Jewish question." The force behind the effort was Louis Darquier de Pellepoix, who succeeded Sezille as head of the CGQJ in May 1942.[18] Darquier delivered many of the talks himself in a "fireside chat" format. The official sponsor was initially the CGQJ, but later the programs came under the jurisdiction of the Union française pour la defense de la race (UFDR), a more broadly based propaganda organization with roots going back to Darquier's prewar Rassemblement antijuif.

The programs were most notorious for their evocation of virtually every stereotype and slander of Jews imaginable, from the charge of dominating the press to fostering sexual immorality.[19] The fact of spreading anti-Semitism via the new medium was telling enough of the changed conditions after the end of the Third Republic, but another feature of the message worth noting was the broader eugenic context of the diatribes. Even the most controversial of actions taken against French Jews – the roundup at the Velodrome d'hiver and deportation in the summer of 1942 – was defended by Darquier later in the year as "the application of a measure which was much more in the province of public hygiene than the anti-Jewish struggle." The protests it evoked in France revealed, according to Darquier, "a profound ignorance of the Jewish problem among the French masses." In the larger picture, he went on,

the settlement of the Jewish problem is not an end in itself; it is only the preparation, a preliminary clearing-away thanks to which there can be reborn tomorrow (and the catastrophic circumstances through which we are passing will aid rather than be an obstacle to) an aristocracy of young men, rid of this Jewish scum, who will be able to conduct France toward its true destiny.[20]

In a similar vein, although expressed in a more anecdotal style, a UFDR broadcast of February 1943 chided its audience in words reminiscent of Charles Richet a generation earlier:

Is it not curious, as we have already said, to note that in the twentieth century more attention is paid to the breeding of an animal race than the protection of the human race?

Very few people do not know about the existence of the English "Stud book" which is the authority on the breeding of thoroughbreds.

Everyone also knows that this book has existed in England since 1791, that is for 150 years, and that it has also existed in France for more than 110 years.

It is because of this genealogical tree, this book of reason, that the thoroughbreds have not only been maintained but improved.

At the same time what has been done for humans? Nothing but stupid anarchy.[21]

Eugenics was not the sole inspiration for the anti-Semitic actions and propaganda of the CGQJ. There was too much opportunism and settling of old scores especially on the part of Darquier and others.[22] Yet even if the scientific, eugenic arguments were only a window dressing, they are a testimony to the continuity of eugenic racial thought, and are indicative at least of the spread of these ideas in France to a much wider audience than ever before thanks to the changed conditions of the Vichy era. Nonetheless, it is perhaps most significant of all that these budding racists were not able to enact a program of eugenic laws to purify the French race *à l'allemand*. The roundup of Jews at the Vel d'hiver for deportation, although done by French police, was on orders from the German high command.[23] Darquier's justification was after the fact and not the result of an all-encompassing French eugenics program. But just because the most extreme racist eugenics program was not established does not mean that other features of prewar eugenics were ignored in France after 1940. In fact, the Vichy government did establish other eugenics-inspired measures that had nothing to do with pressures from across the Rhine; and these were to have a continuing impact after the war.

VICHY AND MEDICAL EUGENICS

It was not just racist anti-Semitism that flourished during the German occupation of France after 1940. There were also many who were genuinely impressed by the overall goal of improving the human race through eugenics, and by this they did not mean the simple removal of Jews. For example, Alfred Fabre-Luce, an impressionable writer in his early thirties, expressed the mood at the time in a book called *Anthologie pour la nouvelle Europe*. He put together this collection of writings early in 1941 because of his conviction that "France did not succumb only to the weight of tanks and planes. This material power was the result of the spiritual power that Adolf Hitler was able to release from his humiliated and battered country." The texts reflected, according to Fabre-Luce, "the history of the spiritual origins of the New Europe," and included French authors such as Sorel, Maurras, and Valery, as well as Nietzsche, Spengler and, of course, Hitler and Mussolini.

Of particular note was an entire section devoted to the subject of "Biological politics," whose ends and means Fabre-Luce described in his preface as follows:

Man can be improved. By concentrating on the progress of individuals? A chimera, says the contemporary biologist Jean Rostand. The child of the twentieth century is the same as the pre-historic child. "Biology ignores culture." The only resource open to us is to imitate nature by aiming towards a selection that this time affects not the body but the seeds. Hence, a definite genetic progression will be possible. But this author only poses the question. He hesitates to accept his own challenge, to treat men as livestock to produce a superman . . .

One man of action, Adolf Hitler, has attempted to realize it. First by eugenics: procreation is for some a duty, for others a shameful act which should be forbidden to them. Because the population can only be brought to a higher level by action of the elite individuals, they should be favored by the suppression of the majority principle and the institution at all ranks of authority and responsibility. Thus, natural selection will be completed and achieved. It is the highest task that politicians can propose.[24]

Although few Frenchmen were willing to go so far as to employ the German measures of selective breeding, many were prepared to take advantage of the change in the French regime to employ other eugenic measures to improve the human race that had been proposed in France since the turn of the century.

If the fruit of four decades of work in eugenics was to be found anywhere in France in the early 1940s, it was in the French medical and health fields. All along, the main institutional support for eugenics had come from the Ecole de médecine. In addition, close ties had developed with the public health and social hygiene movements as well as the natalist movements since the turn of the century. It is therefore not surprising to find a continuing interest in eugenics among health and medical professionals during the Vichy era, even after the formal institutions supporting eugenics ceased to exist. These professionals included doctors engaged in clinical work on specific hereditary diseases, as well as those taking a more general view of the need for a eugenics program in France.[25]

One of the most prolific writers at the time was Raymond Turpin, a pioneer in the study of the genetics of childhood diseases. His interest in eugenics can be dated from the late 1930s, as manifested by his participation in the 1937 Latin Eugenics Congress in Paris, where he presented reports of his research on mongolism, as well as a series of studies on the influence of the age of parents on frequency of stillbirth and characteristics of the newborn.[26] Within a year after the 1940 armistice with Germany, Turpin wrote an article entitled "Eugenics and war," which revealed some surprising conclusions based on the experiences of the previous decades. For example, he reported that according to the results of studies on the First World War, "military service can delay marriages but not reduce in any way the birthrate." Moreover, although the war had increased the incidence of venereal disease by drawing rural youths to the big cities, the problem was more than compensated for by increasing opportunities for education such as campaigns against tuberculosis, alcohol, and venereal disease that started during the war and continued into the 1920s.[27] Overall, however, Turpin agreed with broader assessments of the effects of war going back to Charles Richet's 1907 pacifist writings that claimed war destroyed "the most able men, according to physical, moral and intellectual aptitude."[28] As a result, the proportion of dysgenics also increased because rejects from military service were still free to marry and procreate back home.

This last problem led Turpin to conclude that two of the long-standing goals of eugenicists were more important than ever. The first was the need for "a series of measures favorable to the family," which was necessary as a response to the "continuing crisis of the birthrate." The second was a premarital medical exam, which was immediately necessary because without it, "alcoholics and psychopaths [will] start families with complete freedom and protected by law." And when the inevitable products of their union need care, "society raises the degenerate children at great expense."[29] Turpin repeated this plea in a report for the Comité nationale d'enfance in June 1941 that was more specific about the means. "If a country, of vital necessity, wishes to defend the family, it must give itself the protection of a prenuptial examination of future spouses." Moreover, Turpin clearly identified this action as "the logical departure point of a eugenic policy," which was justified as follows:

It is normal that men should turn towards eugenics because it gives the hope of eliminating the menaces that await their descendents. Puericulture as seen in its largest sense of "homiculture," must utilize all the resources of eugenics, as well as hygiene, obstetrics and pediatrics, and extend their action from a prenuptial certificate of one generation to a prenuptial certificate of the succeeding one. And the family will be the first to benefit from this lasting and concerted effort.[30]

Such ideas were particularly welcome to the new Vichy regime's family and health policies.

Although the Vichy policy was largely conceived by its formulators in political terms, significant elements were shaped by the eugenic, puericulture, and social hygiene movements of the previous decades. Most scholars agree that the ideological inspiration for the emphasis on family – it was engraved as part of the official Vichy slogan along with work and country – was from a different source – namely, an attack on liberalism and its emphasis on the individual.[31] As Marshal Pétain wrote in his September 1940 article for *Revue des deux mondes,* "The rights of the family precede and supersede those of the state and those of the individual." The evils associated with what Vichy critics called "two centuries of anti-family policies" in France were traced directly to the obsession with individual liberty.

Our anti-family, anti-social demagogues have given to man a love of liberty without teaching him how to use this double-edged sword; a man, like a poorly educated child, uses it against himself because liberty only brings true progress if it is voluntarily and solidly anchored to traditional discipline.[32]

The problem with such a position was that its specific program was rather limited. For example, the French were not about to adopt a proposition as radical as the family vote, only some rather innocuous measures such as the requirement that a father of a large family sit on all city councils in large cities,[33] or that a "priority card" be given to mothers of three or more children under the age of fourteen to ensure first access to administrative services, public transport, and shopping.[34] An April 1941 law made divorce more difficult by requiring a three-year waiting period, but this was more a defensive measure to protect marriage than part of an overall family program. It was similar to the record of the regime in championing physical education and sports. As one scholar has noted, "Although the Vichy government favored the practice of gym as a new form of social discipline and as a means of regenerating French youth, . . . as in other aspects of its policies, Vichy promised more than it could deliver."[35]

The promise of large families in these measures does reveal the conscious link between Vichy family policy and the well-entrenched natalist and social hygiene movements that had developed since the turn of the century in France. The purpose of marriage, all agreed, was to have a family; hence the family began when a couple had its first child. Once the focus shifted to children, however, two things followed. First, the question of how many children a couple should have led invariably to the problem of the falling French birthrate with its not so subtle overtones of nationalism, as seen in the following comment from a publication entitled *La Révolution nationale de 1941:*

When we think of the time of Colbert, France was the most populous country of Europe. In 1876 the number of births was still 1,022,000 and in 1938 it was only 612,000 (while in Germany it was 1,492,000 thanks to its family and social policy; and in Italy 1,037,000).[36]

Thus, much of the Vichy legislation fell right in line with natalist measures going back to the First World War.[37]

Second, eugenics specifically entered the picture from the other consequence of the shift in family policy toward the child: an increased emphasis on the importance of health, which in turn led directly to consideration of eugenic measures.

Health is of the greatest importance to well-being; without it no education, no creative activity, no family happiness is possible. A healthy body is indispensable to a healthy spirit. Parents should watch with extreme care the physical health of their children in order to know their potential and their limits. That is why we so strongly want to see the *carnet de santé* play a protective and educative role in families.[38]

The connection between infant health and the physical condition of parents had been one of the basic assumptions of social hygiene and eugenics in France. It also was officially recognized by the Vichy government bureaucracy in July 1940 with the creation of a ministry of youth, family, and health, with Jean Ybarnegaray as head. Although "youth" was soon given a separate ministry, health and family remained officially connected. Specific legislation against alcohol in July and August 1940 was phrased in terms of "saving the race," and in 1941 and 1942 there were additional decrees requiring prostitutes to carry health cards, as well as other measures to combat venereal disease and tuberculosis.[39] But the most far-reaching legislation that was also most consciously connected to prewar eugenics was the Law of December 1942 requiring a premarital physical examination.

THE PREMARITAL EXAMINATION LAW OF 1942

The physical and moral perfection of the race requires that energetic measures be taken in order to effect broad preventative health and social protection.

Thus began the report that prefaced the "Law of 16 December 1942 Relative to the Protection of Maternity and Newborns."[40] The authors of the report were Pierre Laval, along with justice minister Joseph Barthelemy, finance minister Pierre Cathala, minister of agriculture Max Bonnafous, and minister of health Raymond Grasset. There is little question that they were aware of the historic significance of the law. Indeed, the report stated at the outset that the law was intended "to coordinate and complete, without destroying, the work accomplished until now by public organizations and private institutions." True to this goal, the first of eight subsections in the law attempted to coordinate the existing local, regional, and national organizations working on maternal and child care. The main body of the law contained other sections dealing with various stages of infant and maternity development, strengthening and adding measures that in many cases had long been under discussion by health and eugenic leaders. For example, article 3 required at least two medical examinations of expectant mothers during their pregnancy before they could obtain new state allocations such as payment for rest before childbirth or for breastfeeding. Article 4 required every infant to be given a *carnet de santé* at birth, although its form and method of use were to be determined later.

Despite this sense of continuity, another subsection at the beginning of the report boldly declared, "For the first time a eugenic measure appears in French legislation: the certificate of medical examination before marriage which becomes mandatory, without posing any restraint on the possibility of marriage." The last qualification indicated that the authors of the new law were fully informed by the fifteen years of debate and discussion since the French Eugenics Society first proposed the measure. One proof of this is the lack of any provisions to prohibit marriage in the case of negative examination results. Instead, the idea was to "place the future spouses face to face with their consciences and responsibilities," simply by the act of informing them of the state of their health on the eve of marriage. The preface to the law warned, however, that "this measure constitutes only a first step which eventually, and taking into account the results, could be modified in the future." Thus, with statements of confidence in achieving results but with a warning in case of failure, France finally had a premarital examination law.

The specific provisions detailed in article 2 of the law are worth comparing with those that were discussed in the late 1920s and 1930s. For example, the 1942 law retained the simplicity of Pinard's first proposal. The entire description, excluding provisions of penalties and means of defraying costs, stated that

The civil official cannot proceed with the publication of the above mentioned marriage unless each of the future spouses produces a medical certificate less than one month old attesting, with the exclusion of all other indications, that he [or she] has been examined in view of marriage.[41]

One obvious difference from Pinard's proposal was that both future spouses would be examined, a change that had been recommended almost unanimously ever since Pinard's first announcement. In addition, the time period for examination was extended to a month before marriage instead of Pinard's impractical day before. A more significant difference was that the 1942 law described the exam itself in the vaguest possible terms. Earlier, Pinard had at least called for an examination to show "no contagious diseases."

The new Vichy certificate of marriage would thus only be an indication that there had been an examination of each spouse, leaving the question of revealing results or the decision to marry up to their sense of "conscience and responsibility." Slight technical modifications were made to the law the following July that waived the necessity of a certificate for a spouse "in imminent danger of death," and another that extended the period for an exam to three months in the case of military personnel unable to be present at the ceremony.[42] This brought the law in line with a measure passed in wartime to make it easier for soldiers on duty to be married. Although these changes might appear to be the result of pressure to relax an already lax law, serious questions were raised by doctors who worried about the awkward position they would be in when an examination indicated that the future spouse had contracted venereal disease or another serious illness.

One of the first suggestions by these critics appeared in a March 1, 1943, article in *Siècle médical* and proposed that doctors simply not give the certificate of examination to anyone whom they found unfit for marriage. This was possible because there were no penalties prescribed in the law for doctors who refused to participate, even though future spouses and the civil officer were liable to sanctions if they did not conform with the law.[43] Another possibility was pointed out by Henri Gougerot, president of the Société française de prophylaxie sanitaire et morale. Because of new legislation passed in March 1943 concerning venereal disease, doctors were required not only to tell their patients if they were so diagnosed but also to breach confidentiality by informing health authorities of their patient's condition under certain circumstances – if the patient refused treatment, or if the doctor concluded that because of the patient's "profession or style of life [*genre de vie*], the afflicted runs the risk of transmitting the venereal disease to one or more third parties." Although the measure was obviously aimed at prostitutes, Gougerot hypothesized that

If the doctor considers marriage to be a *genre de vie* envisaged by the law, he is thus going to reveal the name and probably recommend, as a corollary to the law, that immediate hospitalization of the patient is required. That will oblige the health authorities to act as soon as the certificate is presented at city hall, thus proving without a doubt that the contagious syphilitic has clearly decided to ignore advice and marry. Would the doctor in this case inform the patient of his decision? Be that as it may concerning this point, the doctor furnishes the necessary document for the marriage and at the same time prohibits the marriage.[44]

The irony of the situation, concluded Gougerot, was that "neither of the two laws relative to the prenuptial certificate and the anti-venereal campaign prohibits marriage of contagious syphilitics; their combined interplay produces the interdiction."

It is difficult to measure the extent of dissatisfaction with the lack of provisions to prohibit marriage in the premarital examination law. When the Société de prophylaxie morale et sanitaire asked physicians to comment on Gougerot's observations about the premarital examination and venereal disease laws, two-thirds responded that they would refuse to give a certificate to a patient with contagious syphilis. Not surprisingly, all said they would notify the patient of his or her condition. In addition, half said they would be willing to divulge the name of the patient to authorities as prescribed by the Law of December 31, 1942, and if hospitalization were necessary they would indicate so to authorities.[45]

The views of the Société de prophylaxie morale et sanitaire were biased because of the organization's immediate concern with halting the spread of venereal disease. Yet ever since the turn of the century the society had presented the problem in terms of its overall effect on the race, thus emphasizing the larger eugenic purposes of the premarital examination. Some of the society's members, in fact, saw the eugenic purposes as much more important. For example, the journal of the society reprinted an article by Raoul Blondel that compared the inadequate premarital examination law with the larger goal it should have served.

It concerns serious matters, that is, to stop the degeneration of the race by prohibiting legal procreation by those whose descendents would likely be only social rejects: syphilitics, alcoholics, epileptics, hardened criminals, not to mention those who are already afflicted with venereal diseases and capable of contaminating their spouses and causing illness that would result in infertility. We recognize immediately that the principle of the mandatory declaration of (so-called social) aptitude for marriage is perfectly justified, and it is the basis of what is today called *eugenics*.[46]

The Vichy premarital examination law was thus introduced with its wider eugenic purposes quite explicitly understood.

THE FOUNDATION OF ALEXIS CARREL

A final example of activity at least partly motivated by eugenic ends that came to fruition in the Vichy period was the work of Alexis Carrel's Fondation pour l'étude des problèmes humaines. However, rather than being the culmination of long-established movements in French society – as was the case with the premarital examination law or racist anti-Semitism – Carrel's organization was largely inspired by his own peculiar ideas that had been nurtured and shaped by over thirty years of work in the United States. The foundation provided a major impetus for a new approach to research in France after the Second World War – government supported, interdisciplinary research in the social sciences outside the established universities.[47] To the extent that eugenic goals were an important part of Carrel's motives, they were carried into the postwar era by such influential proteges as Jean Sutter at the Institut national d'études démographiques. The foundation was, therefore, both another result of the changing times of the Vichy era and an important influence on the survival of eugenics in the postwar period.

Alexis Carrel was one of the most curious figures in twentieth-century French science.[48] It is telling that there is even a legitimate question as to whether he belongs more to American or French research, a fact attested to by Carrel himself, who once noted that he lived "at the same time in the New World and the Old."[49] Born in Lyons in 1873, Carrel received a medical degree from the University of Lyons in 1900. His surgical skill in such techniques as suturing blood vessels brought him early fame but little advancement in the French medical establishment. This prompted him to move, first to Paris and then in 1904 to the United States. Within two years he was invited by Simon Flexner to work at the recently established Rockefeller Institute for Medical Research, where he perfected his surgical skills and began his controversial research on cell and tissue cultivation. Carrel achieved remarkable results in maintaining living cells in vitro, and in 1912 he received the Nobel Prize in Medicine or Physiology. Despite his success in the United States, Carrel returned immediately to France after the outbreak of war in 1914, spending most of his time at a frontline hospital. After the war he returned to the Rockefeller Institute, where he resumed his tissue cultivation research, extending it by the 1930s to a project that purportedly kept whole organs alive outside the body.

This organ culture work was an important development in several respects. First, it was unquestionably a direct precursor of modern heart-lung and organ transplant work. Second, it brought Carrel into contact with Charles Lindbergh, with whom he began a collaboration whose most important scientific product was a sterile glass pump that circulated fluids in the life-support system of tissues and organs in Carrel's laboratory. Lindbergh first met Carrel in 1930 when the aviator was seeking medical help for a sister-in-law with a heart ailment. Carrel explained that despite his world-renowned abilities he had no solution to the problem of isolating and maintaining the heart apart from the body for repair and rejuvenation. This was the direct inspiration for their collaborative project that produced the sterile pump.[50]

Carrel's work with Lindbergh also brought the surgeon/physiologist additional recognition. Such attention was not unusual for Lindbergh, the national hero whose every move had been closely watched and reported by the press since he made his solo flight across the Atlantic in 1927. Naturally the attention spilled over to any contacts or friends, and especially to associates such as Carrel. For his part Carrel seemed to relish the attention, granting interviews and expressing his opinions on all sorts of subjects from politics to extrasensory perception. For example, a newspaper article for the Hearst syndicate dated October 1, 1936 (at the height of the Roosevelt–Landon presidential campaign), carried the headline, "Col. Charles A. Lindbergh May Be President of the United States – in 1940!" The article was based on an interview with Carrel who was identified as "the closest personal friend of the former aviator, who now is devoting his time to aiding Dr. Carel [sic] in intricate studies in medicine, surgery, and experimental medicine."[51]

The nature of Carrel's research also lent itself well to a sensationalist press eager to publish the wildest rumors about potential uses of the new techniques. In the Lindbergh-for-President article, the following was mentioned about Carrel.

Dr. Carel [sic] is now working in his closely guarded laboratory at Rockefeller Institute on the problem of the relation of cells to those of vegetables and plants, with the hope that some time in the future he can build in his laboratory an artificial human being.

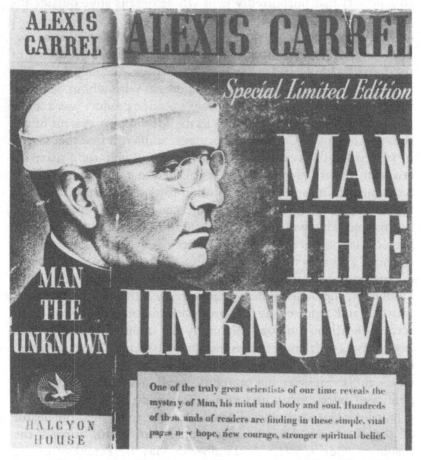

Figure 10.2   Alexis Carrel, Front cover of *Man, The unknown*
(New York: Halcyon House, 1938).

This robot – with blood coursing through his veins, heart beating, brain
vibrating, lungs breathing – would be an assembled man; he would have
the heart of one dead man, the brain of another corpse, the lungs of a
third.[52]

The press was obviously well-attuned to a public conditioned by
the 1930 film version of "Frankenstein."

Carrel's fame, though hardly the equal of Lindbergh's, had also
grown considerably on its own, thanks to the publication in 1935
of *Man, The unknown* (Figure 10.2). This book, which was part

popular science and part mysticism, enjoyed a phenomenal success. Aided by the wide publicity surrounding the announcement of the Lindbergh–Carrel pump in June 1935 – the announcement of the new circulatory pump in the journal *Science* made front-page headlines in the June 21, 1935, *New York Times* – the book's sales after its release in September quickly made it a bestseller. Over 100,000 copies were sold in the first year. Sales were naturally highest in France and the United States, and the book was translated into thirteen languages by 1936.[53]

Another reason for the book's popular appeal was Carrel's candid confession of the limits of scientific knowledge. In a foreshadowing of a whole spate of postwar books challenging the progressive, "Whig" view of science, Carrel described the purpose of the book at the outset as being "to describe the known, and to separate it clearly from the plausible, [and] also to recognize the existence of the unknown and the unknowable."[54] Such a format gave the author carte blanche to impress the reader with the latest discoveries of physiology and medicine, and then abruptly to offer the shocking admission of his own need for faith and prayer. In the words of one reviewer, this mixture of science and religion would please "neither men of science nor men of religion. Scientists will consider such an attempt as puerile or insane. Ecclesiastics, as improper and aborted because mystical phenomena belong only in an indirect way to the domain of science."[55] Disagree though they may, critics still abetted the sales of the book.

The first two chapters of Carrel's book lamented the decline of civilization and the inability of a fragmented, overspecialized science to synthesize the knowledge recently gained about humans in order to correct the problem. The middle chapters, which formed the heart of the book, contained a summary for the layperson of Carrel's view of contemporary research in medicine and physiology. Some of this was straightforward description of laboratory work, but mixed in was a healthy dose of Carrel's own conjectures about such things as telepathy, the power of prayer in healing, and the degeneration of human races from excessive exposure to sunlight.[56]

Carrel's ideas on eugenics, as well as his proposal for an overarching research organization to study human beings, were contained in a long final chapter entitled "The remaking of man." In it he outlined a positive eugenics that concentrated on "promoting the optimum growth of the fit," whose abilities were "hidden under the cloak of degeneration." For example, through Mendelian genetics, he asserted, there was a "probability that the legendary audacity and love of adventure can appear again in the lineage of the feudal lords."[57] As for negative measures, although he favored a premarital medical examination for all, Carrel thought its greatest effect would be its voluntary and educational value. On the other hand, Carrel did pick up some of the more extreme measures proposed by American eugenicists for "defectives and criminals" whom Carrel called "an enormous burden for the part of the population that has remained normal."

It is largely because of such passages that American biographers of Lindbergh have made Carrel into a kind of *eminence fasciste* who

filled his young, philosophically untrained mind with ideas and theories which were only peripherally associated with advanced surgery, but were to have an important bearing on his disciple's attitude towards the National Socialists and their ideology.[58]

Lindbergh himself wrote that Carrel "had the most stimulating mind I ever came to know well." Carrel did not go as far in anticipating Nazi eugenic measures as some of his later critics have implied. In fact, he stated flatly that "the reproduction of human beings cannot be regulated as in animals."[59] Few of the eugenic ideas were original, but their derivation was American rather than French. This is not surprising, because Carrel had worked in the United States since 1905.

Reflecting the attitude of American thinkers going back to Dugdale's study of the Jukes family in 1877, Carrel coldly asked, "Why do we preserve these useless and harmful beings? . . . Why should society not dispose of the criminals and the insane in a more economical manner?" Carrel's answer to his own question was the following passage which, more than any other, has been responsible for his image as a proto-Nazi eugenicist.

Perhaps prisons should be abolished. They could be replaced by smaller and less expensive institutions. The conditioning of petty criminals with the whip, or some more scientific procedure, followed by a short stay in hospital, would probably suffice to insure order. Those who have murdered, robbed while armed with automatic pistol or machine gun, kidnapped children, despoiled the poor of their savings, misled the public in important matters, should be humanely and economically disposed of in small euthanasic institutions supplied with proper gases. A similar treatment could be advantageously applied to the insane, guilty of criminal acts.[60]

This chilling reference to gas chambers was an extreme idea, even for American eugenicists, who by the 1920s generally preferred sterilization as the most effective and humane method of preventing procreation by the "unfit." But the unfit were still thought of as a "burden," and in this sense Carrel reflected the prevailing attitude.[61] Working in New York, Carrel had frequent social and professional contact with a number of scientists who were part of the American eugenics movement such as Henry Fairfield Osborn and Charles Davenport.[62] In November 1933, for example, Carrel wrote to Davenport inquiring about the hereditary transmission of defects. In response, Davenport, the head of the American Eugenics Record Office, offered to send an up-to-date bibliography from *Eugenical news*.[63] Publication of *Man, the unknown* increased contacts in the late 1930s that culminated in a nine-day visit in March 1939 to the Miami Battle Creek sanitarium run by John Harvey Kellogg. Although Carrel intended to study life extension, his letter of thanks afterward talked far more about Kellogg's views on "race betterment" and the degeneracy of the white race.[64]

Carrel's opportunity to introduce these ideas to France came during the special circumstances that existed during the new Vichy regime. The specific details surrounding the creation of the Fondation française pour l'étude des problèmes humaines have been examined in detail by others, including the question of whether or not Carrel was a Nazi sympathizer.[65] As he did when the First World War broke out, Carrel decided to aid his native France again in 1939, although this time he happened to be at his summer home on the coast of Brittany preparing his return to New York at the end of the summer of 1939 when the Second World War began. Without hesitation he decided to remain in France until May 1940, when he went back to New York as the Germans approached Paris. Carrel returned, however, in March 1941 as part of a Rockefeller team to investigate alleged nutritional deficiencies in French children. During the spring and summer he met with Pétain three times to discuss a more ambitious means of dealing with the problem. The result was the creation of the foundation in November 1941.[66]

One of Carrel's models for the foundation was the Rockefeller Institute, where he had worked for over three decades. Since its creation by Simon Flexner shortly after the turn of the century, the institute had gradually assembled a group of eminent researchers who combined their efforts in the study of medicine free from pressures of teaching or hospital service.[67] In *Man, the unknown,* Carrel paid homage to the institute (as well as to its somewhat more limited precursor, the Pasteur Institute), noting that "Flexner did not impose any program on the staff of his institute. He was content with selecting scientists who had natural propensities for the exploration of these different fields." The advantages of this approach were obvious, but a truly comprehensive research enterprise for modern society required, according to Carrel, "an intellectual focus, an immortal brain, capable of conceiving and planning its future, and of promoting and pushing forward fundamental researches, in spite of the death of the individual researchers."[68] What was needed, he went on, were "the lifetimes of several generations of scientists," and an institution capable of undertaking "uninterrupted pursuit for at least a century of the investigations concerning man."

The other model, also American, that Carrel alluded to in his book was the U.S. Supreme Court, whose provisions for longevity of service he found particularly attractive. With appointments for life, Carrel argued, the members would constitute a research institution that

perpetuates itself automatically, in such manner as to radiate ever young ideas. . . . The members of this high council would be free from research and teaching. They would deliver no addresses. They would dedicate their lives to the contemplation of the economic, sociological, psychological, physiological, and pathological phenomena manifested by the civilized nations and their constitutive individuals.[69]

In an address at Dartmouth in 1937, Carrel repeated his view of the "need for a center of collective thought, an institution consecrated to the investigation of knowledge, to the elaboration of a true science of man."[70]

What Carrel created in his 1941 foundation came close to these goals. The laws of November 17, 1941, and January 14, 1942, created the foundation and gave it an initial budget of 40 million francs. They also defined the purpose of the organization very broadly: "the study, in all respects, of the most appropriate measures to safeguard, improve and develop the French population in all its activities."[71] Decision-making, however, was more like a mandarinate than a collective effort, with direction of the foundation placed in the hands of an appropriately titled "regent." As described in the first article of the statutes of the foundation,

The Regent, to whom the highest scientific and administrative direction of the Foundation devolves, sets the programs of work in their grand lines and to a certain extent their details. He prescribes the length of their duration and the order of urgency of their development.

In administrative matters he delegates his powers to the General Secretary who is responsible to him for the execution of his functions.[72]

A steering committee existed only to "assist the Regent with its advice and suggestions in the general governance of the Foundation."

Carrel's working model relied on research teams to study specific problems. These quickly numbered sixteen, broadly defined by stages of human development (hereditary biology, birthrate, childhood development, youth development) or living conditions (housing, nutrition, rural economy, law, etc.). Six departments were supposed to coordinate the work of the research teams, but for all Carrel's talk of synthesis, the teams remained the most important research units.[73] Nonetheless, work within these teams as coordinated by the regent came closer to embodying in practice the group efforts that Carrel had learned at the Rockefeller Institute than any other work in France. It also provided new opportunities for young researchers who would otherwise have been excluded for years, if not indefinitely, from positions in traditional French research institutions. A 1943 report boasted that "the average age of collaborators at the Foundation is around 36 years of age."[74] Shortly after the creation of the foundation, Carrel wrote back to the Rockefeller Institute, "Please tell Dr. Flexner that I have a wonderful opportunity to apply on a large scale what I learned during these many years at the Institute."[75]

Whether through change of mind or lack of time, Carrel's foundation never became a vehicle for championing the extreme, negative eugenic measures he had proposed in the prewar years. In

fact, research never moved beyond the broad basic goal of studying means for improving the French population. Yet a brief look
at the projects undertaken reveals a concern with many of the same
issues that had occupied eugenicists for decades in France, albeit
now from the sharpened and fresh focus that Carrel brought from
the New World as implemented by his youthful research teams.
For example, one of the first projects reported by the foundation
concerned the problem of the child, and the description could not
have been phrased in more classic eugenic terms, at least in France.

The quantity of children is insufficient. The same is true in general of
their quality. This qualitative deficiency is due both to hereditary causes
and the troubles of development which are produced during the intra-
uterine life, at the moment of childbirth and, more often, after birth.[76]

Though phrased in classic terms, the new perspective the foundation researchers used to find a solution of "how to stimulate the
birth of hereditarily well-endowed children" was also apparent from
the start.

Numerous studies have been done, especially in England, America and
Germany on the subject of human genetics. But France has neglected this
research too long. It has, therefore, been necessary to begin by assem-
bling a very extensive foreign bibliography on the heredity of organic
and mental characteristics.[77]

This obviously represents a group out of touch with French eugenic work before 1940, yet other features of the report called for
examining the "conditions of child development" by such traditional measures as nutritional studies or height and weight comparisons of Parisian and provincial children.

Although many more studies were begun on other problems of
school-age children, adolescence, and rural life, the work of the
population and birthrate groups continued to examine the "crisis
of quality and quantity" of the French population. And the eugenic applications were never very far below the surface. In fact,
the second annual report of the foundation cautioned those who
were eager for results, "The implementation of eugenic concepts
is not, for the moment, in the domain of the more or less near
future. Scientific research must still progress without preoccupation of immediate practical applications."[78]

CONCLUSION

In the long run, the importance of the Second World War for eugenics was that Nazi atrocities, instead of ending eugenics in France, gave a new impetus to the study, discussion, and even the implementation of eugenic measures. This was primarily because the war destroyed most of the entrenched positions and institutions of the Third Republic, which had hindered if not openly opposed most change, eugenic or other. The Vichy leaders did not have a detailed eugenic program that they were ready to implement as soon as they took power, but they were certainly sympathetic to the goal of biological regeneration. Moreover, eugenics offered a broad rationale for other pet projects ranging from anti-Semitism to strengthening the family and improving public health. Thus, with the previous obstacles removed, many eugenically inspired or eugenically justified proposals found their way into the "National Revolution" of Vichy France.

In the case of the premarital examination law, it represented the enactment of the first eugenically inspired legislation in the country. Those favoring the most extreme racist eugenic measures also found their Third Republic opponents eliminated after 1940, not to mention the establishment of a friendly occupation regime in Paris eager to support and encourage their ideas. They did not establish any new programs or legislation, but this seems to have been due more to their lack of proposals as specific as the premarital examination than to any inherent Gallic aversion to extreme eugenic measures.

The success of Carrel's foundation illustrates most clearly how much the Vichy era represented a time when old vested interests were eliminated, yet how lacking it was in comprehensive theoretical justifications for the National Revolution. It is not an overestimate to say that Carrel was largely drawn into his new endeavor – out of retirement, from the United States – by the ideological vacuum of Vichy. The speculative, idiosyncratic ideas of *Man, the unknown* rapidly expanded into the full-blown foundation, which became one of the most important institutions carrying eugenic ideas into the postwar period. If the turn of the century had been the germination period of new eugenic ideas, and the interwar years a seedbed, the Vichy era was a hothouse environment of forced growth that tested whether the new ideas would flourish. As will be seen in the next chapter, even if the most virulent racist elements withered and died (at least in the immediate postwar period), the premarital examination and important remnants of Carrel's foundation survived the shock of the postwar period, thus providing a continuity to the present.

11

Conclusion

Several conclusions can be drawn from this study that help our understanding of eugenics in general as well as specific movements for the biological regeneration of France in the twentieth century. The most obvious general conclusion is that eugenics was not simply an Anglo-Saxon phenomenon. A cursory look at any international eugenics congress reveals several participants from other countries of Southern and Eastern Europe and, later on, Latin America and Japan. In France there were organizational, propaganda, and legislative activities that not only supported this international participation, but made eugenics part of the national debate on political and social questions during the first four decades of the twentieth century.

The history of French eugenics also demonstrates that acceptance of Mendelism was not a prerequisite for those whose goal was the biological improvement of the human race. In fact, Mendelian eugenics only appeared in France in the 1930s as part of one of the more extreme proposals for immigration restriction. Although in this case it confirmed the link between Mendelism and harsher negative measures, it was exceptional. The French Eugenics Society, which was founded in 1912, deserved its reputation as the home of a neo-Lamarckian eugenics whose main emphasis was on positive measures. One key reason for the development of this emphasis was the population problem. The decline of the French birthrate in the nineteenth century, and the fear of depopulation at the turn of the century, worked against proposals for negative measures (even though aimed at the "unfit") if they might be a general hindrance to marriage or procreation. As a result, most eugenicists chose to emphasize the positive measures that could increase the quality of all offspring. This had broad support in France because of the widespread belief in the inheritance of acquired characteristics. Accordingly, those wishing to improve the quality of future generations could do so by improving the environment and health of the present generation. The idea had logical as well as emotional appeal.

In addition to those encouraging propagation by the fit and – thanks to neo-Lamarckism – making the unfit healthier, there were many Frenchmen who wished to eliminate dysgenic elements by use of negative measures such as prohibition of marriage, sterilization, or immigration restriction. The call for the latter came as early as the 1880s in the writings of Georges Vacher de Lapouge. The fact that the early formal structure of a French Eugenics Society was largely in the hands of neo-Lamarckians and *puericulteurs* should not obscure the existence of men such as Charles Richet and others who were French voices that could command a following if conditions were right.

The First World War was one development that made important changes in the conditions that had surrounded the beginning of eugenics in France. Initially, however, the war's effect was to strengthen French eugenicists in their resolve to follow the same program as before the war. The war losses and added fear of depopulation made social hygiene a popular idea that appeared to tie eugenics to the even broader range of medical and health reform programs that emerged in the postwar years. The problem was that there were too many groups and policies for the eugenicists to control. With many of their issues usurped, French eugenicists were already rethinking their position before the 1930s made many new approaches possible. The most concrete proof of this was the campaign for a premarital examination law begun by the French Eugenics Society in 1926.

Another reason for the change in French eugenics before the 1930s was a turnover in the participants. As the founding generation of the French Eugenics Society either died or retired from public life, it was replaced by newcomers with different backgrounds whose new approach to eugenics soon became apparent in the meetings and publications of the mid-1920s. The very organization of the society also changed in the 1920s when institutional affiliation shifted from the Ecole de médecine to the Ecole d'anthropologie. These changes did not result in a dramatic shift from one interpretation of eugenics to another; rather they provided an opportunity for new and different ideas to be heard.

Developments outside France had important effects on eugenics in the 1930s. The earliest was a change in the policy of the Catholic church, which produced the first organized opposition to the movement. Prior to the 1930 papal encyclical, French Catholics, along with their natalist allies, attempted to reach an accommodation with what they perceived as a milder eugenics program advocated by their compatriots. Strains in this alliance would have developed in any case, as a result of some of the new ideas being proposed by eugenicists in response to the Great Depression of the 1930s. For example, increasing unemployment changed perceptions of the population problem, and produced calls for the elimination of anti-Malthusian legislation and the implementation of negative eugenic measures such as immigration restriction. Among these measures, debate about the use of sterilization was perhaps most novel. Although the immediate inspiration for discussion was the action by eugenicists in the United States and Germany, serious discussion about sterilization was most telling of how conditions in France had changed. Yet, despite the increasing calls for negative eugenic measures, the positive program continued to have its advocates in the 1930s, and even picked up important new support from the French left after its decision to participate in the Popular Front coalition. By 1939, a natalist, eugenic family program was an official part of the French Communist Party platform.

Eugenics in France did not produce new biological research or statistical studies as did its counterpart movements in England, the United States, Russia, or Germany. The most fruitful new work it can be credited with indirectly inspiring was on inherited childhood diseases. Hence, it would be a misnomer to call eugenics a "science" or even a "pseudoscience" in the French context. It was certainly an attempt to apply the new scientific study of human evolution toward a social end; therefore, eugenics was a sensitive barometer of much broader trends in the twentieth century that transcended narrow political or ideological boundaries. How else can one explain the fact that eugenics was part of the vocabulary of groups ranging from the far left to the extreme right in the French political spectrum? The French communists' family program deliberately picked up eugenic ideas as part of remaking its image of respectability. Right-wing eugenicists were hard-headed and deliberately provocative in proposing sterilization and immigration restriction, but their goals could also be encompassed within the broad definition of eugenics. The common elements shared by these groups were a concern over biological decline in modern society, a view of the problem in scientific or hereditarian terms, a heightened sense of nationalism, and an expectation of a governmental role in remedying the situation.

EUGENICS IN FRANCE SINCE THE SECOND WORLD WAR

As shown in the previous chapter, the Second World War provided the opportunity for increased study and discussion of eugenics as well as the establishment of the first eugenic measures in France. The Vichy regime and the Nazis with whom it was associated did not, however, permanently discredit eugenics. There was an important continuity after the war, although the process was very different from what happened in the First World War, when there had merely been a suspension of activities by the French Eugenics Society. There was no organizational carryover after 1945 and almost no reprise of activity by eugenicists from the 1930s. René Martial disappeared except for the publication of an anthropological monograph on Madagascar in the early 1950s.[1] Georges Schreiber survived the war, but only wrote one article on a eugenic subject, singing the praises of the premarital examination legislation he had championed for such a long time. A few politicians marginally associated with eugenics, such as Justin Godart, finished out their careers with vigorous denunciations of the Vichy regime and convenient memory lapses concerning their interwar support for social hygiene measures. Raymond Turpin achieved the most fame in the postwar period despite his frequent writings on eugenics during the Vichy period. This was because, unlike Martial, he had avoided the racial aspects of eugenics; and independently his reputation in the postwar era was made in medical genetics, as was the case with researchers in England, the United States, and even Germany who had shown an interest in eugenics before 1945.[2]

The only prewar eugenicist who survived the war long enough and who was in an influential enough position to qualify him as a continuing voice of French eugenics was Just Sicard de Plauzoles. He regained his posts as general secretary of the Société de prophylaxie morale et sanitaire and director of the Institut Fournier.

He also remained as editor of the institute's journal in which he continued to publish articles on such topics as eugenics, immigration, criminal degeneration, and overpopulation until his death in 1968. Sicard was isolated, however, because of the anachronistic nature of the organization and his advanced age (he was 96 when he died). Moreover, his articles were largely reminiscences and even repetitions of the prewar period, citing literature from thirty years past; hence, his eugenics after 1945 represents more an epilogue than a story continued.[3]

The survival of the premarital physical examination law after the end of the Vichy regime is the most obvious example of continuity of eugenic ideas after 1945. As indicated in the previous chapter, the 1942 enabling legislation contained a clear statement that the law could be broadened at a later time. The possibility of extending this first step into a full-blown French eugenics program was ended abruptly, however, with the fall of the Vichy regime and its replacement by the provisional government in 1944. Any new legislation passed by Vichy was suspect, especially any requirement that could be seen as an infringement on individual rights. Yet, after a year of study, the provisional government of Charles de Gaulle proclaimed its own statute on maternity and early childhood requiring a certificate of medical examination before marriage that at first glance looked strikingly similar to the Vichy ordinance.

The civil officer cannot proceed with the publication of the above-mentioned marriage, or in cases which forego the publication, with the celebration of a marriage, unless each of the future spouses produces a medical certificate less than two months old attesting, with the exclusion of all other indications, that the interested party has been examined in view of marriage.[4]

Aside from extending the time period of the examination to two months, the ordinance thus far was unchanged. In subsequent sections, however, the law was much more explicit about what doctors should do in their examination, ranging from the specific requirement of an x-ray for tuberculosis and a blood test for venereal disease, to the general catch-all admonition that

the attention of the doctor must be particularly focused on chronic or contagious afflictions which are liable to have dangerous consequences for the spouse or descendents.[5]

The reason for this new emphasis on the medical benefits of the exam can be found in the very different justifications of the *"exposé des motifs"* of the law.

Infant mortality has reached such alarming figures today in France that vigorous measures must immediately be taken to halt it. . . .

At a period in its history when France has the vital need to increase its population, the first duty of public authorities is to safeguard the existence of its children who come into the world; and the present ordinance appears in this regard, as a veritable measure of public health.[6]

There was no mention of the word eugenics, no mention of the protection of the race. The only such reference left was the need to examine patients for diseases with consequences for descendents. The 1942 premarital examination law that had been introduced for eugenic reasons was to be retained by the provisional government and the Fourth Republic solely on natalist and patriotic grounds.

Yet this was hardly the final word on the premarital examination, which continued to be discussed and debated in the postwar period.[7] Despite disagreements, the examination has proven remarkably popular among physicians. A 1953 survey of 665 rural doctors (living in towns of less than 2,000 inhabitants) by Jean-Jacques Gillon found that 74 percent of respondents considered the premarital examination valuable, and over 20 percent thought more should be done in the exam.[8] Nor did the eugenic justifications disappear among the general public. A survey taken in 1959 of 200 people (drawn from employees of the French railroads) found that the premarital examination law was both very well known – 95 percent knew generally that there were medical formalities before marriage – and well accepted – only 2.5 percent wished to eliminate it.[9] Perhaps most interesting was the fact that 59 percent thought the government should be able to delay marriage in case of illness. Moreover, although only 37 percent thought the government should also have the general power to prohibit marriage when groups with specific afflictions were mentioned, a much higher percentage felt that marriage should be outlawed by the state (Table 11.1).

Shortly after the 1942 premarital examination was instituted, health minister Raymond Grasset explained the reason for its mildness by the fact that in France "the scientific study of the facts of heredity are less honored than in foreign countries." Even the

Table 11.1. *French public opinion on prohibition of marriage (1959)*

Group	Percentage who thought government should refuse the right to marriage
Severe alcoholic (*profondement alcoolique*)	78
Repeat criminal (*malfaiteur recidiviste*)	47
Mentally ill or epileptic (*atteint de maladie mentale ou d'epilepsie*)	73[a]

[a] 56% of those polled thought sterilization of this group was justified.
Source: Freour et al., "Certificat prenuptial et l'opinion," *Hygiène mentale,* 48 (1959), 225.

medical community, he noted, was ignorant of medical genetics.[10] This meant that according to postwar opinion in France, either the public attitude toward questions of genetics and state control had changed greatly, or opinion had always been more favorably disposed toward eugenic measures than advocates realized. One thing is certain – the desire to improve the population biologically (or to prevent procreation by the unfit) continued to be a desired goal.

The survival of eugenics in the postwar period was more than simply the carryover of old ideas such as the premarital exam. It also depended on the introduction of new ideas and the attraction of new followers. In this respect, Carrel's foundation served as a stimulus both for new ideas and for the recruitment of new people who carried the eugenic perspective into the postwar years. In effect, it introduced a whole new generation of demographers and geneticists to eugenic ideas. For example, in a March 1945 issue of the *Cahiers* of the foundation, Robert Gessain and Paul Vincent wrote an article entitled "A few quantitative and qualitative aspects of the French population," which expressed the need for the French public "to admit the truth that it can foster the development of its potential by a true eugenics."[11] Alfred Sauvy, the father of postwar French demography, whose Institut national d'études démographiques (INED) absorbed part of the foundation in 1945, was also sympathetic to this perspective. During the war he wrote of his concern about the quality of the French population, and hypothesized that an increased quantity of the population could stimulate an improvement in its quality. His logic reflects a curious combination of neo-social Darwinism and neo-Lamarckism.

Numbers create pressure and pressure increases the quality. In turn the exceptional qualities of a few are reflected in the quality of the masses through teaching by example. The formation of an elite depends upon numbers and contributes to the improvement of the whole.[12]

When Sauvy created INED, he took with him a number of the foundation researchers, including both Gessain and Vincent.[13] In addition, article 2 of the October 24, 1945, ordinance creating the institute contained the following statement of purpose:

The National Institute of Demographic Studies is charged with studying demographic problems in all their respects.

To this end the Institute collects useful documentation, conducts inquiries, undertakes experiments and monitors experiments conducted in foreign countries, studies all the material and moral means capable of contributing to the quantitative growth and the qualitative improvement of the population, and assumes the diffusion of demographic knowledge.[14]

Like the provisional government's justification of the premarital examination, this statement of purpose represented the modification of a Vichy position but still retained many of its essential features.

Another Carrel foundation researcher who joined Sauvy at INED was Jean Sutter, who became the most articulate spokesman for eugenics in France during the postwar period.[15] Sutter had worked on the nutrition research group of the foundation that conducted the famous "100,000 children" study. Taking its name from the size of the sample studied, this research became one of the most frequently cited studies in France of social science research in the postwar period.[16] When he started at INED, Sutter took up the study of genetics with particular attention to the question of the "quality" of the population, and he continued that interest to the end of his career. His publications in INED's *Population* included studies of qualitative influences ranging from abortion to immigration.[17] Sutter authored an entire volume in 1950 on eugenics. A 1958 article, "The evolution of the height of polytechnicians," could just as easily have been a chapter in Galton's *Men of genius*, and one of his last articles was entitled "Social and genetic influences on life and death," published in the 1968 volume of *Eugenics review*.[18]

From a theoretical perspective, Sutter also deserves credit for finally introducing contemporary Mendelian population genetics to postwar French eugenics, analagous to what had occurred in England and the United States in the 1930s.[19] This fact points up the lack of ties between the pre-Second World War eugenics movement in France and Sutter, or between any of the foundation and INED researchers after the war. Even Carrel, although he spent every summer at his house in France during the 1920s and 1930s, had apparently not been in contact with any active French eugenicists, with the exception of Charles Richet, but that was on a matter relating to the nomination of a Nobel laureate.[20] The postwar eugenics that derived from Carrel's foundation, like the foundation itself, was largely rooted in the United States. Sutter's book on eugenics was an admission of the lack of continuity and a conscious effort to establish a link to the prewar tradition. He was helped by the fact that the problems of birthrate, immigration, and the quality of the population were the same problems that had plagued France before 1940; hence, they provided a continuity of context despite the new hereditarian assumptions. An additional feature of Sutter's revamped eugenics was that because of its basis in Mendelian genetics, his postwar writings on eugenics enjoyed a greater prestige, not just compared with prewar French eugenics but even with the postwar English and American movements, which had used these ideas to support their programs during the 1930s. Sutter had no such earlier baggage to discredit him.

Regardless of the new hereditarian assumptions, the result was continuity of eugenics in France after the Second World War, in fact much more so than in Germany or the United States. Only in the case of anti-Semitism had activities in the Vichy era discredited racial eugenics to the point of being unthinkable in the postwar era. But even here, the persistence of colonial and post-independence immigration to France eventually resurrected the biological eugenic racism of the 1930s.[21] Does this mean that eugenic thought might have ended had Carrel not returned to France, or if the provisional government had let the premarital examination law lapse? Perhaps for a time. But certain broader continuities are apparent from this examination of eugenics in France that fit the general observations of Foucault about bio-power since the end of the eighteenth century: the perception of biological (and related social) problems in the population, increased attention to and knowledge of science (in particular the workings of human heredity), and a persistent desire by government to use that scientific knowledge to correct the biological problems. To the extent that eugenics is the product of these longer-range trends, it is not surprising that eugenic thought in France survived even so traumatic an episode as the Second World War.

Notes

CHAPTER I

1   On Fischer and his institute, see Paul Weindling, "Weimar eugenics:
    The Kaiser Wilhelm institute for anthropology, human heredity and
    eugenics in social context," *Annals of science*, 42 (1985), 303–18. I am
    grateful for background information on the Maison de la chimie from
    Jean-François Picard. For more on German eugenics, see n. 2–5.

2   On Verscheurer, see K. D. Thomann, "Otmar von Verscheurer – ein
    Hauptvertreter der faschistischen Rassenhygiene" in *Medizin im Faschis-
    mus*, ed. Achim Thom and Horst Spaar (Berlin: Akademie der ärztliche
    Fortbildung der DDR, 1983), 36–52. For a collaborationist account of
    his talk, see Gerard Mauger, "Le Professeur Von Verscheurer: Theori-
    cien et pionnier du 'Front de l'humanité aryenne,' " *Ethnie française* (1942),
    13–14. A series of six such talks were sponsored by Karl Epting's no-
    torious Institut allemand, a self-styled cultural and propaganda center
    in Paris with branches in the major provincial cities. In presenting Ver-
    scheurer to the audience, Epting noted that prewar attempts to bring
    him and Fischer to speak in Paris on German race doctrine had been
    rebuffed. See Epting, "L'Institut allemand français," *Ethnie française* (1942),
    13. The six talks on health and biology were published under Epting's
    editorship with the title *Etat et santé* (Paris: Fernand Sorlot, 1942).

3   Eugen Fischer, "Le problème de la race et la législation raciale alle-
    mand," in *Etat et santé*, 81.

4   Ibid., 102, 104, 106.

5   Ibid., 110.

6   Briand, "Une conference du Professeur Eugen Fischer à Paris," *Revue
    anthropologique*, 51(1941), 195–96.

7   An extensive literature has developed on eugenics, especially in the past
    ten years. One good bibliographic overview, now somewhat dated, is
    by Lyndsay A. Farrall, "The history of eugenics: A bibliographic re-
    view," *Annals of science*, 36(1979), 111–23. Americans were the first to
    produce critical studies by nonparticipants, beginning with Mark H.
    Haller, *Eugenics: Hereditarian attitudes in American thought* (New Bruns-
    wick: Rutgers University Press, 1963); Donald Pickens, *Eugenics and the
    progressives* (Nashville: Vanderbilt University Press, 1968); and Kenneth
    Ludmerer, *Genetics and American society* (Baltimore: Johns Hopkins Uni-

versity Press, 1972). British studies appeared somewhat later, well after Farrall's thesis, "The origins and growth of the English eugenics movement, 1862–1925." (PhD dissertation, Indiana University, Bloomington, 1970). A monograph by Geoffrey Searle, *Eugenics and politics in Britain, 1900–1914* (Noordhoff: International Publishing, 1976) and a special issue on "Eugenics in Britain" in the *Annals of science*, 36(1979), 111–69, did much to stimulate interest in that country. German eugenics has only recently been studied in depth. Sheila Weiss has written on one of the founders of German eugenics, *Race hygiene and national efficiency: The eugenics of Wilhelm Schallmayer* (Berkeley: University of California Press, 1987), and broader recent studies are by Peter Weingart, "The rationalization of sexual behavior: The institutionalization of eugenic thought in Germany," *Journal of history of biology*, 20 (1987), 159–93, and Paul Weindling, *Health, race and German politics between national unification and Nazism, 1870–1945* (New York: Cambridge University Press, 1989).

It is telling that a review by Horace Judson appearing in the *New Republic* (August 1985) of a recent major work on British and American eugenics, Daniel J. Kevles, *In the name of eugenics* (New York: Knopf, 1985), stated that eugenics "has been a movement in large part peculiar to England and the United States." Although one of the fundamental purposes of my book is to disprove this statement, it is true of scholarship *about* the history of eugenics. A recent estimate by Barry Mehler in "A history of the American Eugenics Society, 1921–1940," (PhD dissertation, University of Illinois, 1988), is that 90 percent of the published literature has been on the British and American movements.

8   C. B. S. Hodson, "Lucien March: An appreciation," *Eugenics review*, 25(1933), 261. This obituary was about a Frenchman who constituted an exception to the rule.

9   Kevles, 91–112; Jeremy Noakes, "Nazism and eugenics: The background to the Nazi sterilization law of 14 July 1933," in *Ideas into politics*, ed. Roger J. Bullen et al. (London: Croom Helm, 1984), 75–94; Kurt Nowak, *"Euthanasie" und Sterilisierung im Dritten Reich* (Göttingen: Vandenhoeck Ruprecht, 1984); and Gerhard Baader, "Das 'Gesetz zur Verhütung erbkranken Nachwuchses' – Versuch einer kritischen Deutung," in *Zusammenhang. Festschrift für Marielene Putscher*, ed. Otto Baue and Otto Glanden (Köln: Wienland, 1984), 865–75.

10   For a summary of the extensive literature on Galton, see Kevles, 3–19; 383–85.

11   On the significance and debate over the German term, see Loren R. Graham, "Science and values: The eugenics movement in Germany and Russia," *American historical review*, 82(1977), 1138–40. On puericulture, which was defined by Adolphe Pinard as "knowledge relative to the reproduction, the conservation and the amelioration of the human species," see Chapter 3.

12   In this sense it was fundamentally "reactionary" and almost always conservative in that advocates were primarily interested in preserving

an existing state of affairs. There was a great deal of talk about improving the biological status of the population in all eugenic movements, but this utopian strain was rarely the motivation at the base. For an example of the lengthy and at times unproductive debate among scholars on the "conservative" versus "progressive" nature of eugenics, see the exchange in the *Historical journal*, Michael Freeden, "Eugenics and progressive thought: A study in ideological affinity," 22(1979), 645–71; Greta Jones, "Eugenics and social policy between the wars," 25(1982), 717–28; and Freeden, "Eugenics and ideology," 26(1983), 959–62.

13 On Russia, see also Graham's, *Between science and values* (New York: Columbia University Press, 1981). Other works include Werner Kienreich, "Die Wiener Gesellschaft für Rassenpflege im Lichte ihrer 'Nachrichten,' " *Psychologie und Gesellschaftskritik*, 3(1979), 61–73; Niels Roll-Hansen, "Eugenics before World War II. The case of Norway," *History and philosophy of the life sciences*, 2(1981), 269–98. A new volume compares movements in Brazil, Russia, Germany, and France, *The wellborn science*, ed. Mark B. Adams (New York: Oxford University Press, 1990). Zenji Suzuki, "Genetics and the eugenics movement in Japan," *Japanese studies in the history of science*, 14(1975), 157–64, unfortunately tries too hard to fit the Japanese movement into the Anglo-Saxon mold. For example, the high percentage of medical doctors in the Japanese Eugenics Society (53 of 75 founding members), which Suzuki describes as an anomaly, is quite consistent with the French and German movements, where medical men predominated. See Chapter 4 for more. The thesis by Mehler is a hopeful sign that newer studies of American eugenics will take this broader view.

14 This is particularly ironic because the proceedings of the three international eugenics congresses were published and widely distributed. In fact, they have recently been reprinted by Garland Press as *Problems in eugenics: First International Eugenics Congress, 1912* (New York: Garland Press, 1984); *Eugenics, genetics and the family: Second International Eugenics Congress, 1921*, vol. 1 (New York: Garland Press, 1985); *Eugenics in race and state: Second International Eugenics Congress, 1921*, vol. 2 (New York: Garland Press, 1985); and *A decade of progress in Eugenics: Third International Congress of Eugenics, 1932* (New York: Garland Press, 1984).

15 Francis Galton, *Inquiry into human faculty and its development* (New York: Macmillan, 1883), 24–25.

16 The most recent example is Kevles, 19, 57–59. Noakes, 77 also uses this reasoning, but cautions, "It would be a mistake, however, to explain the eugenics movement simply in terms of the context of scientific ideas."

17 For more, see Chapter 3. There is beginning to be an appreciation of the continuity of Lamarckism in England, as reflected in Peter J. Bowler, "E. W. MacBride's Lamarckian eugenics and its implications for the social construction of scientific knowledge," *Annals of science*, 41(1984), 245–60. Bowler would see the example as less of an anomaly if he had looked more broadly at eugenics outside Britain and the United States.

18   See, for example, the contributions of Lion Murard and Patrick Zyl-
      berman in their *L'Haleine des faubourgs* (Fontenay-sur-bois: Recherches,
      1977) and their earlier *Petit travailleur indefatigable* (Paris: Recherches,
      1976). See also Jacques Donzelot, *The policing of families* (New York:
      Pantheon, 1979). Examples of British studies inspired by Foucault are
      David Armstrong, *Political anatomy of the body* (Cambridge, England:
      Cambridge University Press, 1983) and Bryan S. Turner, *The body and
      society* (Oxford: Oxford University Press, 1984).

19   Michel Foucault, *The history of sexuality* (New York: Pantheon, 1978),
      142–45, 149–150. Foucault's extended treatment of discipline is *Disci-
      pline and punish* (New York: Pantheon, 1977). For a bibliographic guide
      through the enormous literature that has accumulated on Foucault, see
      Joan Nordquist, *Michel Foucault: A bibliography* (Santa Cruz: Reference
      and Research Services, 1986). Two analyses of bio-politics are Hubert
      L. Dreyfus and Paul Rabinow, *Michel Foucault: Beyond structuralism and
      hermeneutics,* 2nd ed. (Chicago: University of Chicago Press, 1983), 133–
      42, 168–73; and Martin Hewitt, "Bio-politics and social policy: Fou-
      cault's account of welfare," *Theory, culture and society,* 2(1983), 67–84.

20   There have been only a handful of articles on French eugenics, such as
      Lion Murard and Patrick Zylberman, "La cité eugénique," in *L'Haleine
      des faubourgs,* 423–53, that explicitly follow Foucault's lead; but Jacques
      Léonard, "Eugénisme et darwinisme," in *De Darwin au darwinisme: Sci-
      ence et ideologie,* ed. Yvette Conry, (Paris: J. Vrin, 1983), 187–208, and
      Léonard, "Le premier congrès international d'eugénique et ses conse-
      quences françaises," *Histoire des sciences médicales,* 17(1983), 141–46, not
      only ignore Foucault but minimize the importance of eugenics in France.

21   Rosanna Ledbetter, *A history of the Malthusian league, 1877–1927* (Co-
      lumbus: Ohio State University Press, 1976), 203–206; Richard Allen
      Soloway, "Neo-Malthusians, eugenists, and the declining birthrate in
      England, 1900–1918," *Albion* 10 (1978), 264–86.

22   Francis Ronsin, *La grève des ventres* (Paris: Aubier, 1980); Alain Corbin,
      Les filles de noce (Paris: Aubier, 1978) recently translated as *Women for
      hire:* (Cambridge: Harvard University Press, 1990); Institut national de
      la statistique et des études economiques, *Pour une histoire de la statistique,*
      2 vols (Paris: INSEE, 1978, 1986); Joy Harvey, "Races specified, evo-
      lution transformed," (PhD dissertation, Harvard University, 1983);
      Elizabeth Williams, "The science of man: Anthropological thought and
      institutions in nineteenth-century France," (PhD dissertation, Indiana
      University, 1983).

23   On the change in British eugenics, see G. R. Searle, "Eugenics and
      politics in Britain in the 1930s," *Annals of science,* 36(1979), 159–69;
      Kevles, 113–19, 164–75; and Garland Allen, "From eugenics to popu-
      lation control," *Science for the people* (1980), 22–28.

CHAPTER 2

1   C. P. Blacker, *Eugenics: Galton and after* (London: Duckworth, 1952) is
      an example of an "inside" history by a long-time secretary of the En-

glish Eugenics Society. The most highly publicized debate is between Freeden and Jones, as cited in Chapter 1, n. 12. Loren Graham also considers this question in "Science and values: The eugenics movement in Germany and Russia," *American historical review*, 82(1977), 1159–63.

2 Garland Allen, "Genetics, eugenics and society: Internalists and externalists in contemporary history of science," *Social studies of science*, 6(1976), 113. The remark was made in reference to Donald K. Pickens, *Eugenics and the progressives* (Nashville: Vanderbilt University Press, 1968).

3 Edward Shorter and Charles Tilly, *Strikes in France 1830–1968* (New York: Cambridge University Press, 1974), 48, 72, 107–18. Michelle Perrot, *Les grèves en France, 1870–1890*, 2 vols. (Paris: Mouton, 1974), 1: 51, documents a rise in the frequency of strikes during the 1880s, but she describes the climate of the period as "more rebellious than revolutionary."

4 See, for example, Richard A. Soloway, "Counting the degenerates: The statistics of race degeneration in Edwardian England," *Journal of contemporary history*, 17(1982), 137–64; or more generally, Geoffrey Searle, *The quest for national efficiency* (Oxford: Oxford University Press, 1971).

5 Mark Haller, *Eugenics: Hereditarian attitudes in American thought* (New Brunswick: Rutgers University Press, 1963), 21–39; 95–110; Daniel J. Kevles, *In the name of eugenics* (New York: Knopf, 1985), 70–84.

6 For general background, see Hans-Ulrich Wehler, *Das Deutsche Kaiserreich* (Göttingen: Vanden hoeck und Ruprecht, 1977) and Richard J. Evans, ed. *Society and politics in Wilhelmine Germany* (New York: Barnes and Noble, 1978). On specific manifestations of decline, see Evans, "Prostitution, state and society in imperial Germany," *Past and present*, no. 70(1976), 212–14; and James S. Roberts, *Drink, temperance, and the working class in nineteenth century Germany* (Boston: Allen and Unwin, 1984).

7 See the special issue of *Journal of contemporary history*, note 4, which was devoted to "Decadence," ed. Eugen Weber, 1–218, with articles also on Austria, Italy, Germany, and Russia at the turn of the century.

8 The significance of the Commune has been debated to this day. For a balanced assessment see Stewart Edwards, *The Paris Commune 1871* (London: Eyre and Spottiswood, 1971).

9 Eric C. Hansen, *Disaffection and decadence: A crisis in French intellectual thought, 1848–1898* (Washington, DC: University Press of America, 1982), 8–16; Koenraad W. Swart, *The Sense of decadence in nineteenth century France* (The Hague: Martinus Nijhoff, 1964), 144–52. For more specifically on the right, see Zeev Sternhell, *La droite revolutionnaire, 1885–1914; les origines françaises du fascisme* (Paris: Editions du Seuil, 1978).

10 For a sampling of the extensive literature on the subject, see David Landes, "French entrepreneurship and industrial growth in the nineteenth century," *Journal of economic history*, 9(1949), 45–61; Rondo Cameron, "Economic growth and stagnation in France, 1815–1914," *Journal of modern history*, 30(1958), 1–13; Charles Kindleberger, *Economic growth in France and Britain, 1851–1950* (Cambridge: Harvard University Press,

1964); and François Caron, *An economic history of modern France* (New York: Columbia University Press, 1979).

11   Claude Digeon, *La crise allemande de la pensée française, 1870–1914*. (Paris: PUF, 1959), Allan Mitchel, *German influences in France after 1870* (Chapel Hill: UNC Press, 1979); and his more recent *Victors and vanquished* (Chapel Hill: UNC Press, 1984). For more specifically on science, see Harry W. Paul, *The sorcerer's apprentice: The French scientists' image of German science, 1840–1919* (Gainesville: University of Florida Press, 1972).

12   Swart, 160–72. For background, see A. E. Carter, *The idea of decadence in French literature, 1830–1900* (Toronto: University of Toronto Press, 1958).

13   Swart, 69–70, 162–63. On the *fin-de-siècle* mood, see Steven Brush, *The temperature of history* (New York: Burt Franklin, 1978), 103–20; and George Mosse's introduction to Max Nordau, *Degeneration* (New York: Howard Fertig, 1968), 1–44.

14   It was not the only one available, given the discoveries and models of explanation that science provided by 1900. For example, the nineteenth-century physicist Rudolf Clausius had developed the Second Law of Thermodynamics as a corollary to Helmholtz's Law of Conservation of Energy, which concluded that heat (or other energy) tended to move from a higher level to a lower level. Based on this assumption, there were some who concluded that the universe was "running down." Those wishing to apply this perspective to the late nineteenth century could see specific manifestations in the fatigue and exhaustion (or "neurasthenia") of the population. On the application of this model, see Brush, 61–76; Anson Rabinbach, "The body without fatigue: A nineteenth-century utopia," in *Political symbolism in modern Europe*, ed. Seymour Drescher, et al. (New Brunswick, NJ: Transaction, 1982), 42–62; Theodore Zeldin, *France 1848–1945*, (New York: Oxford University Press, 1977), 2: 839–44; and Robert A. Nye, *Crime, madness, and society in modern France* (Princeton: Princeton University Press, 1984), 148–54.
    The proposals for countering this condition also reflected the physical model of decline, such as Taylorism, time-work discipline, and efficiency. This is the thesis of Lion Murard and Patrick Zylberman, *Petit travailleur indéfatigable* (Paris: Recherches, 1976). For an example of the impact of Taylorism on a future eugenicist, see René Martial, "Organisation scientifique des usines ou méthode de F. W. Taylor," *Revue d'hygiène et de police sanitaire*, 35(1913), 146–68. For background and a broader context, see Patrick Fredenson, "Un tournant Taylorien de la société française, 1900–1914,"*Annales ECS*, 42 (1987), 1031–60.

15   For a broad view of developments, see Foucault's first volume on the history of sexuality, *Volonté de savoir* (Paris: Gallimard, 1976), 177–211. Treatments in more depth can also be found in Nye, and the Murard and Zylberman volume, *Petit travailleur*. A recent historical survey of the history of the demographic question in France is Angus McLaren, *Sexuality and social order* (New York: Holmes and Meier, 1983), 9–27.

16   Francis Ronsin, *La grève des ventres* (Paris: Aubier, 1980) p. 24. See also

Louis Chevalier, *Labouring classes and dangerous classes* (Princeton: Princeton University Press, 1981), 161–85.

17 Nye, 132–70; Zeldin, 2: 823–75. For background on the medical profession in the nineteenth century, see Zeldin, 1: 23–42 and the series of books by Jacques Léonard, *La vie quotidienne du médicin de province au 19e siècle* (Paris: Hachette, 1977); *France médicale: médecins et malades au XIXe siècle* (Paris: Gallimard, 1978); and *La médecine entre les savoirs et les pouvoirs; histoire intellectuelle et politique de la médecine française au XIXe siècle* (Paris: Aubier Montaigne, 1981).

18 Zeldin, 1: 23–42.

19 Zeldin 2: 823ff.

20 Roger L. Williams, *The mortal Napoleon III* (Princeton: Princeton University Press, 1971); Murard and Zylberman, *Petit travailleur*, 51–53.

21 Paul Broca, "Sur la pretendu dégénéresence de la population française," *Revue des cours scientifiques de la France et à l'étranger*, 4(1866–67), 305. For other examples of literature in this vein, see J. Boudin, "De l'acroissement de la taille et des conditions d'aptitude militaire en France," *Mémoires de la société d'anthropologie de Paris*, le sér. 2(1865), 221–59; and the bibliographies of Jacques Bertillon, "La taille en France," *Revue scientifique* (1885), 481–88, and M. Champouillon, "Etude sur le developpement de la taille et de la constitution de la population civile dans l'armée," *Receuil des mémoires de médecine chirurgicale et pharmacie militaire*, 3e sér., 22(1869).

22 Broca, 306. A recent reworking of the statistics offers an explanation for the divergence of opinion. One reason Broca could make the case for improvement was that his figures began at such a low starting point. See J.-P. Aron, "Taille, maladie et société: Essai d'histoire anthropologique," in J.-P. Aron, P. Dumont, E. Leroy-Ladurie, *Anthropologie du conscrit français d'après les comptes numériques et sommaires du recruitment (1819–1820)* (Paris: Mouton, 1972). For the later period, see M. C. Chamla, "L'accroissement de la stature en France, 1880–1960," *Bulletin de la Société d'anthropologie*, 11e sér. (1964), 201–78.

23 Yves Malinas, "Zola et les hérédités imaginaires," *Ouest médicale*, 24 (1971), 551.

24 Robert F. Byrnes, "The French publishing industry and its crisis in the 1890s," *Journal of modern history*, 23(1951), 234–35, claims that sales of the book were a stimulus to the entire French publishing industry. Because other novels of Zola and authors such as Daudet achieved similar success, one should be cautious about drawing conclusions as to the public's agreement with the particular viewpoint of the novel. Large sales were more likely the result of the emergence of a new mass reading public of the day. See Michael R. Marrus, "Social drinking in the belle epoque," *Journal of social history*, 7(1974), 117–18.

25 For an introduction to the medical concept of degeneration, see Brush, pp. 103–111; Colin Martindale, "Degeneration, disinhibition, and genius," *Journal of the history of the behavioral sciences*, 8(1972), 177–82; and Richard D. Walter, "What Became of the Degenerate? A brief history

of a concept," *Journal of the history of medicine*, 11(1956), 422–29. On the influence of Morel in America, see Charles E. Rosenberg, "The bitter fruit: Heredity, disease and social thought in nineteenth century America," *Perspectives in American history*, 8(1974), 217–22.

The most extensive treatment of Morel is an unpublished thesis by Ruth Friedlander, "Bénédict-Augustin Morel and the development of the theory of degeneresence," (PhD dissertation, University of California, 1973). Morel is of greatest interest to historians of science because his theory was evolutionary, and it was published two years before Darwin's *Origin of species*. There was, however, only a limited similarity between the ideas of the two men. For example, although Morel consciously sought to destroy the notion that man was not created according to Genesis, his focus was only on humans and never had the breadth of scope of Darwin's. Also, his theory of degeneration focused much more attention on adaptations and changes produced in human evolution that resulted in negative effects on the population. Hence, his concept described a fall from a higher state, as opposed to Darwin's concept of evolutionary change from lower to higher forms.

26   Etienne Rabaud, "Origine et transformation de la notion de dégénéré," *Revue de l'école d'anthropologie*, 17(1907), 37.

27   The author is Henri Sauval, as quoted in Chevalier, p. 148.

28   As quoted in ibid., 155.

29   Chevalier, 337.

30   Chevalier, 338–39. For a study of one of the most important mining centers, see Donald Reid, *The miners of Decazeville* (Cambridge: Harvard University Press, 1983).

31   Murard and Zylberman, *Petit travailleur*, 105–08, 121–91; Gareth Stedman Jones, *Outcast London*, (Oxford: Clarendon Press, 1971), 127–51.

32   Jones, 283.

33   Barrows, "After the Commune: Alcoholism, temperance and literature in the early Third Republic," in *Consciousness and class experience in nineteenth-century Europe*, ed. John M. Merriman (New York: Holmes and Meier, 1979), 205–18.

34   Ibid., 208.

35   A. Brière de Boismont, "De la proportion toujours croissante de l'alienation mentale sous l'influence de l'alcool," *Bulletin de l'association française contre l'abus des tabacs et des boissons alcooliques*, 4(1872), 18, as quoted in Barrows, "After the Commune", 209. See also Jacqueline Lalouette, "Discours bourgeois sur le débats de boisson aux alentours de 1900," in *L'haleine des faubourgs*, ed. by Murard and Zylberman (Fontenay-sur-bois: Recherches, 1978), 320–21.

36   Barrows, *Mirrors*, 67, n. 54, quotes a range from 1,700 to 4,100 arrests per month for drunkenness in 1888 out of an average of 8,000. See also Barrows, "After the Commune," 211–212. There is some dispute, however, as to exactly when awareness of the alcohol problem reached the general public. Marrus, 118, for example, argues that only in the

late 1880s and 1890s was there the kind of publicity that reached the masses of society.

37 In addition to Lalouette, and Marrus, see Jacques Borel, *Du concept de dégénérescence à la notion d'alcoolisme dans la médecine contemporaine* (Montpellier: Causes et Cie., 1968).

38 On the alcohol problem itself as opposed to perceptions of it, see P. E. Prestwich, "French workers and the temperance movement," *International review of social history*, 25(1980), 35–52; and Sully Ledermann, *Alcool, alcoolisme, alcoolisation*, 2 vols (Paris: PUF, 1956–64).

39 Nye, *Crime*, 228–32.

40 Valentin Magnan and Paul-Marie Légrain, *Les dégénérés* (Paris: Rueff, 1895) 84.

41 Gerard Jacquemet, "Médecine et 'maladies populaires' dans le Paris de la fin du XIXe siècle," in *L'haleine des faubourgs*, 360–61.

42 "Enquête sur la déscendance de 442 familles ouvrières tuberculeuses," *Revue de médecine*, 32(1912), 900–44, as cited in Jacquemet, 362.

43 Examples of popular and scientific manifestations include a series of articles comprising a stinging critique in a popular medical tabloid, *Médecine moderne*, by the iconoclast physician Madelaine Pelletier: "Qu'est-ce que la dégénérescence?" 16(1905), 281–82; "La prétendue dégénérescence des hommes de génie," 17(1906), 25–26; and "Les dégénérés dans l'armée," 18(1907), 36–37. For criticism by more established members of the scientific and medical community, see Rabaud, 37–46; and Charles Capdepont, "La doctrine de la dégénérescence et ses contradictions," *Revue de stomatologie*, 15(1908), 26–30, 129–33.

44 The author is Henri Wallon (1875), as quoted in Gordon Wright, *France in modern times*, 3rd. ed., (New York: Rand McNally, 1982), 221.

45 The standard work on the acquisition of empire remains Henri Brunschwig, *French colonialism, 1871–1914, myths and realities*, (London: Pall Mall Press, 1966). For more on perceptions in France, see William H. Schneider, *An empire for the masses: The French popular image of Africa, 1870–1900* (Westport, CT: Greenwood Press, 1982).

46 Swaart, 193–212; Eugene Weber, *The nationalistic revival in France, 1905–1914* (Berkeley: University of California, 1959).

47 William H. Schneider, "Colonies at the 1900 world's fair," *History today*, 31(1981), 31–36.

48 Richard D. Mandell, *Paris 1900* (Toronto: University of Toronto Press, 1967), 68–69.

49 March 26, 1904, p. 1. On other 1900 retrospectives, see Jan Marius Romerein, *The watershed of two eras: Europe in 1900* (Middletown, CT: Wesleyan University Press, 1978) and Eugen Weber, *France fin-de-siècle* (Cambridge: Harvard University Press, 1986).

50 April 26, 1904, 1.

51 April 2, 1904, 6.

52 April 2, 1904, 5.

53 April 9, 1904, 1.

54 April 9, 1904, 2.

55 March 26, 1904, 2

56 Swaart, 187.

57 On the English background, see Bruce Haley, *The healthy body and Victorian culture* (Cambridge: Harvard University Press, 1978). For a general introduction to France, see Richard Holt, *Sport and society in modern France* (Hamden: Archon, 1981), and more specifically, Eugen Weber, "Gynmastics and sport in *fin-de-siècle* France: Opium of the classes?," *American historical review*, 76(1971), 70–98. An excellent social biography of the most famous French sport enthusiast is by John J. MacAloon, *The great symbol: Pierre de Coubertin and the origin of the modern Olympic games* (Chicago: University of Chicago Press, 1981). For the potential link of sport to eugenics, which did not materialize until later, see Robert A. Nye, "Degeneration, neurasthenia and the culture of sport in *belle epoque France*," *Journal of contemporary history*, 17(1982), 51–68.

58 Hayward, "The official social philosophy of the French Third Republic: Léon Bourgeois and solidarism," *International review of social history*, 6(1961), 19–48. For background, see also his "Solidarity: The social history of an idea in nineteenth century France, *International review of social history*, 4(1959), 261–84; as well as John A. Scott, *Republican ideas and the liberal tradition in France, 1870–1914* (New York: Columbia University Press, 1951), 157–86; and Maurice Hamburger, *Léon Bourgeois, 1851–1925* (Paris: M. Rivière, 1932). For a more recent testimony to the influence of solidarism, see Zeldin, 1: 654–79. For an analysis of solidarism's relationship to social Darwinism, see Linda L. Clark, *Social Darwinism in France* (Birmingham: University of Alabama Press, 1984), 67–75.

59 On Fouillé, see Scott, pp. 159–69. Fouillé's fullest statement is *Science sociale contemporaine* (Paris: 1880). For other influences on the origins of solidarism, see Hayward's 1959 article and Clark, 54–57.

60 On public health, see Hayward, "Official social philosophy," and following. An example of the economic theory is Charles Gide, "Solidarité économique," in *Essai d'une philosophie de solidarité*, ed. Alfred Croiset (Paris: Felix Alcan, 1902). On mutual aid societies, see Zeldin, 1: 660–65.

61 Bourgeois, "Lettres sur le mouvement social," *Nouvelle revue*, 93(1895), 645.

62 It was Perrier's acceptance of evolution in 1879 that more than anything else accounts for his subsequent biological theories. Although credit has recently begun to be given to Perrier by scholars for his role in publicizing Darwin's ideas in France, he has traditionally been better known for his Lamarckian view of heredity. See Yvette Conry, *L'introduction du darwinisme en France au XIXe siècle* (Paris: Vrin, 1974), 42–44; 382–87; Robert E. Stebbin, "France" in *The comparative reception of Darwin*, Thomas Glick, ed. (Austin: University of Texas Press, 1974), 139–41. His support for "transformism," as it was called, should not be minimized, for he was one of the first French biologists in the post-Darwin

period to accept the idea of species change and evolution. His steadfast support of the theory of acquired hereditary characteristics, however, has hurt his reputation among twentieth-century Anglo-Saxon scientists. His most significant disagreement with Darwin was over the Malthusian-inspired idea of competition for scarce resources as the driving force of natural selection. In its place, Perrier argued, one should substitute the idea of cooperation and association, which he claimed not only produced change but the evolution of more complex, better adapted organisms that were fitter to survive.

63 Henri Milne-Edwards, *Leçons sur la physiologie et l'anatomie comparaée*, 14 vols. (Paris: Masson, 1857–1881).

64 Perrier, *Colonies animales et la formation des organismes* (Paris: Masson, 1881). The publication of this book caused quite a stir in scientific circles. For Perrier's account, see preface to Armand de Quatrefages, *Les émules de Darwin* (Paris: Félix Alcan, 1894), lxviii–lxxiii.

65 Perrier, 701–702; emphasis in the original.

66 Ibid.

67 Alfred Espinas, *Les sociétés animales* (Paris: Félix Alcan, 1877). On the Germans, see Paul Weindling, "Theories of the cell state in imperial Germany," in *Biology, medicine and society, 1840–1940*, Charles Webster, ed. (Cambridge, England: Cambridge University Press, 1981), 99–155.

68 Bourgeois, "Lettres sur le mouvement social (1ère lettre)," *Nouvelle revue*, 93(1895), 395.

69 Perrier, *Colonies animales et la formation des organismes*, 2nd ed. (Paris: Mason, 1897), xxxii.

70 Foucault, 183–91.

71 Of course, the fundamental difference was over the optimal population size. If it had been large and growing, one assumes the neo-Malthusians would have been opposed to a laissez-faire policy. Unfortunately, the traditional names of the movements have focused on process and not ends, thus adding to the confusion. The point here is that in a larger sense both favored "controlling" the movement of the size of the population to a higher or lower level.

72 Michael Freeden, "Eugenics and progressive thought," *Historical journal*, 22(1979), 663–64, comes to the same conclusion about eugenics in Britain.

73 Frances Ronsin, "Liberté – natalité. Reaction et répression anti-malthusiennes avant 1920," in *Haleine des faubourgs*, 365–93; Catherine Valabreque, *Contrôle des naissances et planning familial* (Paris: Table Ronde, 1960), 46–54; John T. Noonan, *Contraception*, (Cambridge: Harvard University Press, 1965) pp. 387–91; 410–19. See also Ronsin's book, *La grève des ventres* and Angus McLaren, *Sexuality and social order*, mentioned earlier. The best bibliography of the literature of the day remains D. V. Glass, *Population policies and movements in Europe* (Oxford: Oxford University Press, 1940), 154–218, 441–49.

74 For a more complete list, see Glass, 442–43.

75 Ronsin, *Grève des ventres*, 164–89; McLaren, 77–89. For background,

see Léon Gani, "Jules Guesde, Paul Lafargue et les problèmes de population," *Population*, 34(1979), 1023–43. André Armengaud, "Mouvement ouvrier et néo-malthusien au début du XXe siécle," *Annales de demographie historique*, 3(1966), 7–21, makes a convincing case that there was support for the neo-Malthusians quite high up in the syndicalist hierarchy. For the experience in England, see Rosanne Ledbetter, *A history of the Malthusian league, 1877–1927* (Columbus: Ohio State University Press, 1976), 87–119.

76 Désiré Descamp, "Le problème de la population," *Revue socialiste*, (1896), 283. On earlier socialists, see McLaren, 80–85.

77 Scholarship on Robin has been uneven. McLaren's recent "Revolution and education in the late nineteenth century: The early career of Paul Robin," *History of education quarterly*, 21 (1981), 317–35 is a welcome scholarly addition to the biography by Robin's son-in-law Gabriel Giroud under the pseudonym G. Hardy, *Paul Robin, sa vie, ses idées, son action* (Paris: Mignolet et Storz, 1937). On Giroud and other figures in the movement, see Jeanne Humbert, "Gabriel Giroud," *Grande reforme* (1946), and "Deux grandes figures du mouvement pacifiste et néo-Malthusien: Eugène Humbert, Sebastian Faure," *La voix de la paix* (1970), 3–11.

78 Jacques Bertillon, *La dépopulation de la France* (Paris: Félix Alcan, 1911), 210, 216–17.

79 As cited in Bertillon, 213–14.

80 *Bulletin de la société d'anthropologie*, 7(1896), 139–40, 143, 210–12, 224.

81 For similar earlier arguments to the society, see Chapter 3.

82 For more on puericulture and the founding of French eugenics, see Chapter 3 and William H. Schneider, "Puericulture and the style of French eugenics," *History and philosophy of the life sciences*, 8(1986), 265–77.

83 *Régénération*, no. 10, March 1902.

84 McLaren, *Sexuality and social order*, 106–107.

85 G. Castet, "Les eugénics," *Le Malthusien*, 23(Oct. 1910), 180.

86 *Le Malthusien*, no. 42(May 1912), 331–32.

87 Among the longer articles in the journal were Edmond Potier, "Le congrès eugénique," no. 46 (September 1912), 361–64; Sicard de Plauzoles, "Procréation rationnelle" (November 1912), 315–18; Albert LeComte, "La tâche des eugénistes" (December 1912), 385–87; Remy Perrier, "L'eugénique et l'amélioration de la race humaine" (June 1913), 435–36; and Perrier, "Precéptes eugéniques," (May 1914), 521–23.

88 *Le Journal* (March 29, 1912) as cited in *Le malthusien*, (May 1912), 331.

89 See Richard A. Soloway, "Neo-Malthusians, eugenists, and the declining birthrate in England, 1900–1918," *Albion*, 10(1978), 264–86. On the United States, see James Reed, *From private vice to public virtue: The American birth control movement and American society since 1830* (New York: Basic Books, 1978), 134–39; and Linda Gordon, "The politics of population: Birth control and the eugenics movement," *Radical America*, 8(1974), 61–97.

90 For an introduction and bibliography of the extensive literature on the subject, see John Joseph Spengler, *France faces depopulation: Postlude edition, 1936–1976* (Durham, NC: Duke University Press, 1979).

91 The standard history is by Robert Talmy, *Histoire du mouvement familiale en France, 1896–1939*, 2 vols. (Paris: Union nationale des caisses des allocutions familiales, 1962). See also Glass, 154–218. More recent scholarship promises a much needed reexamination of the subject. See J. M. Winter, "The Fear of Population Decline in Western Europe, 1870–1940," in *Demographic patterns in developed societies*, ed. P. W. Hiorns (London: Taylor and Francis, 1980), 173–97, which also indicates that the French were not alone in their fear of depopulation. See also P. E. Ogden and Marie-Monique Huss, "Demography and pronatalism in France in the 19th and 20th centuries," *Journal of historical geography*, 8(1982), 283–98 and Françoise Thébaud, "Le mouvement nataliste dans la France de l'entre-deux-guerres: L'Alliance nationale pour l'accroissement de la population française," *Revue d'histoire moderne et contemporaine*, 32(1985), 276–301.

92 Broca, 307–309.

93 André Armengaud, *La population française aux XIXe siècle* (Paris: PUF, 1971), 12–13, 48–49.

94 Bertillon, "Sur la natalité en France," *Bulletin de la société d'anthropologie* (1891), 366–85, and *La dépopulation de la France*. On Bertillon, including a bibliography of his works, see Terry N. Clark, "Jacques Bertillon," in the *International encyclopedia of the social sciences* (1968). Bertillon's daughter wrote a biography of his more famous brother, the anthropologist Alphonse, which also contains interesting background on the family. See Suzanne Bertillon, *La vie d'Alphonse Bertillon* (Paris: Gallimard, 1941).

95 See, for example, Chevalier, pp. 161–258.

96 Richet, "Accroissement de la population française," *Revue des deux mondes*, 3e sér., vol. 50(1882), 900–32; 51: 587–616. For more on early years, see Talmy, 1: 53–65.

97 For England, see Soloway, "Neo-Malthusians," and his book, *Birth control and the population question in England, 1877–1930* (Chapel Hill: UNC Press, 1982).

98 Richet, "Faut-il laisser la France périr?," *Revue bleue* (1896), 620–22.

99 That Zola should wish to offer a solution to the problems he so laboriously and graphically described in his earlier series is not surprising. But that the first of the four-book series should be about "fecundity," thus taking precedence over "work," "truth," and "justice" is, for our purposes, even more telling of the importance of the population question at the time. For more, see David Baguley, *Fecondité d'Emile Zola* (Toronto: University of Toronto Press, 1973).

100 For an example of the warm reviews Zola's new work received, see Gustave Kahn, "Fecondité," *Revue blanche*, 20(1899), 285–93. On Brieux, see the introduction by George Bernard Shaw to *Three plays by Brieux*, (New York: Brentanos, 1911) in which Shaw calls Brieux the equal of

Ibsen. An even better analysis of the setting in which Brieux wrote is
William H. Scheifley, *Brieux and contemporary French society* (New York:
G. P. Putnam's Sons, 1917), and the article by Claude Sulleron, "La
littérature au XIXe siècle et la famille," in *Renouveau des idées sur la
famille*, ed. Robert Prigent, (Paris: PUF, 1954), 60–80.

101   Glass, 441–42. See also Winter, 176–79.
102   For more on the limited successes of 1913–14, see Talmy, 1: 159–66.
For the 1939 legislation, see Talmy, 2: 232–41 and Thébaud, 299, who
puts it more diplomatically, "The successes obtained were not equal to
the activities undertaken."
103   *Revue de l'alliance nationale pour l'accroissement de la population française*
[hereafter cited as *Revue de l'alliance*], (1900), 117. Once again, for a
close parallel in England see Soloway, *Birth control*, 22–24. There were
two English study commissions: the official 1911 Fertility of Marriage
Commission and the unofficial 1913 National Birthrate Commission.
104   Talmy, 1:105–22.
105   Reprinted in *Revue de l'alliance*, (1902), 322–30.
106   They found no significant difference between the sterility rate in France
and other countries, which led them to the rather unspectacular conclusion, "To remedy the drop in births in France, one can only count on
means that will change the preference of French families and encourage
them to have more children than they want today." *Annales de gynécologie et d'obstétrique*, 59(1903), 24. For more on puericulture, see Chapter
3.
107   McLaren, *Sexuality and social order*, pp. 44–64. Even the church was
divided, hence the delay until 1930 before eugenics was condemned. In
addition to McLaren, 31–43, see Jean Stengers, "Les pratiques anti-
conceptionnelles dans le mariage aux XIXe et au XXe siècle: Problèmes
humaines et attitudes religieuses," *Revue belge de philologie et d'histoire*,
49(1971), 1161 and Noonan, 399–403.
108   Dr. Klotz-Forest, "La prophylaxie anticonceptionnelle est-elle legi-
time?" *Chronique médicale*, 11(1904), 689–99.
109   They were published under the title, "Referendum de la 'chronique
médicale' sur la prophylaxie anti-conceptionnelle," *Chronique médicale*,
12(1905), 97–144.
110   *Chronique médicale*, 12(1905), 119–32.
111   Ibid. On the Severine/Richet exchange, see *Revue philanthropique*, 1(1897),
337–41, 492–96.
112   *Chronique médicale*, 12 (1905), 128.
113   Ibid., 137.
114   Ibid., 138.
115   The history of French social hygiene is yet to be written. Even the
related history of public health has been studied primarily for the first
half of the nineteenth century. See, for example, Erwin H. Ackerknecht, "Hygiene in France, 1815–1848," *Bulletin of the history of medicine*, 22(1948), 117–55; Ann F. La Berge, "Public health in France and
the French public health movement, 1815–1848" (PhD dissertation,

University of Tennessee, 1974); or more recently, William Coleman, *Death is a social disease: Public health and political economy in early industrial France* (Madison: University of Wisconsin Press, 1982). Some recent exceptions to these are Ann-Louise Shapiro's "Private rights, public interest and professional jurisdiction: The French public health law of 1902," *Bulletin of the history of medicine*, 54(1980), 4–22, and Martha Lee Hildreth, *Doctors, bureaucrats and public health in France, 1888–1902* (New York: Garland, 1987). A more systematic study by Murard and Zylberman has already produced "De l'hygiène comme introduction à la politique expérimentale (1875–1925)," *Revue de synthèse*, 3e sér., 115(1984), 313–41 and their broader, "La raison de l'expert ou l'hygiène comme science sociale appliquée," *Archives europeénes de sociologie*, 26(1985), 58–89.

116 This has been studied much more thoroughly in Germany than any other country. See Dieter Tutzke, *Alfred Grotjahn* (Leipzig: G. Teubner, 1979); Paul Weindling, "Die preussische Medizinalverwaltung und die 'Rassenhygiene': Anmerkungen zur Gesundheitspolitik der Jahre 1905– 1933," *Zeitschrift für Sozialreform*, 20(1984), 675–87; and Gerhard Baader, "Sozialhygienische Theorie und Praxis in der Gewerbehygiene in Berlin der Weimarer Zeit," *Koroth*, 8(1985), 24–37. On the American social hygiene movement, see James F. Gardner, Jr., "Microbes and morality: The social hygiene crusade in New York City, 1892–1917" (PhD dissertation, Indiana University, 1974).

117 Emile Duclaux, *Hygiène sociale* (Paris: Félix Alcan, 1902), i–ii; 109. For more on this aspect, see Murard and Zylberman, "De l'hygiène," 313– 41. For a different view of the Pasteurians, see Bruno Latour, *Les microbes. Guerre et paix* (Paris: A. M. Metailie, 1984).

118 Barrows, "After the Commune," 205–218; repeated and elaborated in her *Mirrors*, 61–72. See also, Prestwich, 39–40; Lalouette, 315–47; Marrus, 115–41; and Nye, *Crime, madness and politics*, pp. 155–58.

119 Prestwich, 40; Gerard Jacquemet, "Médecine et 'maladies populaires' dans le Paris de la fin du XIXe siècle," in *Haleine des faubourgs*, 354–55. Lalouette, 316–17, analyzed an 1873 membership list of 382 members and found 120 in medicine.

120 Jacquemet, 350–51; Marrus, 117–18. There were 586 theses on syphilis and 908 on tuberculosis during these same years.

121 Prestwich, 41.

122 Borel, 53–55.

123 On Légrain, see Jacquemet, 355; Nye, 156–57; and Prestwich, 41–43. The most comprehensive, if rambling, account of these anti-alcohol campaigns is by Borel, 51–90.

124 Légrain, *L'hérédité et l'alcoolisme* (Paris: O. Doin, 1889), xxxiv.

125 Légrain, *Dégénérescence social et l'alcoolisme* (Paris: Masson, 1895), p. xxvii.

126 Ibid., xvii–xviii. On the substance of the campaign to link alcoholism and degeneration, see Borel, 11–49 and Nye, 156–57.

127 Prestwich, 42–43.

128 Duclaux, 121.
129 Jacquemet, 358–59. As will be seen later, André Couvreur made tuber-culosis one of the subjects in his widely read novel, *La graine* published in 1903. Thomas Mann's *Magic mountain* (1924) is usually considered the first treatment in depth of tuberculosis in classic literature. For an indication of the persistent fatalism toward tuberculosis in the United States even after Koch's discovery, see Rosenberg, 204–205.
130 Jacquemet, 359.
131 *Xe congrès international d'hygiène et de démographie à Paris en 1900. Compte rendu* (Paris: Masson, 1901), 753–56.
132 On the importance of Bourgeois to the tuberculosis movement, see Murard and Zylberman, "La santé publique en France sous l'oeil de l'Amérique," *Revue historique*, 276(1986), 374.
133 One can hardly say, however, that syphilis was an unknown affliction. Soon after the discovery of the Americas, the disease took a permanent place not only in the medical annals of Europe but in popular culture as well. The variety of popular names – running to several pages – is a vivid testimony to public awareness of the ravages of venereal disease. See Alfred W. Crosby, *The Columbian exchange* (Westport, CT.: Green-wood Press, 1972), 124–125.
134 For an excellent overview, see Alain Corbin, *Les filles de noce* (Paris: Aubier, 1978), 15–53.
135 For a summary of the organization's work, see Corbin, 390–402.
136 *Bulletin de la société de prophylaxie sanitaire et morale*, 1(1901), 1.
137 Ibid., 16–24. Corbin, 391–92. Among the future eugenicists were Pinard, François Hallopeau, André Honnorat, Edouard Jeanselme, Louis Landouzy, and Charles Richet.
138 Corbin, 391.
139 Henri Cazalis, *Science et mariage* (Paris: A. Doin, 1900). It was also the title of a shorter article in the *Revue scientifique*, 38(1900), 609–16. On Cazalis, whose literary name was Jean Lahor, see Laurence A. Joseph, *Henri Cazalis: sa vie, son oeuvre, son amitié avec Mallarmé* (Paris: A.-G. Nizet, 1972). *Science et marriage* was not the first proposal for a medical screening before marriage. Most immediately prior was a call by a feminist congress in 1896 for each future spouse to present a certificate of good health at city hall before obtaining a marriage license. Lucien Grellety, "Psychologie du mariage – l'examen des jeunes mariés," *Revue de psychiatrie, neurologie et hypnologie*, 1(1890), 202–204.
140 *Bulletin de l'académie de médecine*, 3 sér., 43(1900), 618–19.
141 Scheifly, 384–85.
142 "Damaged goods," in *Three plays by Brieux*, (New York: Brentanos, 1911), 243–44.
143 Scheifly, 376–77.
144 Hippolyte Mireur, *L'avarie, Etude d'hygiène sociale*, 7, as quoted in Corbin, 397. Cazalis claimed it sold 30,000 copies by 1903. See "Garanties sanitaires du mariage," *Bulletin de la Société de prophylaxie sanitaire et morale*, 3(1903), 285.

145 See vol. 3(1903), 271–324, 339–85, 392–420, 470–88, 531–54.
146 Scheifley, 384–85; Corbin, 395–402. See also Victor Margueritte, *Prostituée* (Paris: E. Pasquelle, 1907). Among works in English that were influenced by Brieux was Upton Sinclair's, *Sylvia's marriage* (Chicago: John C. Winston, 1914).
147 Vol. 10(1903), 449–95.
148 Duclaux, *Hygiène sociale* (Paris: Félix Alcan, 1902)
149 *L'Alliance d'hygiène sociale* (Paris: Musée social, 1904), 3.
150 *Annales d'hygiène publique,* 4e sér., 2(1904), 262–79; 6(1906), 337–57; 8(1907), 66–73.
151 Dr. Gautrez, *11e Congrès de l'alliance d'hygiène sociale* (Clermont-Ferrand, 1921), 5, as cited in Eugène Montet, "Pour l'hygiène sociale," *Annales d'hygiène publique* n.s., 4(1923), 3–4.

CHAPTER 3

1 Clémence Royer, "Preface" in her translation of Charles Darwin, *L'origine des éspèces* (Paris: Guillaume et Masson, 1862), lxvi. For biographical information on Royer, see following. On the broader impact of Darwin, see Yvette Conry, *L'introduction du darwinisme en France* (Paris: Vrin, 1974).
2 The publication of Galton's *Hereditary genius* preceded Candolle's book by a few years, but Candolle vigorously insisted on the independence of his work, which he claimed had begun in 1833. Candolle letter to Galton, January 2, 1873, in *Life, letters and labours of Francis Galton*, ed. Karl Pearson (Cambridge, England: Cambridge University Press, 1924), 2:136. Galton subsequently published *English men of science: Their nature and nurture* (New York: Macmillan, 1874), with an acknowledgment in the preface that it was directly inspired by Candolle's book. Later Galton recalled, "I thought that a somewhat similar investigation might be made with advantage into the history of English men of science," as quoted in Pearson, 2:134. The complete correspondence between Galton and Candolle is contained in ibid., 135–56. For an indication of the continuing interchange between the two men, see Raymond E. Fancher, "Alphonse de Candolle, Francis Galton, and the early history of the nature–nurture controversy," *Journal of the history of the behavioral sciences*, 19(1983), 341–52.
3 On Lapouge's self-confessed reliance on Galton and Candolle, see *Sélections sociales* (Paris: A. Fontemoing, 1896), vi–vii, 461–64.
4 No less an authority than Lapouge called Royer "the first to state in her translation of the *Origins* that the discovery of Darwin would have more importance from a social point of view than from that of biology." *Sélections sociales*, vi. For a recent analysis, see Claude Blanckaert, "L'anthropologie au feminin: Clémence Royer (1830–1902)," *Revue de synthèse*, 105(1982), 28, who calls hers "one of the first French testimonials in favor of eugenics and social Darwinism." On the latter, see Linda L. Clark, *Social Darwinism in France* (Montgomery: University of Ala-

bama Press, 1984), 12–16. For a different side of Royer, see Joy Harvey, "Strangers to each other: Male and female relationships in the life and work of Clémence Royer," in *Uneasy careers and intimate lives: Women scientists, 1789–1978*, ed. Pnina Abir-Am and Dorinda Outram (New Brunswick: Rutgers University Press, 1987), 147–71.

5 This was very similar to the discussions of natalists, according to scholars of French feminism. For example, see Karen Offen, "Depopulation, natalism and feminism," *American historical review*, 89(1984), 653–54, 670–71. An exception to this was the important participation of women in Robin's neo-Malthusian movement.

6 Lxix–lxx; also cited in *Chronique médicale*, 13(1906), 477–78.

7 Ibid., also cited in Joy Harvey, "Races specified, evolution transformed," PhD dissertation, Harvard University, (1983), 270.

8 Harvey, "Races," 272.

9 Paul Broca, "Les sélections," *Memoires d'anthropologie* 3(1877), 244–45. The comments were first made in an 1873 article in *Revue anthropologique*. For background, see Harvey, "Races," 272–75.

10 Tarboureich, *La cité future* (Paris: Stock, 1902), 205–307.

11 *Régéneration* (September 1902), 105.

12 Alfred Pichou, "L'élite," *Revue internationale de sociologie* 14(1896), 583–84. Of note is the conservative, defensive tone of the proposal.

13 Ibid., 584–85.

14 *Chronique médicale*, 12(1905), 265–66; 13(1906), 476–78. In addition to the *Revue internationale de sociologie* article cited in note 12, see Pichou, "La religion de l'élite," *Chronique médicale*, 14(1907), 597–618. These articles also signaled the beginning of a cumulative awareness of eugenic ideas. For example, the 1905 article on Pichou in *Chronique médicale* featured a long quote from Royer's 1862 preface to Darwin, and on the occasion of the 1912 London eugenics congress, the same journal noted the earlier proposals of Pichou. See *Chronique médicale* 19(1912), 606.

15 The most extensive work based on the papers of Lapouge has been by Jean Boissel, "Autour du gobinisme," *Annales du CESERE*, 4(1981), 91–120; "Georges Vacher de Lapouge: Un socialiste revolutionnaire Darwinien," *Nouvelle école*, 38(1982), 59–84; and "A propos de l'indice céphalique," *Revue d'histoire des sciences*, 35(1982), 289–317. See also Guy Thullier, "Un anarchiste positiviste: Georges Vacher de Lapouge," in *L'idée de race dans la pensée politique française contemporaine*, ed. Pierre Guiral and Emile Temine (Paris: Editions du CNRS, 1977), 48–65; Andre Bejin, "Le sang, le sens, et le travail," *Cahiers internationaux de sociologie*, 72 (1982), 325–45; Gunter Nagel, *Georges Vacher de Lapouge: Sozialdarwinismus in Frankreich* (Freiburg: Schulz Verlag, 1975); and Clark, 143–54, which utilizes material in the ministry of public instruction archives. For an exhaustive bibliography, see Henri de la Haye Jousselin, *Georges Vacher de Lapouge (1854–1936). Essai de bibliographie* (Paris: n.p., 1986); and for recent interpretations, see Pierre-André Taquiett ed., *G. Vacher de Lapouge et l'anthroposociologie en France* (Paris: Editions du CNRS, in press).

16 For example, see Jean Colombat, *La fin du monde civilisé* (Paris: Vrin, 1947).
17 Thullier, 53; Boissel, "Georges Vacher de Lapouge," 61–62.
18 See Thullier, 57 on Lapouge's application for a chair at the Museum of Natural History in 1909.
19 Vacher de Lapouge, *L'aryen et son rôle social* (Paris: A. Fontemoing, 1899), 464–81.
20 Cited in Clark, 153.
21 The complete text was published as "L'anthropologie et la science politique–leçon d'ouverture du cours libre d'anthropologie de 1886–87," *Revue d'anthropologie* (March 15, 1887), 136–57.
22 This is essentially the heart of his book *Sélections sociales*.
23 Lapouge, "La dépopulation de la France," *Revue d'anthropologie* (1887), 69–80. For background, see Nagel, 63–68.
24 Lapouge, *Sélections sociales*, 472–73.
25 See Jean Rostand, *Biologie et humanisme* (Paris: Gallimard, 1964), 161–65.
26 For a complete list see the bibliography in Jousselin and Lapouge's own *Resumé des travaux scientifiques* (Poitiers: Société d'imprimerie et de librairie, 1909), which he compiled for his application for the chair at the museum.
27 See, for example, Thullier, 53–57, and Clark, 144–45. The most devastating attack was by Léonce Manouvrier of the Ecole d'anthropologie who challenged Lapouge's claims of scientific proof in craniometry. See Manouvrier, "L'indice céphalique et la pseudo-sociologie," *Revue anthropologique*, 9(1899), 233–59, 280–96.
28 Benjamin Weill-Hallé, "La puericulture et son evolution," *Presse médicale*, 37(1929), 217. Alfred Caron, *L'hygiène des nouveau-nés dans ses rapports avec le developpement physique et moral des individus au point de vue de l'amélioration de l'éspèce* (Paris: Plon, 1858), and *Introduction à la puericulture et l'hygiène de la prémière enfance* (Paris: n.p., 1865). Caron, *Puericulture ou la science d'élever hygiéniquement et physiologiquement les enfants*, 2nd ed. (Rouen: E. Orville, 1866).
29 Weill-Hallé, 217.
30 Victor Wallich, "Au propos de l'histoire de la puericulture," *Annales de gynécologie et d'obstétrique*. 2e sér., 3(1906), 20.
31 Weill-Hallé, 217; Wallich, 19.
32 For more on Pinard's background, see Chapter 4.
33 Wallich, 23–24.
34 Pinard, "De la conservation et l'amélioration de l'espèce," *Bulletin médical*, 13(1899), 141.
35 His classic study was "Note sur l'allaitement des nouveaux-nés," *Bulletin de l'academie de médecine*, 3e sér., 28(1892), 99–114.
36 Philippe Ariés, *Centuries of childhood* (London: Jonathan Cape, 1962); André Armengaud, "L'attitude de la société à l'égard de l'enfant au XIXe siècle," *Annales de démographie historique*, 10(1973), 303–12. George Sussman, *Selling mother's milk* (Champaign-Urbana: University of Illi-

nois Press, 1982) also points to more concrete economic facts accompanying this broad trend to explain the passage of laws on wet nursing. For more specific criticisms of Pinard, see Offen, and Mary Lynn McDougall, "Protecting infants: The French campaign for maternity leaves, 1890–1913," *French historical studies,* 13(1983), 94–96.

37 Pinard, "De l'assistance des femmes enceintes," *Revue d'hygiène* 12(1890), 1102.

38 Ibid., 1107–08, 1111–12.

39 Pinard, "Note pour servir à l'histoire de la puericulture intra-uterine," *Bulletin de l'academie de médecine,* 3e sér., 34(1895), 593–94; *Revue scientifique,* 28(1890), 109. Strauss claimed priority of a few months for his refuge in an article entitled "Puericulture," which appeared in *Revue des revues.*

40 Pinard, "Note pour servir," 595. The definitive study was produced by Pinard's student Charles Bachimont, *Documents pour servir à l'histoire de la puericulture inter-uterine* (medical dissertation, University of Paris, 1898).

41 Pinard, "Note pour servir," 597. In the article from the December talk he stated simply, "A woman during gestation must not be overburdened." *Revue d'hygiène,* 17(1895), 1096.

42 Pinard, "A propos du developpement de l'enfant," *Revue scientifique,* 34(1896), 111.

43 Jacques Bertillon immediately seized upon the idea, even carrying it one step further by calling for an "industrialization" of child care in a nursery of factory proportions and layout. See "Puericulture à bon marché," *Revue d'hygiène,* 19(1897), 311–20. For Pinard's rebuttal, see ibid., 655–64. For indications of the wider impact of Pinard's revived puericulture, see Linda Clark, *Schooling the daughters of Marianne* (Albany: SUNY Press, 1984), 83–84, 94–96; McDougall, 94–96; and Offen, 653–54, 670–71.

44 Strauss, "La puericulture," 140. See McDougall, 79–105 for background on the campaign.

45 Wallich, 19.

46 *Congrès international d'hygiène scolaire,* 3(1910), 620.

47 Some examples are Virginie Alexandresco, "Enseignement officiel et particulier de la puericulture et vulgarisation de l'hygiène infantile en Roumanie," *Annales de médecine et de chirurgerie infantile,* 11(1907), 474–79; G. Arostegul, "Puericultura," *Gaceta medica catalana* 28(1905), 275–300; Maria Martinetti, "Sulla puericultura intrauterina," *Rivista di igiene e sanita pubblica* 12(1901), 940–53; "La puericultura en Mexico," *Gaceta medica de Mexico* 2e sér., 3(1903), 201–221. After the war and during the 1920s, additional articles were published on puericulture in Tunisia, Peru, Puerto Rico, Argentina, and Switzerland.

48 Pinard, "De la conservation," 144.

49 For an informed geneticist's view of the importance of Darwin to the history of heredity, see François Jacob, *The logic of life,* (New York: Random House, 1982), 172–77. It was not Darwin's ideas about heredity but rather their implications that added to the rising interest. For a survey of the growth of importance of heredity to social thought irre-

spective of Darwin, see Charles Rosenberg, "The bitter fruit: Heredity, disease and social thought in nineteenth-century America," *Perspectives in American history,* 8(1974), 189–235.

50 Ernst Mayr, *The growth of biological thought* (Cambridge, MA: Belknap Press, 1982), 633–41.

51 Peter J. Bowler, *The eclipse of Darwinism* (Baltimore: Johns Hopkins Press, 1983), 38–39; R. G. Swinburne, "Galton's law – formulation and development," *Annals of science,* 21(1965), 15–31; P. Froggatt and N. C. Nevin, "Galton's law of ancestral heredity – its influence on the early history of genetics," *History of science,* 4(1971), 1–27.

52 Among the more relevant of the many works on Zola are Henri Massis, *Comment Emile Zola composait ses romans* (Paris: Fasquelles, 1906); Henri Martineau, *Le roman scientifique d'Emile Zola* (Paris: Baillière, 1907); and a series of articles by Yves Malinas entitled "Zola et les hérédités imaginaires," *Ouest médical,* 24(1971), 549–59, 1105–09, 1323–37, 1403–10, 1477–83, 1615–21, 1785–90, 1937–46, 2101–16. Malinas subsequently published this work as *Zola et les hérédités imaginaires* (Paris: Expansion scientifique française, 1985).

53 Martineau, 87. Malinas notes that these were essentially the same as Darwin's categories.

54 These examples are taken from a list by Zola reproduced in Martineau, 85–86.

55 Emile Zola, *Docteur Pascal* (Paris: Garnier-Flammarion, 1975), 147–67.

56 See Rosenberg, 203; Bowler, *Eclipse of Darwinism;* and Bowler's more recent, *Theories of human evolution: A century of debate* (Baltimore: Johns Hopkins University Press, 1986). For more on the influence of neo-Lamarckism on eugenics, see William Schneider, "Towards the improvement of the human race: The history of eugenics in France," *Journal of modern history,* 54(1982), 270–75. The complicated question of the mechanism of heredity was further confused at the end of the nineteenth century by the development of the terms "neo-Darwinism" and "neo-Lamarckism," which were not only different from each other but quite different in important respects from the ideas of their namesakes. The main reason for the "neo" labels was Weismann's theory of continuous germ plasm, which challenged the inheritance of acquired characteristics that both Darwin and Lamarck had assumed. Of course, it was ultimately the acceptance of Weismann's new idea, subsequently corroborated by Mendel and the whole new science of modern genetics, that has made neo-Lamarckian ideas of the inheritance of acquired traits such a curiosity today. In addition, the long delay before any French researchers began working on the neo-Darwinian synthesis – the 1930s to be exact – has added to the anomaly of twentieth-century French biology. See Ernest Boesiger, "Evolutionary biology in France at the time of the evolutionary synthesis," in *The evolutionary synthesis* (Cambridge: Harvard University Press, 1982), ed. Ernst Mayr and William Provine, 322–28; and Camille Limoges, "A second glance at evolutionary biology in France," in Mayr and Provine, 309–21. This study does

not propose to resolve these questions or remake the image of French science, but it does underscore the fact that in terms of the science of the day, neo-Lamarckism, with its presumption of the inheritance of acquired characteristics, was the norm at the beginning of the twentieth century. Hence, it should not be surprising that Zola assumed it nor that Pinard incorporated it into his proto-eugenic idea of puericulture.

57 See the special issue on "Les néo-Lamarckiens français" in *Revue de synthèse*, 95–96(1979), 279–468; and for its continuing importance into the twentieth century, see Denis Buican, *L'Histoire de la génétique et de l'evolutionnisme en France* (Paris: PUF, 1984). On neo-Lamarckism and eugenics in the Soviet Union, see Loren Graham, "Science and values: The eugenics movement in Germany and Russia," *American historical review*, 82(1977), 1162–64. The best first-hand account of Lysenko is Zhores A. Medvedev, *The rise and fall of T. D. Lysenko* (New York: Praeger, 1969).

58 *Bulletin médical*, 13(1899), 141–46.

59 Ibid., 141. The quote is from an 1816 text by Gardien, *Traité complet d'accouchment et des mal des filles, des femmes et des enfants.*

60 Pinard, "Preservation," 144.

61 Ibid., 144–45.

62 Ibid., 145.

63 Interview with Pinard's grandson, Roger Couvelaire (October 1983); Pinard, "Preservation," 145–46.

64 *Bulletin de l'académie de médecine*, 3e sér., 43(1900), 618.

65 See Cazalis' remarks in *Bulletin de la société de prophylaxie sanitaire et morale*, 3(1903), 283. See also, ibid., 324–25, 372–79.

66 *Chronique médicale* 10(1903), 490–91.

67 Pinard, "Rapport sur un arrêté municipal pris par M. Morel de Villiers, médecin et maire de la commune de Villiers-le Duc (Côte-d'Or)," *Bulletin de l'académie de médecine*, 3e sér., 51(1904), 222–36; "Note sur les causes de la faible mortalité infantile dans la ville du Creusot," *Annales de gynécologie et d'obstétrique*, 62(1905), 523–30.

68 Pinard, "Des aptitudes du mariage envisagées au point de vue physique, moral et social," *Revue pratique d'obstétrique et de paediatrique*, 19(1906), 2.

69 Ibid., 8–10, 12.

70 Ibid., 14.

71 Ibid., 16. See also the report by Pinard and Charles Richet cited in Chapter 2.

72 Ibid., 16.

73 *Régénération*, 2e sér., no. 17(June 1906), 160.

74 M. Jarach, "Cours de puericulture," *Revue Pedagogique*, 42(1903), 67–68; 43(1904), 270–72.

75 Clark, *Schooling the daughters*, 83–84, cites archives of the publisher Armand Colin that indicate sales of nearly 100,000 copies of Pinard's book.

76 Fruhinsholz, 399–400. The quote is from Pinard.

77 March, "Deux congrès internationaux. L'hygiène sociale," *Revue politique et parlementaire*, 74(1912), 531–51. The Pearson book was translated as *La grammaire de la science* (Paris: Félix Alcan, 1912). On the importance of March's translation, see Alain Desrosiers, "Histoires de formes: Statistiques et sciences sociales avant 1940," *Revue française de sociologie*, 26(1985), 294–97. For more on March's background, see Chapter 4.

78 March, "Pour la race. Infertilité et puericulture," *Revue du mois*, 10(1910), 552–53.

79 Ibid, 585.

80 Papillaut, "Galton et la biosociologie," *Revue anthropologique*, 21(1911), 56–65. On Papillaut's international perspective see his report, "Le VIe congrès d'anthropologie criminelle," *Revue de l'ecole d'anthropologie [Revue anthropologique]*, 19,(1909), 28–40.

81 Pinard, "De l'eugénnetique," *Bulletin médical*, 26(1912), 1123–24.

82 Ibid., 1125. Emphasis in original.

83 Ibid., 1126.

CHAPTER 4

1 *Problems in eugenics. Papers communicated to the First International Eugenics Congress held at University of London, July 24–30, 1912* (London: Eugenics Education Society, 1912), xii–xiii. For a brief account of the French at the congress, see Jacques Léonard, "Le prémier congrès international d'eugénique et ses consequences française," *Histoire des sciences médicales*, 17(1983), 141–46.

2 *Journal*, May 10, 1912; July 25, 1912; July 26, 1912; July 27, 1912; July 28, 1912; *Journal des débats*, July 26, 1912, July 27, 1912; *Le matin*, July 25, 1912; July 27, 1912; July 30, 1912.

3 All of the papers with translations can be found in *Problems in eugenics*.

4 Frédéric Houssay, "Eugénique, sélection et determinisme des tares," in *Problems in eugenics*, 157.

5 Valentin Magnan and Alfred Filassier, "Alcoolisme et dégénérescence," in *Problems in eugenics*, 361. For background on Magnan, see Jacques Borel, *Du concept de dégénérescence à la notion d'alcoolisme dans la médecine contemporaine* (Montpellier: Causse et Cie, 1968), pp. 21–23, 36. Magnan is even more famous because of the students he trained, such as the founder of the French anti-alcoholic league, Paul-Marie Légrain (mentioned in Chapter 2), and the psychiatrist René Charpentier.

6 Magnan and Filassier, 362.

7 *Problems in eugenics*, 34.

8 Ibid., 21. For Manouvrier's earlier work, see Chapter 3 and Robert A. Nye, "Heredity or milieu: The foundation of modern European criminological theory," *Isis*, 67(1976), 341–44, 349–51.

9 *Problems in eugenics*, 33.

10 Houssay, 155.

11 *Eugénique*, 1(1913), 42.

12   *Eugénique*, 1(1913), 47.

13   Ibid., 13. As noted in Chapter 1, France was not the only country where the naming of the new field prompted a debate. See Loren R. Graham, "Science and values: The eugenics movement in Germany and Russia in the 1920s," *American historical review*, 82(1977), 1138–39. For England, see Michael Freeden, "Eugenics and progressive thought: A study in ideological affinity," *Historical journal* 22(1979), 645–46.

14   *Eugénique*, 1(1913), 53.

15   Lucien March, "Dépopulation et eugénique," *Eugénique*, 1(1913), 36–40. March had first heard of the Eugenics Record Office at the London eugenics congress in July. When a meeting of the International Congress of Hygiene and Demography brought him to the United States in September 1912, he wrote to Charles Davenport to arrange a visit to Cold Spring Harbor. See American Philosophical Society, Davenport Papers, March letter to Davenport, September 4, 1912.

16   Soloway, 122–23, finds physicians comprising one-quarter of the officers and council members of the Eugenics Education Society and 10 percent of its overall membership. For more extensive treatment of doctors in German eugenics, see Paul Weindling, "Die Preussische Medizinanverwaltung und die 'Rassenhygiene,' " *Zeitschrift für Sozialreform*, 20(1984), 675–87.

17   Weindling, 677. This is also based on copies of material supplied by Sheila Weiss from the Ploetz family archives. Mackenzie, 504, finds only five women in the leadership of the British movement.

18   *Revue anthropologique*, 51(1941), 195–96.

19   See *Eugénique*, 2(1914–22), 87, and inside back cover for an example of the subscription notice.

20   *Eugénique*, 3(1922–26), 89.

21   The exact figures are:

Year	Dues (in francs)	Total budget (in francs)
1913	2,020	4,153
1914	1,860	2,944
1920	1,224	1,911
1921	1,310	2,267
1922	1,093	2,143
1923	1,236	4,447
1924	1,056	3,287
1925	940	4,162

22   *Eugénique*, 2(1914–22), 87. Juliette Reinach was the mother of the deputy Joseph Reinach and the sister-in-law of Baron Jacques Reinach who was implicated in the Panama Scandal. The participation of Jews in the French eugenics movement, although ironic given later developments, was not unique. They were also in German and American organizations, at least in their early years, and some Jews pointed with pride to

the eugenic character of many Jewish customs. See, for example, Max Reichler, *Jewish eugenics* (New York: Bloch Publishing, 1916).

23 Eugène Apert et al., *Eugénique et sélection* (Paris: Félix Alcan, 1922). The importance of royalty income is evident from the fact that in 1923 the royalties of 1,900 francs exceeded membership dues of 1,236 francs.

24 *Eugénique*, 3(1922–26), 244–45.

25 *Lois et décrets* [hereafter cited as J. O.] (1925): 353.

26 *Eugénique*, 2(1914–22), 91.

27 MacKenzie, 503; Haller, 20, 73.

28 For an excellent study of why grass-roots organizations were inimical to the French setting, see Robert J. Bezucha, "The moralization of society: The enemies of popular culture in the nineteenth century," in *The wolf and the lamb: Popular culture in France*, ed. Jacques Beauroy, Marc Bertrand, and Edward T. Gargan (Saratoga: Anima Libri, 1976), 175–87.

29 J. O. Documents parlementaires. Chambre (1926), 31. The speech he gave introducing the bill was reprinted in *Eugénique*, 3(1922–26), 195–204. The *Dictionnaire des parlementaires français*, 1889–1940, 7, 270–71, calls Pinard's election to the Chamber "the consecration of a particularly brilliant scientific and medical career."

30 *Eugénique*, 2(1914–22), 123, 246; 3(1922–26), 35.

31 *Academie des sciences. Comptes-rendus des séances*, 115(1892), 1049; 157(1913), 1370; 160(1915), 16.

32 Lucien Cuénot, *Invention et finalité en biologie* (Paris: Flammarion, 1941), 126, called Perrier an "ultra-Lamarckian." See also Robert E. Stebbins, "France" in *The comparative reception of Darwinism*, Thomas F. Glick, ed. (Austin: University of Texas Press, 1972), 139–41; and Yvette Conry, *L'introduction du darwinisme en France au XIXe siècle* (Paris: Vrin, 1974), 382–85. Perrier is also the subject of an article by Claude Blanckaert, "Edmond Perrier et l'étiologie du 'polyzoisme' organique," *Revue de synthèse*, 95–96(1979), 353–76, a special issue devoted to French neo-Lamarckians.

33 Stebbins, 140–41.

34 *A travers le monde vivant* (Paris: Flammarion, 1916), *La vie en action* (Paris: Flammarion, 1918), and *Les origines de la vie et de l'homme* (Paris: Flammarion, 1920).

35 Martial Dumont and Pierre Morel, *Histoire de l'obstétrique et de la gynécologie* (Lyon: SIMEP Editions, 1968), 74–75. There is no full-length biography of Pinard, but among the best short accounts are P. Bar, "Adolphe Pinard," *Gynécologie et obstétrique*, 29(1934), 497–512; and Albert Fruhinsholz, "Adolphe Pinard, puericulteur français," *Médecine de France*, 21(1951), 3–9.

36 Fruhinsholz, 3.

37 Archives Nationales, AJ 16, carton 6519, "Dossier personnel d'Adolphe Pinard". The visit was in January. Alexis was born in August, and the Czar later made a generous donation to Pinard's Baudelocque Clinic. There is an irony in the fact that the infant's inherited hemophilia was

318   Notes for pp. 101–105

as unaffected by Pinard's puericulture as Pinard's Lamarckism was
uneffected by this striking example of Mendelian inheritance.

38 In addition to published material cited earlier, the following is also based
on interviews with two of Pinard's grandsons – Pierre Morax and Roger
Couvelaire. Couvelaire authored an unpublished biography of Pinard
entitled "Epigrammes familiales et violons imaginaires."

39 Pinard, "Note pour servir à l'histoire de la puericulture intra-uterine,"
Bulletin de l'academie de médecine, 3e sér., 34(1895), 593–97.

40 See Pinard, *La puericulture du premier âge*, 6th ed. (Paris: Armand Colin,
1913). See Chapter 3 for background.

41 Bar, 507.

42 There is a good deal of biographical material on Richet, but it is very
uneven and incomplete. A lengthy entry in the *Dictionary of scientific
biography* is a good introduction, and Richet himself published at least
two autobiographical accounts of his life, *Souvenirs d'un physiologiste*
(Yonne: J. Peyronnet, 1933) and "Charles Richet, autobiographie," in
Les biographies médicales, ed. P. Busquet and Maurice Genty (Paris: J.-B.
Ballière, 1932), 5:157–88. Richet is also the subject of a short medical
thesis by Marilisa Juri, *Charles Richet, physiologiste, 1850–1935* (Zurich:
Juris Druck, 1965). The following is also based on interviews with two
Richet grandsons – Gabriel and Denis Richet. From among the family
papers, they were kind enough to show me an unpublished autobiog-
raphy, "Souvenirs sur moi et les autres," written shortly after the First
World War, and later used by Richet as the basis of part of his autobiography, *Souvenirs d'un physiologiste*.

43 An ardent republican, Richet liked to cite the fact that after the coup
d'état of 1851, it was in his grandfather's court that Louis Napoleon
had to justify his military takeover. See Richet, "Autobiographie,"
157.

44 *Le peuple*, December 5, 1935.

45 The obituaries of Richet invariably referred to his breadth of interests
as being "encyclopedic," the product of a "universal curiosity." Henri
Roger, "Charles Richet," *Presse médical*, 43(1935), 2045; M. Archard,
"Décès de M. Charles Richet," *Comptes rendus de la société de biologie*,
120 (1935), 927; André Meyer, "Notice nécrologique sur M. Charles
Richet (1850–1935)," *Bulletin de l'académie de médecine*, 115(1936), 53.
Gustave-Roussy, secretary general of the Academy of Medicine chose
Richet as the subject of his annual eulogy in 1945 and compared him to
such Renaissance men as Leonardo da Vinci, Erasmus, and Vesalius,
because of "the diversity of the fields where his intelligence satisfied
itself." Gustave Roussy, "Charles Richet (1850–1935)," *Bulletin de l'a-
cadémie de médecine*, 129(1945), 720. André Meyer's 1935 obituary concluded with a long quote from Diderot's *Encyclopédie* entry for "genius," a term he thought particularly appropriate for Richet.

46 Richet, *Souvenirs d'un physiologiste*, 147–50. The article was "Du som-
nambulisme provoqué," *Journal de l'anatomie et de la physiologie normale
et pathologique de l'homme et des animaux*, 11(1875), 348–78.

47 *Souvenirs,* 152–53. Other scientists Richet introduced to psychism included Camille Hammarion and the Curies.

48 Roussy, 730; Roger, 2044.

49 *Souvenirs,* 139.

50 Letter in Richet family papers. Bertha von Suttner, of course, had received the Peace Prize herself in 1905.

51 The article was published in *Revue de tuberculose* (1912). See also Landouzy, "Aperçus de médecine sociale," *Revue de médecine* 25(1905), 955–77, and "A propos de l'hérédité et de sa signification clinique," *Revue pratique d'obstétrique et de gynécologie* (1906), 94–96. An example of the biographical notices at his death is Maurice Letulle, "L'oeuvre de Landouzy," *Presse médicale,* 26(1917), 265–67.

52 See especially his report to the Senate, *Commission de la dépopulation. Sous-commission de la natalité. Rapport sur les causes professionelles de la dépopulation* (Melun: Imprimerie administrative, 1905). On March and the Statistique générale, see Michel Huber, "Quarante années de la Statistique générale de la France, 1896–1936," *Journal de la société statistique de Paris,* 38 (1937), 179–89. Huber also wrote an obituary notice that includes an extensive list of March's published work, "Lucien March, 1859–1933," *Journal de la société statistique de Paris,* 32(1933), 269–80.

53 Lucien March, "La comité eugénique internationale permanente," *Eugénique,* 1(1913), 146–60; "Les infirmités mentales en Angleterre et l'act de 1913," *Eugénique,* 2(1914–22), 108–18; P.-L. Ladame, "L'alcool et l'eugénique. Alcoolisme et divorce," *Eugénique,* 1(1913), 177–91; and C. W. Saleeby, "Les progrès de l'eugénique," *Eugénique,* 2(1914–22), 1–16.

54 Adolphe Landry, "Eugénique," *Revue bleu* (1913), 779–83.

55 J. Laumonnier, "Eugénique," *Larousse mensuel* (July 1912), 454–55.

56 Adolphe Pinard, "De l'eugénetique," *Bulletin médical,* 26(1912), 1123–24.

57 For an example of a review, see Georges Bohn's in *Mercure de France* (1919), 506–508. Edouard Jordan's, "Eugénisme et morale," *Cahiers de la nouvelle journée,* 19(1931), 1–176 was the most thorough critique of eugenics in France, and used Richet's book as a point of departure.

58 Charles Richet, *La sélection humaine* (Paris: Félix Alcan, 1919), 15.

59 Ibid., 29.

60 Ibid., 30.

61 Ibid., 32.

62 In fact, whole chapters were devoted to each of these topics. See 113–30.

63 Ibid., 62.

64 Ibid., 89–93.

65 Ibid., 64–65.

66 Ibid., 170.

67 Ibid., 191–93.

68 Ibid., 189.

69 Ibid., 166–67.

CHAPTER 5

1   In addition to the references cited in Chapter 2, n. 115, see Just Sicard de Plauzoles, *Principes d'hygiène sociale* (Paris: Editions médicales, 1927), 44.

2   *Larousse du XXe siècle* (1930), 3: 1108; *Alliance d'hygiène sociale* (Paris: Musée sociale, 1904), 3.

3   Emile Duclaux, *Hygiène sociale* (Paris: Félix Alcan, 1902), 5.

4   The term was first used by Gordon Wright to describe the Second World War in *Ordeal of total war, 1939–1945* (New York: Harper and Row, 1968); but textbooks such as Joseph R. Strayer and Hans W. Gatzke, *The mainstream of civilization*, 4th ed. (New York: Harcourt Brace Jovanovich, 1984), 699, now apply the term to the First World War.

5   The literature on the subject is vast, beginning with Michel Huber's *La population de la France pendant la guerre* (Paris: PUF, 1931). For a more recent interpretation, see Colin Dyer, *Population and society in twentieth century France* (New York: Holmes and Meier, 1978), 5–63. For repercussions among natalists, see J. M. Winter, "The fear of population decline in western Europe, 1870–1940," in *Demographic patterns in developed societies*, ed. R. W. Hiorns (London: Taylor and Francis, 1980), 173–97.

6   Charles Richet, "Mémoires sur moi et les autres" (unpublished manuscript), Chapter 7, 37.

7   Ibid., Chapter 7, 90. Richet filled a page in his "Mémoires" with the names of close friends whose sons also died in the war.

8   Dyer, 50.

9   *Eugénique*, 2(1914–22), 247. The words are those of Georges Papillaut.

10 Robert Talmy, *Histoire du mouvement familiale en France, 1896–1939* (Paris: Aubenas, 1962), 2: 5–6.

11 Ibid., 2: 14–37. For other natalist activity in the 1930s, see Françoise Thébaud, "Le mouvement nataliste dans la France de l'entre-deux-guerres," *Revue d'histoire moderne et contemporaine*, 32(1985), 298–91.

12 See Francis Ronsin, "Liberté – natalité. Réaction et répression anti-malthusien avant 1920," in *Haleine des faubourgs*, ed. Lion Murard and Patrick Zylberman (Fontenay-sur-bois: La recherche, 1978), 388–91; and Ronsin, *Grèves des ventres* (Paris: Aubier Montaigne, 1980), 137–47; 193–208.

13 Quoted in Ronsin, "Liberté – natalité," 390.

14 For a complete list of these measures, see France. Ministère de la santé. Bulletin du secretariat d'état à la santé, *Receuil des textes officiels concernant la protection de la santé publique* (Paris: Imprimerie Nationale, 1942).

15 Lucien March, "Some attempts toward race hygiene in France during the war," *Eugenics review*, 10(1918), 198–200.

16 Ibid., 204.

17 Ibid., 201–202.

18 Talmy, 1:212–17. On Bréton, see *Dictionnaire des parlementaires français*.

19 Talmy, 1:217–20.

20 Talmy, 1:211–17.
21 France. Archives nationales. Série AJ 16 (hereafter cited as AN AJ 16), folder 6558, letter from ministère de la santé to ministère de l'instruction publique, February 5, 1920; accord signed April 29, 1922.
22 Cited in France. *Journal officiel*, Dec. 1924. The date of creation was September 7, 1920.
23 AN AJ 16, 6559, letter from Marfan to dean of Faculty of Medicine, November 6, 1918.
24 Fernand Cattier, "Enseignement de la puericulture," *Revue pedagogique*, 85(1924), 132–38.
25 Linda Clark, *Schooling the daughters of Marianne* (Albany: SUNY Press, 1984), 96.
26 AN AJ 16, procès-verbaux du Conseil de la faculté de médecine, 6276 (December 11, 1924). A compromise was worked out in 1928 whereby Pinard remained ceremonial director and Weil-Hallé the assistant director, AN AJ 16, 6277 (December 8, 1927); AN AJ 6559, convention signed between the Ecole de puericulture and the Faculté de médecine, March 30, 1928. At the death of Pinard, Weil-Hallé assumed the title of director, but only after the statutes were changed so that the director did not also have to be a member of the faculty. The dean wrote Weill-Hallé, "I am happy to see terminated so favorably this affair so long in suspense." Weill-Hallé thus never became a member of the faculty. A final irony was that Weill-Hallé was forced to resign as director of the Ecole de puericulture in 1940 because of the law of October 3, 1940 banning Jews from holding government posts, and Alexandre Couvelaire, Pinard's son-in-law, took over from him. See AN AJ 16, 6559, "Ecole de puericulture – personnel et credits." For Weill-Hallé's version of the creation of the Ecole de puericulture, see "La puericulture et son evolution," *Presse médicale*, 37 (February 16, 1929), 217–20; and "L'Ecole de puericulture," *Revue française de puericulture*, 1(1933), 21–41.
27 AN AJ 16, 6559.
28 *Revue de l'alliance nationale contre la dépopulation* (1916), 125.
29 Ibid.
30 Ibid., 189–90.
31 J. Dassonville and L. DeGeuser, *Les lauréats des prix Cognacq-Jay* (Paris: Eds. Spes, 1926).
32 Foundation Ungemach – acte de donation (Jan. 7, 1920), in Archives municipale, ville de Strasbourg (hereafter cited as AMVS), dossier J 427–2997.
33 See also *Illustration* (March 30, 1929), 339–40, and for lavish pictures, see *Répertoire de l'architecture: La cité jardin*, ed. Jean Virette (Paris: Editions de Bonadona, n.d.). For another foreign view, see *New York Times*, August 30 and September 27, 1931.
34 AMVS, Dossier J, 427–2997, minutes of foundation council, December 13, 1924.
35 Ibid., November 16, 1925.

36 AMVS, dossier J, 427–2997, "Renseignements eugéniques."

37 Anthony Sutcliffe, *Towards the planned city: Germany, Britain, the United States and France, 1780–1914* (New York: St. Martins, 1981), 126–62, 189–94. Sutcliffe also offers an excellent introduction and comparison with the broader movement, as does Daniel Schaffer, *Garden cities for America* (Philadelphia: Temple University Press, 1982) and Dugald MacFadyen, *Sir Ebenezer Howard and the town planning movement* (Manchester: Manchester University Press, 1970).

38 Sutcliffe, 146–52.

39 See Larry V. Thompson, " 'Lebensborn' and the eugenic policy of the 'Reichsfuhrer-SS'," *Central European history*, 4(1971), 54–77; and Georg Lilienthal, *Der Lebensborn* (Stuttgart: G. Fischer, 1985).

40 AMVS, dossier J, 427–2997, minutes of foundation, February 2, 1929; October 31, 1920.

41 Paul Popenoe and Roswell Johnson, *Applied eugenics* (New York; MacMillan 1920), 339.

42 I am grateful to Daniel Kevles for first pointing this out. See the correspondence of C. P. Blacker and Dachert in Contemporary Medical Archive Centre (London), and *Nations Unies. Cycles d'études sociales européennes, Division des activités sociales* (November 26–December 10, 1949). As planned, Ungemach Gardens was turned over to the city in 1950, and remains that way to the present.

43 *Eugénique*, 2(1914–22), 248.

44 Ibid., 247.

45 Quoted in *Eugénique*, 3, 200.

46 *Eugénique*, 3(1924), 204. For a review of the book, which was called *Eugénique et sélection*, ed. Eugène Apert (Paris: Félix Alcan, 1922), see *Mercure de France* (1923): 482–86.

47 The pages of the English *Eugenics review* and the American *Eugenical news* carried a running discourse on this problem throughout the war years. Examples of the English articles are Theodore Chambers, "Eugenics and the war," 6(1914–15), 272–90; Leonard Darwin, "Eugenics during and after the war," 7(1915–16), 91–106; E. B. Poulton, "The disabled sailor and soldier and the future of our race," 9(1917–18), 218–22; and J. A. Lindsay, "The eugenic and social influence of the war," 10(1918–19), 133–44. Lucien March even joined the debate with "Some attempts towards race hygiene in France during the war," 10(1918–19), 195–212.

48 Richet, *Le passé de la guerre et l'avenir de la paix* (Paris: Ollendorff, 1907), 87–88.

49 Perrier, "Eugénique et biologie," in *Eugénique et sélection*, 2.

50 Ibid., 20.

51 Apert, "Eugénique et santé nationale," in ibid., 60.

52 Ibid., 69. He had first offered this reassurance during the war in an article for *Monde médical* (November 15, 1916). French eugenicists did not, however, see these effects of the war as a grotesque repetition on

humans of Weismann's original experiments cutting tails off mice without producing a tailless offspring.

53 Ibid., 60.
54 This was a reference to the common assumption at the time that fresh air was a cure for tuberculosis and other diseases. Apert's mention of housing makes the lack of awareness of Ungemach Gardens all the more ironic.
55 Ibid., 72–73.
56 Lucien March, "Natalité et eugénique," ibid., 97–98.
57 Georges Schreiber, "Eugénique et mariage," ibid., 172–82.
58 For new members at meetings from May 1922 to December 1923, see *Eugénique*, 2(1914–22), 53, 131,149.
59 Ibid., 247.
60 The best and most complete description of the program is a medical thesis by one of the participants, Alexandre Bruno, *Contre la tuberculose. La mission Rockefeller en France et l'effort français* (Paris: Villages sanatoriums de hautes altitudes, 1925). More widely published accounts can be found in Charles Nordmann, "La croisade des américains contre la tuberculose en France," *Revue scientifique*, 47(1918), 457–68; and Linsly R. Williams, "La fondation Rockefeller dans la lutte contre la tuberculose en France," *Revue du musée social* (1922), 33–64. The first results of a recent reassessment of the subject by Murard and Zylberman are "L'autre guerre (1914–18): France sous l'oeil de l'Amérique," *Revue d'histoire*, 276(1986), 367–98; and "La mission Rockefeller en France et la création du comité national de defense contre la tuberculose (1917–23)," *Revue d'histoire moderne et contemporaine*, 34(1987), 257–81.
61 Letter from Warwick Greene to Jerome Greene, July 13, 1916, Rockefeller Foundation Archives (hereafter referred to as RA), RG 1.1, series 500T, folder 247.
62 Report by Wallace C. Sabine, August 4, 1916. RA RG 1.1, series 500T, folder 247. The sending of Sabine to investigate conditions in France was the first response of the foundation's board of directors to Greene's recommendation.
63 *Bulletins des textes officiels concernant la protection de la santé publique*, 4(1911–20), 386, 451, 453–56.
64 Examples of these and others liberally illustrate the Bruno book. A more complete collection of posters can be found in RA, RG 1.1, series 500T France, map cabinet drawer 7, folders 1 and 2.
65 November 30, 1918, as cited by *Rockefeller Foundation annual report* (1918), 27–28.
66 Williams, 36–37.
67 Williams, 50–54; *Rockefeller annual report* (1918), 25–27.
68 *Rockefeller annual report* (1925), 290–91.
69 November 30, 1918, as cited in *Rockefeller annual report*, (1918), 27–28.
70 On Gunn, see *Dictionary of American biography*, suppl. 3, 323–25.

71 LRW [Linsly R. Williams], "Memoire on hygiene in France," March 6, 1922, RA, RG 1.1, 500L, box 13 folder 131.

72 LRW, "General remarks concerning the present situation of the ministry of health and statements concerning the more important needs as visualized by the minister," August 17, 1922, ibid.

73 Gunn letters to Russel, September 2, September 9, 1924, plus attachments of Godart decrees, RA, RG 1.1, 500L, box 13, folder 151.

74 January 6, 1926 attachment to Gunn letter to Russel, December 21, 1925, RA, RG 1.1, 500L, box 13, folder 152.

75 *J. O. Lois et décrets,* (December 9, 1924), 10803.

76 RA, RG 1.1, 500L, box 13, file 151.

77 *J. O. Lois et décrets. Annexe.* (November 11, 1926), 926.

78 *J. O. Lois et décrets. Annexe II* (August 20, 1932), 763–67.

79 The number of representatives from these organizations on the council of the propaganda service ran to twenty-five.

80 *J. O. Lois et décrets. Annexe,* (August 26, 1933), 927–28.

CHAPTER 6

1 For an introduction to the politics of the late Third Republic, see Philippe Bernard and Henri Dubief, *The decline of the Third Republic, 1914–1938* (Cambridge, England: Cambridge University Press, 1985).

2 Yvonne Carniol-Dreyfus, "Le certificat d'examen médical prenuptial," *Prophylaxie sanitaire et morale,* 26(1954), 124–29. The article was based on a 1953 law thesis at Dijon.

3 *Société de prophylaxie sanitaire et morale. Bulletin,* 3(1903), 271–324, 339–85, 392–420, 470–88, 531–54; "Le mariage, doit-il être réglementé?" *Chronique médicale,* 10(1903), 449–95.

4 Georges Schreiber, "Examen médical prenuptial devant la société française d'eugénique," *Vie médicale,* 7(1926), 2412, which cited a talk by René Sand at the 1926 meeting of the International Eugenics Federation in Paris. The British were also interested in the American marriage laws, as indicated by R. Newton Crane, "Marriage laws and statutory experiments in the United States," *Eugenics review,* 2(1910), 61–73. No less a figure than Charles Davenport had whetted the European appetite for information about the American marriage laws in his talk at the 1912 London eugenics congress, "Marriage laws and customs," in *Problems in eugenics* (London: Eugenics Education Society, 1912), 151–55.

5 Charles Richet, *Sélection humaine,* (Paris: Félix Alcan, 1919), 176.

6 Richet, "Sélection humaine," in *Eugénique et sélection,* ed. Eugéne Apert (Paris: Masson, 1922), 49–50. The talk was originally given at the University of Utrecht, but was reprinted in the volume from the 1920–21 Eugenics Society conferences. Curiously enough, Richet learned to swim only at a very advanced age, but he was obviously quite proud of his lately acquired ability.

7 Schreiber, "Eugénique et mariage," in ibid., 163.

8   Ibid., 164–66. For more on these policies from a broader perspective, see Colin Dyer, *Population in twentieth-century France* (New York: Holmes and Meier, 1978), 29–56.
9   Schreiber, "Eugénique et mariage," 175, 182.
10 *Problems in Eugenics*, 151–55.
11 *Revue anthropologique*, 31(1921), 452–59.
12 For examples, see *Eugénique*, 2(1914–22), 190–91; 3(1922–26), 57–58, 97, 176. In the last part of the 1920s when a law was under discussion in France, a survey of legislation in other countries was an almost mandatory preface to any serious examination of the subject.
13 *Eugénique*, 3(1922–26), 52–53.
14 Ibid., 87.
15 Ibid., 88.
16 Ibid., 136.
17 Ladislaus Haskovec, "Le certificat médical prematrimonial," *Institut international d'anthropologie. 2e session de Prague, 14–21 septembre 1924* (Paris: Noury, 1926), 455–59.
18 Henri Vignes, "Certificat de mariage ou vulgarisation des notions d'eugéniques," ibid., 459–96.
19 Ibid., 460.
20 Ibid., 472–78.
21 See, for example, Paul Thomas, "Le certificat d'aptitude matrimoniale," *Vie médicale*, 5(1924), 1621–22; L. Boulanger, "Au sujet du certificat d'aptitude matrimoniale," *Vie médicale*, 6(1925), 297–302.
22 *Eugénique* 3(1922–26), 249.
23 *Eugénique*, 3(1922–26), 281. On the Musée social, see Sanford Elwitt, "Social reform and social order in late nineteenth century France: The musée social and its friends," *French historical studies*, 11(1980), 431–51; and Anthony Sutcliffe, *Towards the planned city* (New York: St. Martins, 1981), 148–52.
24 C. B. S. Haldane, "Report of the meeting of the International Federation of Eugenics Organizations," *Eugenical news*, 11(1926), 137–39. Talks were given by Maurice Letulle, Louis Heuyer, and Léon Bernard as well as by Schreiber.
25 J. O. Lois et décrets, (November 16, 1942). It is, of course, just as significant that the premarital examination law did not herald the beginning of extensive eugenic laws in France. One reason was that the initiators of the legislation made the measure mild enough and broad enough to rally support from public health lobbyists; hence, without follow-up, it would remain a public health measure. The eugenic excesses of the Nazis insured that subsequent legislation was not forthcoming.
26 *Eugénique*, 3(1922–26), 267–68.
27 These papers, along with some from the July congress of the International Eugenics Federation meeting, were published in a book, *Examen médicale en vue de mariage* (Paris: Flammarion, 1927). Schreiber summarized both conferences in *Bulletin médical*, 41(1927), 170–74.
28 Ibid.

29 Louis Forest, "L'utilité de l'examen médical en vue de mariage," in *Examen médical*, 35.

30 Louis Heuyer, "Conditions de santé à envisager au point de vue du mariage dans les maladies mentales et nerveuses et les intoxications," in *Examen médical*, 135–36.

31 March, "Conclusions générales," in *Examen médical*, 244.

32 *Eugénique*, 3(1926), 285.

33 *Vie médicale*, 7(1926), 2414.

34 Comité national d'études sociales et politiques, *Mariage et certificat prénuptial* (June 4, 1928), 29.

35 Ibid., 28–29.

36 J. O. Documents parlementaires. Chambre, (January 1927).

37 June 1, 1927, 579.

38 Just Sicard de Plauzoles, "Le droit à la vie saine," *Cahiers des droits de l'homme*, 27(1927), 103. This and subsequent league positions are summarized in *Prohphylaxie antivénérienne*, 1(1929), 318–20.

39 Siredey repeated his objections in the Comité nationales d'études sociales et politiques session on the premarital examination, 30–33.

40 J. O. *Documents parlementaires. Chambre*, (1927), no. 3585, annexe no. 5172, 372.

41 Ibid., 377.

42 Ibid., 376.

43 Ibid., 378.

44 Ibid.

45 *Revue anthropologique*, 38(1928), 300.

46 Ibid., 302.

47 *Bulletin de la société médicale de S. Luc. S. Côme et S. Damen*, 35(1929), 41. For another example of a more widely read critical account, see Henri Bouquet, "Chronique," *Monde médical*, 38(1928), 425–28.

48 Comité nationales d'études sociale et politiques, 23–33.

49 *Revue anthropologique*, 39(1929), 311.

50 Edgar Leroy, "Le certificat prénuptial à la campagne," *Mouvement sanitaire*, 6(1930), 76.

51 Louis Verwaeck and Jules LeClercq, "Le certificat prénuptial," *Annales de médecine legale*, 9(1929), 297–337.

52 Ibid., 337.

53 See, for example, Sicard de Plauzoles, "Le certificat prénuptial," *Prophylaxie antivénérienne*, 1(1929), 347–52; F. Legueu, "Le certificat prénuptial," *Progrès médical*, 44(1929), 2273–78; Edgar Leroy, "Le certificat à la campagne," *Mouvement sanitaire*, 9(1930), 75–83. In addition, see summaries of such articles as F. Imianitoff, "L'examen médical prénuptial," *Le scalpel*, (February 1, 1930); "Le certificat prénuptial," *Le quotidien* (July 27, 1930), and Edouard Jordan, *Eugénisme et morale*, (Paris: Blond and Gay, 1931), 52–88.

54 *Prophylaxie antivénérienne*, 2 (1930), 321. Jordan reproduced an interview by Couvelaire in a July 1930 issue of *Oeuvre*, Jordan, 54–56.

55 *Revue anthropologique*, 40(1930).

56 The president of the commission was Eugenics Society member Georges-Risler, and two vice presidents were Louis Forest and Louis Queyrat, both of whom spoke at the 1926 conference on the premarital examination.

57 J. O. *Documents parlementaires. Sénat*, (1932), 31.

58 The theses included G. Brandenburg, "Du certificat d'aptitude du mariage," (Paris, 1926); Bouessel du Bruy, "De la necessité du certificat prenuptial" (Paris, 1927); Laure Biardeau, "Le certificat prénuptial," (Paris, 1930); Jacques Etienne, "Du certificat prénuptial," (Paris, 1931); Nicholas Popovsky, "Contribution à l'étude des législations français qui pourra intervenir à l'occasion d'un examen pré-nuptial" (Paris, 1932); André Raynaud, "Contribution à l'étude du certificat prénuptial," (Marseilles, 1933); Pauli Flloko, "Protection de la race et le certificat prénuptial," (Paris, 1934); Max Gebuhrer, "Contribution à la question du certificat prénuptial," (Strasbourg, 1935); Juan Anias, "Contribution à l'étude du certificat prénuptial," (Paris, 1935); Jacques Conray, "L'examen prenuptial," (Lyons, 1938).

59 *Siècle médical* (July 15, 1928), 1.

60 Ibid. Of course, with the final qualifying clause, the statement was entirely true of Schreiber's attitude, but the headline and main clause calling him an "opponent" had a different effect.

61 André Toledano, "La question eugénique," *Revue de l'alliance nationale pour l'accroisement de la population française*, (1928), 53.

CHAPTER 7

1 See, for example, G. R. Searle, "Eugenics and politics in Britain in the 1930s," *Annals of science*, 36(1979), 159–69. Daniel Kevles, *In the name of eugenics* (New York: Knopf, 1985), 113–28, argues that the Depression strengthened the positions of both eugenicists and their opponents.

2 Autobiographical sketches by Louise Hervieu are contained in *Le malade vous parle* (Paris: Editions Nol, 1943). For an account of a conference organized by the Louise Hervieu Foundation with church and government officials in attendance (including Léon Blum), see "Le carnet de santé," *Prophylaxie antivénérienne*, 10(1938), 216–30. For an example of legislative measures proposed, see that of Jean Bernex in J. O. *Documents parlementaires. Chambre*, (1938), 530–31.

3 "Le carnet de santé," *Prophylaxie antivénérienne*, 11(1939), 437–44; 15(1943), 53–61.

4 See, for example, J. Laumonnier, "Eugénique," *Larousse mensuel*, no. 65(July 1912), 455; and Adolphe Landry, "Eugénique," *Revue bleue*, (1913), 782.

5 *Revue anthropologique*, 37(1927), 255–26.

6 Kenneth Ludmerer, *Eugenics and American society* (Baltimore: Johns Hopkins University Press, 1972), 127. On the overall political consequences of the Depression, see Julian Jackson, *The politics of depression*

in France. 1932–1936 (Cambridge, England: Cambridge University Press, 1985).

7   *Foules d'Asie* (Paris: A. Colin, 1930). Other examples of this 1930s version of the "Yellow Peril" are Henri Toulouse, "Le problème humaine," *Le journal* (November 2, 1931), p. 1; and Charles Richet, *Au secours* (Paris: Peyronnet, 1935), 111–22. For the influence of the Dennery book, see Gaston Bouthoul, *La population dans le monde* (Paris: Payot, 1935), especially the chapter entitled "La situation démographique en Europe et Asie," 69–87; or Just Sicard de Plauzoles, "L'avenir de l'éspèce humain. La surpopulation, c'est la guerre," *Prophylaxie antivénérienne,* 7(1935), 69–99. An example of a natalist response to this view is Paul Haury, "Une natalité suffisante, est-ce la guerre?" *Revue de l'alliance nationale contre la dépopulation,* 35(1934), 33–40.

8   Dennery, 238–39, as cited in Bouthoul, 87–88.

9   Ibid., 235. On the objectivity of Bouthoul's perspective, see J. M. Winter, "The fear of population decline in western Europe, 1870–1940," in R. W. Hiorns, ed., *Demographic patterns in developing societies* (London: Taylor and Francis, 1980), 176.

10 Bouthoul, 18.

11 Sicard de Plauzoles, 81; Toulouse, 1.

12 For the effects of the Depression on the natalists see Talmy, 1: 179–214. Françoise Thébaud's analysis of the Alliance nationale generally ignores the political activity and effect of the Depression, but she concludes, nevertheless that "The successes achieved were not equal to the activities undertaken." Thébaud, "Le mouvement nataliste dans la France de l'antre-deux-guerres: L'alliance nationale pour l'accroisement de la population française," *Revue d'histoire moderne et contemporaine,* 32(1985), 299.

13 Bouthoul, 234. In reality the figures were 40 million for France and slightly more than 60 million for Germany in the mid-1920s.

14 *Bulletin de l'academie de médecine,* 113(1935), 143. For a full account plus rejoinders, see 143–47, 219–27, 492–504, 516–19, and Paul Haury, "Le destin des races blanches," *Revue de l'alliance nationale contre la dépopulation* 36(1935), 267–72.

15 A. Laffont and J. Audit, "Eugénique," *Encyclopédie médico-chirurgicale* (Paris: Masson, 1934) 6–2: 10. This 24-page article is an excellent summary of favorable medical opinion of the day. On the Association d'études sexologiques, see n. 29.

16 "Hommage à Just Sicard de Plauzoles," *Prophylaxie antivénérienne,* 7(1938), 343–64.

17 *Cahiers des droits de l'homme* [hereafter cited as *Cahiers*] (1936), 308.

18 *Eugénique,* 3(1922–26), 53, 169–70.

19 France. AN AJ16, dossier 6273, "Procès-verbaux de la faculté de médecine," (November 17 and December 22, 1921).

20 *Prophylaxie antivénérienne,* 5(1933), 137–38.

21 *Principes d'hygiène* (Paris: Editions médicales, 1927).

22 Ibid., 16. See also the opening lecture of the 1927–28 social hygiene lectures entitled "La production du capital humain. L'avenir de la France,"

reprinted in ibid., 121–50. For the nineteenth-century precursors of this concept, see Lion Murard and Patrick Zyleberman, *Le petit travailleur indéfatigable* (Paris: Recherches, 1976).

23 Ibid., pp. 83–89.

24 Just Sicard de Plauzoles, "L'avenir et la préservation de la race: L'eugénique," *Prophylaxie antivénérienne*, 4(1932), 199–201.

25 Ibid.

26 Ibid., 210.

27 Plauzoles gives a table of figures for Paris, Vienna, London, and Berlin, but with no source cited. Henri-Jean Marchand, "L'évolution de l'idée eugénique" (medical dissertation, Bordeaux, 1933), 48–49, suggests that Sicard's source was Rainer Fetscher, *Grundzüge der Rassenhygiene* (Dresden: Deutsche Verlag für Volkswohlfahrt, 1924).

28 Sicard de Plauzoles, "L'avenir et la preservation de la race," 216.

29 The organization published a journal beginning in 1932 entitled *Bulletin de la société de sexologie*. For other accounts of its founding, see *Prophylaxie antivénérienne*, 3(1931), 596–607 or Justin Godart, "A l'association d'études sexologiques," *Siècle médicale*, 7(1933), 10.

30 There are only a few, brief biographical notices on Toulouse, such as Henri Piéron's "Nécrologie – Dr. Edouard Toulouse," *BINOP*, 2e sér., 3(1947), 95–96; L. Marchand, "Edouard Toulouse (1865–1947)," *Annales médico-psychologiques*, 105(1947), 359–60; and André Plichet, "Necrologie – Edouard Toulouse," *Presse médicale*, 55(1947), 442. A medical dissertation by Sage Michel, "La vie et l'oeuvre d'Edouard Toulouse" (Marseilles, 1979) is a disappointment, containing little more than a summary of the obituaries. There is an entry for Toulouse in *Nouvelle histoire de la psychiatrie*, Jacques Postel and Claude Quétel, eds. (Toulouse: Privat, 1983), 722–23.

31 Paris: Société des éditions scientifiques, 1896. Toulouse did a second study in the series in 1910 on Henri Poincaré.

32 Toulouse, "L'organisation technique de la prophylaxie mentale," *Annales médico-psychologiques*, 76(1920), 510–12.

33 Toulouse has left a very complete record of the steps along the way to creating the hospital. One very detailed account is "The organization of the psychiatric hospital and its role in social life," *Proceedings of the First International Congress on Mental Hygiene, Washington, DC, May 5–10, 1930*, ed. Frank E. Williams (New York: International Committee for Mental Hygiene, 1932), 295–352. For a later, equally detailed version in French, see, "L'hôpital psychiatrique Henri Rousselle," *Prophylaxie mentale*, 11(1937), 1–59.

34 Toulouse, "Prophylaxie et assistance," *Informateur des alienistes*, 10(1920), 323–25; 327–28. Unlike the history of mental testing in the United States, there is very little written on its history in France. For one aspect, see William H. Schneider, "Henri Laugier, the science of work and the workings of science," *Cahiers pour l'histoire du CNRS*, 5(1989), 7–34.

35 Quoted in E. Gauthier, "Vocational guidance [in France]," *International Labour Review*, 5(1922), 710.

36   *Comment former un esprit* (1908); *Comment se conduire dans la vie (1910);*
     Comment conserver sa santé (1914).

37   Toulouse, "L'organisation technique," 510. See n. 32.

38   *Mélanges pour la cinquantenaire de l'hôpital Henri Rousselle, 1922–1972*
     (Tours: Laboratoire Sandoz, 1973), 10.

39   Toulouse, "Le problème sexologique," *Bulletin de l'Association d'études*
     sexologiques, 1(1932), 2–3.

40   Godart, 10

41   On the early years of the league, see Henri Sée, *Histoire de de la ligue des*
     droits de l'homme, 1898–1926 (Paris: Ligue des droits de l'homme, 1927).

42   See Sicard's articles in the *Cahiers,* "Une thèse interdite," (1929), 539;
     or for the broader program, "Le droit à la vie saine," (1927), 103.

43   Just Sicard de Plauzoles, "Le droit à la vie saine," *Cahiers,* (1922), 447–
     58; "Les droits de l'enfant," ibid., (1923), 150–51; "Le secret médical,"
     ibid., (1928), 603–10. The question of the conflict between the child's
     rights and mother's rights was debated at length by various committees
     of the league in subsequent years. See *Cahiers* (1927), 469–70; "Allaite-
     ment obligatoire," ibid., (1929), 14, 229–30; "Commission de la vie
     saine," ibid., (1928), 160.

44   Ferdinand Buisson, "Les droits de l'enfant," *Cahiers,* (1921), 99–104.

45   Sicard, "Une thèse interdite," *Cahiers,* (1929), 539.

46   Ibid.

47   Victor Basch, "La prophylaxie anticonceptionelle," *Cahiers,* (1932), 413–
     14.

48   *Cahiers,* (1933), 99–107; (1934), 579; 713.

49   *Cahiers,* (1936), 76.

50   To say that Basch subscribed to eugenic ideas does not imply right-
     wing or fascist connections. On the contrary, he, along with Sicard and
     Godart suffered at the hands of the Nazis. See Henri Nogueres, *Histoire*
     de la résistance en France, vol. 4 (Paris: Robert Laffont, 1976), 296–97,
     for a graphic description of the assassination of the eighty-year-old Basch
     and his wife by the *milice* [Vichy secret police] in 1944. The attachment
     of the non-communist left to eugenic proposals in the 1930s indicates
     the broad appeal of the ideas.

51   Godart, 10. In late 1932, Toulouse also helped organize a Société de
     biotypologie, whose stated goal was

     > l'étude scientific des types humains par la recherche des corrélations
     > entre les diverses caractères morphologiques, physiologiques, psy-
     > chologiques, pathologiques, psychiatriques et l'application de ces
     > données dans les diverses branches de l'activité humaine: eu-
     > génique, pathologie, psychiatrie, pédagogie, orientation et sélec-
     > tion professionnelle, organisation rationnelle du travail humain,
     > prophylaxie criminelle.

     "Statuts de la Société de biotypologie," *Biotypologie,* 1 (1932/33), 40.
     This was hardly the first attempt at a systematic examination and clas-

sification of humans as a prerequisite to better mating and procreation in the future. In fact, its founders consciously identified with Galton's school of biometrics created at the beginning of the century. For more on the French biotypologists who, like their English counterparts, followed a path from questionable scientific beginnings to legitimate statistical and human biological research, see Schneider, "Henri Laugier" 29–31.

52 Kelves, 108–12. For the broader context, see Judith K. Grether, "Sterilization and eugenics: An examination of early twentieth century population control in the United States," (PhD dissertation, University of Oregon: 1980).

53 See, for example, Félix Heger-Gilbert, "La stérilisation des fonctions genitales," *Bulletin de la société française sanitaire et morale*, 28(1928), 65–74; Marie-Thérèse Nisot, "La stérilisation des anormaux," *Mercure de France*, 209(1929), 595–608. On the U.S. legislation, see Georges Schreiber, "La stérilisation humain aux Etats-Unis," *Revue anthropologique*, 39(1929), 260–81; G. Ichok, "L'hygiène à l'étranger. La stérilisation des indésirables aux Etats-Unis d'Amérique," *Revue d'hygiène*, 52(1930), 271–76; and J. Penel, "La stérilisation eugénique en Amérique," *Hygiène mentale*, 25(1930), 173–88.

54 Paul Schiff and Pierre Mareschal, "Hérédité psychopathique et stérilisation eugénique," *Annales médico-legales*, 89(1931), 77.

55 Etienne Levrat, "Stérilisation et eugénique," *Toulouse médical*, 31(1930), 1–11.

56 See, for example, J. Hamel, "La stérilisation des aliénés et des criminels," *Siècle médicale*, 7(1933), 6.

57 Schreiber, "Stérilisation aux Etats-Unis," 260–81.

58 Ibid., 265.

59 Ibid., 265–66.

60 Georges Heuyer, "Conditions de santé à envisager au point de vue du mariage dans les maladies mentales et nerveuses et les intoxications," in *Examen médicale en vue de mariage*, Schreiber, ed. (Paris: Flammarion, 1927), 132–36.

61 Schreiber, "Stérilisation," 267.

62 Henri Vignes, "Stérilisation des inadaptés sociaux," *Revue anthropologique*, 42(1932), 228–44.

63 For an example of moderate newspaper opinion, see Henri de Varigny's scientific column for the *Journal des débats*, (January 23, 1930). Of course, criticisms continued, such as Penel, "La stérilisation eugénique en Amerique," and Frantz Adam, "Que faut-il penser de la stérilisation des aliénés? La doctrine française," *Siècle médical*, 3(1929).

64 To be fair to the others, none was a geneticist. All the rest were doctors (Apert, Briand, Drouet, Schreiber, and Turpin), anthropologists (Papillaut and Paul-Boncour) or psychologists (Biot and Jeudon).

65 For examples, see Henri Vignes, "Les indications de la loi allemande de stérilisation eugénique," *Presse médicale*, 42(1934), 825–27, 971–73; Fer-

dinand Pièchaud and Henri Marchaud, "La loi allemande de stérilisa-tion," *Journal de médecine de Bordeaux*, 11(1934), 103–104; and G. Swarc, "La stérilisation sexuelle et l'eugénique," *Hygiène mentale*, 29(1934), 228–34.

66 Georges d'Heucqueville, "Points de vue sur la stérilisation chirurgi-cale," *Annales de médecine legale*, 15(1935), 214.

67 Dr. Lowenthal, "La lutte contre la dégénérescence: Stérilisation et cas-tration," *Paris médical*, 95(1935), 250–54.

68 M. Tisserand, "A propos des mesures appliqués depuis quatres ans en allemand pour veiller à la protection de la race," *Concours médical*, 61(1939), 1087–89, 1161–62. For Schreiber's comments, see *Revue anthropolo-gique*, 45(1935), 78–92.

69 *Revue de l'alliance nationale contre la dépopulation* (1934), 101. Although natalists condemned the sterilization measures, they evinced an overall "fascination" with the Nazi regime. See Thébaud, 296–97.

70 D. Raymond, "La dépopulation et la misère de l'enfance," *Cahiers du bolchevisme*, 13(1936), 108.

71 Lucien Cuénot, "Eugénique," *Revue lorraine d'anthropologie*, 8(1935–36), 22.

72 John T. Noonan, *Contraception* (Cambridge: Harvard University Press, 1965), 424–25; Richard A. Soloway, *Birth control and the population ques-tion in England, 1877–1930* (Chapel Hill: University of North Carolina Press, 1982), 254.

73 Jordan, "Le certificat médical prenuptial," *Pour la vie*, (June 1926).

74 "Eugénique et morale catholique," *Interdiocesaine*, (1930), 115.

75 Ibid., 116.

76 Ibid.

77 Mgr. Dubourg, "Le véritable eugénisme," in *L'église et l'eugénisme* (Paris: Editions mariage et famille, 1930), 224.

78 Ibid., vi.

79 Jordan repeated his support in "Eugénisme et morale," *Cahiers de la nouvelle journée*, 19(1931), 88, which was otherwise a highly critical at-tack on eugenics.

80 Arnould, "L'examen médical prenuptial," in *L'église et l'eugénisme*, 124.

81 For other examples of the pre-encyclical view, see Jordan's articles in *Pour la vie*, June 1926; January, March, June, and July 1928; or Jean Pieri, "La stérilisation," in *L'église et l'eugénisme*, 73, and Edouard Jor-dan, Abbé Viollet, and Chanoine Tiberghien, *Eugénisme stérilisation: Leur valeur morale* (Paris: Association du mariage chrétien, 1929).

82 Edouard Jordan, "Eugénisme et morale," 173.

83 Charles Richet, *Sélection humaine* (Paris: Félix Alcan, 1919).

84 Richet, 17.

85 Richet, 89–93, 164–65.

86 Jordan, "Eugénisme et morale," 172.

87 Ibid., 172.

88 "Encyclical letter . . . on Christian marriage," *Sixteen encyclicals of Pope Pius XI* (Washington: National Catholic Welfare Conference, n.d.), 22.

89 Ibid., 23–24.

90 Quoted in René Brouillard, "Causerie de morale," *Etudes. Revue catholique d'intérêt general,* 207(1931), 441.

91 Brouillard, 440, 454. The reference was to the Varigny article, "Ou en est l'eugénique." For another criticism of this press coverage, see Charles Grimbert, "Les psychopathies ou anomalies mentales et l'eugénisme," *Revue de philosophie,* 30(1930), 140.

92 Brouillard, 578–82.

93 Broullaird, 597–600.

94 Brouillard, 597.

95 Examples in the Jesuit review *Etudes* were André Toulemon, "Le suffrage dit 'universel' et la natalité," 231(1937), 588–602; Edouard Jordan, "Natalité dirigée," 231(1937), 762–742; René Bied-Charreton, "Le problème national No. 1: Dénatalité et dépopulation," 239(1939), 471–89. A volume published from the Congrès de la natalité of the Catholic Church held in the fall of 1931, although it included contributions by Jordan and Viollet, contained no reference to eugenics. See *Où en-sommes-nous? La doctrine familiale de l'église catholique* (Paris: Editions du mariage et famille, 1932).

96 Jordan, "Natalité dirigée," 770.

97 Ibid., 771.

98 Fernand Boverat, "Qualité et quantité," *Bulletin de l'Alliance nationale contre la dépopulation,* (Jan. 1931), 399–403. For the review of Nisot's book, see (Feb. 1928), 53.

99 Fernand Boverat, "Eugénisme. Dangers des mesures preconisées pour éviter la naissance des enfants anormaux," ibid., (March 1933), 69–73.

100 Ronsin, 164–84; Angus McLaren, *Sexuality and social order* (New York: Holmes and Meier 1983), 177–89.

101 On prewar socialist concerns about alcoholism, see E. Quillent, "A la santé du proletariat. L'action antialcoolique," *Revue socialiste,* 30(1914), 519–26. See also P. E. Prestwick, "French workers and the temperance movement," *International review of social history,* 25(1980), 44–52. On the lack of interest by the left in contraception, see also Talmy, 2:179–80. For background on the communist/socialist split in France, see Edward Mortimer, *The rise of the French communist party, 1920–1947* (London: Faber and Faber, 1984).

102 Tilly Abeau, "Les ravages de l'Article 317 contre l'avortement," *Cahiers du bolchevisme,* 6(1931), 791.

103 J. O. *Documents parlementaires. Chambre. Annexe* (1933), no. 1705, 865–74.

104 Ibid., 866.

105 Ibid., 871.

106 Ibid., 872.

107 Maurice Thorez, "Rapport à l'assemblé communiste du Paris (October 7, 1935)," *Oeuvres* (Paris: Editions sociales, 1952), 9:196.

108 Ibid., 197.

109   *L'Humanité* (November 17, 1935), 1. For more on Vaillant-Couturier, see Mortimer, 70–71, and the *Dictionnaire des parlementaires français*.

110   Ibid. (November 18, 1935), 2. Of course, that the editor chose these two as examples is in itself a testimony to their prominence as advocates for the biological regeneration of France.

111   See November 19, 21, 22, 23, 24, 25, 27, 30; December 3, 5, 8, 9, 11, 15, 16, 19, 22, 31, 1935; January 1, 2, 6, 1936.

112   November 22, 24, 1935.

113   November 30, December 8, 21, 1935.

114   January 2, 1936.

115   The italics are Vaillant-Couturier's.

116   J. O. *Documents parlementaires. Chambre. Annexe* (1936), no. 259; no. 1415, 938–40.

117   D. Raymond, "La dépopulation et la misère de l'enfance" *Cahiers du bolchevisme*, 13(1936), 101–109; André Chipau, "La lutte contre les taudis," ibid., 13(1936), 1250–57.

118   Thorez, "Rapport au huitième congrès du parti communiste (January 22–25, 1936)," *Oeuvres*, 11:41.

119   Levy, "Le problème de la santé publique en France," *Cahiers du bolchevisme*, 14(1937), 55.

120   Ibid., 57.

121   Thorez, *Oeuvres*, 16:84–92. Reference to this speech is also made in Levy, "Pour une politique de protection de la famille et de l'enfance," *Cahiers du bolchevisme*, 16(1939), 363.

122   Ibid., 367.

123   Thorez, "Rapport à la conference du parti communiste (July 10, 1936)," *Oeuvres*, 12:89.

124   See, for example, *Revue de l'alliance nationale contre la dépopulation*, 37(1936), 35–42. Catholics were more negative, calling it a "false mirage." See J. de Bivort de la Sandée, "Le communisme et la famille," *Etudes*, 233(1937), 52–62.

125   Thorez, "La main tendue aux catholiques et aux croix de feu" (May 25, 1936), *Oeuvres*, 12:22–23, made the following appeal, "Nous te tendons la main, catholique, ouvrier, employé, artisan, paysan, nous qui sommes des laïcs, parce que tu es notre frère, et que tu es comme nous accablé par les mêmes soucis." For the Catholic reception, see G. Fessard, *La main tendue: Le dialogue catholique-communiste, est-il possible?* (Paris: Bernard Grasset, 1937); and Paul Christophe, *1936: Les catholiques et le front populaire* (Paris: Desdée, 1979). See also Mortimer, 259–60.

126   Thorez, "Rapport au comité central du parti communiste (October 17, 1935)," *Oeuvres*, 10:82.

127   Ibid., 83.

128   Ibid., 84.

129   Levy, "Pour une politique de protection de la famille et de l'enfance," *Cahiers du bolchevisme*, 14(1937), 373.

130   See Mortimer, 255–64, for communist appeals to patriots as well as the Catholic church.

131   *Revue anthropologique* 46(1936), 190–91; 48(1938), 249. Raymond Tur-
       pin, ed., *Premier congrès latin d'eugénique (1–3 août 1937)*. *Rapport* (Paris:
       Masson, 1938).

CHAPTER 8

1   For more on these powerful concepts, see Ashley Montagu, *Man's most
     dangerous myth*, 5th ed. (New York: Oxford University Press, 1974);
     and Bernard Seeman, *The river of life* (New York: W. W. Norton, 1961).
2   Jean Colombat, *La fin du monde civilisé: Les prophèties de Vacher de La-
     pouge* (Paris: Vrin, 1946), 9; Guy Thullier, "Un anarchiste positiviste:
     Georges Vacher de Lapouge," in *L'idée de race dans la pensée politique
     française contemporaine*, ed. Pierre Guiral and Emile Temine (Paris: Edi-
     tions du CNRS, 1977), 57. In addition to the citations in Chapter 3, see
     Gunter Nagel, *Georges Vacher de Lapouge: Ein Beitrag zur Geschichte des
     Sozialdarwinismus in Frankreich* (Freiburg: H. F. Verlag, 1975), and an-
     other Boissel article covering Lapouge's later life, "Georges Vacher de
     Lapouge: Un socialiste revolutionnaire darwiniste," *Nouvelle école*,
     38(1982), 59–83.
3   Allen Chase, *The legacy of Malthus* (New York: Alfred Knopf, 1977),
     279–81; Margaret Sanger, *Margaret Sanger: An autobiography* (New York:
     Norton, 1938), 372–73. For the text of Lapouge's address to the New
     York eugenics congress, see, "La race chez les populations mélangées,"
     in *Eugenics, genetics and the family: Scientific papers of the Second Interna-
     tional Congress of Eugenics* (Baltimore: Williams and Wilkins, 1923), 1–
     6.
4   The literature on the Dreyfus affair is enormous, one of the most recent
     accounts being by Jean-Denis Bredin, *The affair* (New York: George
     Braziller, 1986). Studies more specifically on anti-Semitism associated
     with the affair, include Michael R. Marrus, *The politics of assimilation*
     (New York: Oxford University Press, 1971), 10–27, and William Her-
     zog, *From Dreyfus to Petain* (New York: Octagan Books, 1976, first
     published 1947), 25–58. A special study on the role of the Catholic
     church is Pierre Sorlin, *'La Croix' et les juifs* (Paris: Grasset, 1967). On
     the consequences of the affair for Jews in France, see Paula Hyman,
     From Dreyfus to Vichy: The remaking of French Jewry, 1906–1939 (New
     York: Columbia University Press, 1979). For broader background on
     racist ideas in Europe generally, see Jacques Barzun, *Race, a study in
     superstition*, 2nd ed. (New York: Harper and Row, 1965) and Leon Po-
     liakov, *The aryan myth*, (New York: New American Library, 1977).
5   William B. Cohen, *The French encounter with Africans* (Bloomington:
     Indiana University Press, 1980); William H. Schneider, *An empire for the
     masses: The French popular image of Africa, 1870–1914* (Westport, CT:
     Greenwood Press, 1982).
6   Raymond F. Betts, *Assimilation and association in French colonial theory,
     1890–1914* (New York: Columbia University Press, 1961); Martin
     Deming Lewis, "One hundred million Frenchmen: The 'assimilation'

theory in French colonial policy," *Comparative studies in society and history*, 4(1962), 129–53.

7   These two views of Broca can be found in Francis Schiller, *Paul Broca: Founder of French anthropology, explorer of the brain* (Berkeley: University of California Press, 1979) and the more critical chapter in Stephen Jay Gould, *The mismeasure of man* (New York: W. W. Norton, 1981), 73–112.

8   Gould, 85.

9   Quoted in Gould, 83.

10 Ibid., 88.

11 Barzun, 133–75; Poliakov, 272–325.

12 J. Laumonnier, "Le retour au type dans les métissages humains," *Eugénique*, 2(1914), 46–49.

13 See, for example, Eugène Apert, "Le problème des races et immigration en France," *Eugénique*, 3(1921), 152; or Georges Bohn's review in *Mercure de France* (1919), 506–508. As seen in Chapter 7, Edouard Jordan's "Eugénisme et morale" used Richet's book as a point of departure for a highly critical rebuke of eugenics.

14 Charles Richet, *Sélection humaine* (Paris: Félix Alcan, 1919), 58.

15 Ibid., 59.

16 Ibid., 88–93.

17 Ibid., 33–34, 60–78.

18 Ibid., 59.

19 Ibid., 79–80.

20 Ibid., 92–93.

21 The classic study of the day was Georges Mauco, *Les étrangers en France* (Paris: Armand Colin, 1932). More popular in its audience and attitudes surveyed was Raymond Millet, *Trois millions d'étrangers en France* (Paris: Librairie de Medicis, 1938). Two recent studies are Jean-Charles Bonnet, *Les pouvoirs publiques français et l'immigration dans l'entre-deux-guerres* (Lyons: Centre d'histoire économique et sociale de la région lyonnaise, 1976), and Gary S. Cross, *Immigrant workers in industrial France* (Philadelphia: Temple University Press, 1983).

22 *Eugénique*, 3(1922–26), 87.

23 Ibid., 134.

24 Eugène Apert, "Le problème des races," *Eugénique*, 3(1923), 152.

25 Ibid., 155–57.

26 *Eugénique*, 3(1922–26), 210.

27 Barzun, 116–32; Poliakov, 264; Gould, 98–100.

28 Franz Boas, "Changes in bodily form of descendants of immigrants," from *Abstract of the report on changes in bodily form of descendants of immigrants* (Washington: Government Printing Office, 1911), reprinted in *Frontiers of anthropology*, ed. Ashley Montagu (New York: G. P. Putnam's Sons, 1974), 321–22. For an example of the significance of Boas's study, see M. S. Goldstein, "Franz Boas, 1858–1942," *American journal of physical anthropology*, 56(1981), 491–93.

29 In this regard, the title of the review article on Boas's work by Société

d'anthropologie member Adolphe Bloch is telling, "Sur un prétendue découverte anthropologique aux Etats-Unis," *Bulletin de la société d'anthropologie*, 6e sér. 2(1911). Bloch includes himself among the authors who anticipated Boas's work. See Bloch, "De la transformation d'une race dolichocéphalique en une race brachycéphalique, et vice-versa," *Bulletin de la société d'anthropologie*, 5e sér, 2(1901), 73–83.

30 Alfred Binet, "Recherche sur la technique de la mensuration de la tête vivante," *L'année psychologique*, 7(1900), 403, as quoted in Gould, 147.

31 Paul Rivet, "Les données de l'anthropologie," in *Nouveau traité de psychologie*, ed. Georges Dumas (Paris: Félix Alcan, 1930), 1:61.

32 Ibid., 1:61–62.

33 Ludwig and Hanna Hirszfeld, "Essai d'application des méthodes sérologiques au problème des races," *Anthropologie*, 29(1919), 505–37.

34 For a review of the literature plus background on applications, see William H. Schneider, "Chance and social setting in the application of the discovery of blood groups," *Bulletin of the history of medicine*, 57(1983), 545–62.

35 Hirszfeld and Hirszfeld, 533. These percentages differ from those on Table 8.1 because they do not include the AB type. The Hirszfelds counted individuals with AB blood in both the A and B types.

36 Ibid., 535.

37 Louis H. Snyder, "Human blood groups: Their inheritance and racial significance," *American journal of physical anthropology*, 9(1926), 244; Paul Steffan and Siegmund Wellisch, "Die geographische Verteilung der Blutgruppen," *Zeitschrift für Rassenphysiologie*, 2(1930), 114–45; 3(1931), 184–7; 5(1932), 180–85; 6(1933), 28–35; A. L. Kroeber, "Blood group classification," *American journal of physical anthropology*, 18(1934), 378; Raymond Dujarric de la Rivière and Nicholas Kossovitch, *Les groupes sanguins* (Paris: J.-B. Ballière, 1936), 108ff; William C. Boyd, "Blood groups," *Tabula biologicae*, 17(1939), 113–240; A. E. Mourant, Ada C. Kopec and Kazamiera Domaniewska-Sobczak, *The distribution of human blood groups and other polymorphisms*, 2nd ed. (London: Oxford University Press, 1976), 6.

38 Schneider, "Chance and social setting," 558.

39 Frigyes Verzar and Oskar Weszecky, "Rassenbiologische Untersuchungen mittels isohaemagglutinen," *Biochemische Zeitung*, 126(1921), 33–39; Sabin Manuila and Georges Popoviciu, "Recherches sur les races roumanes et hongrois en Roumanie par l'isohemagglutination," *Comptes-rendus de la société de biologie*, 90(1924), 542–43, 1069–73.

40 For a summary of early German literature on blood group anthropology, see Ludwik Hirszfeld, *Konstitutionsserologie und Blutgruppenforschung* (Berlin: Springer, 1928), trans. in *Selected contributions to the literature of blood groups and immunology*, 3, pt. 1(1969), 105–108. A whole journal devoted to blood group research was published in Germany beginning in 1928, the *Zeitschrift für Rassenphysiologie*. This was predated, however, by a similar journal in Russia (bilingual in Russian and German), which appeared in 1927 with the title *Zentralblatt für Blutgrup-*

penforschung. For a summary indication of the extent of Russian work, see Boris Vishnevski, "Anthropology in the U.S.S.R. in the course of 17 years (1917–34)," *American journal of physical anthropology*, 21(1936), 10–11.

41   The earliest article on American blacks was by J. H. Louis and D. L. Henderson, "The racial distribution of isohaemagglutination groups," *Journal of the American medical association*, 79(1922), 1422–24; the first work on American Indians came shortly thereafter, A. F. Coca and O. Diebert, "A study of the occurrence of the blood groups among the American Indians," *Journal of immunology*, 8(1923), 487–93. Examples of early British work are James Hunter Harvey Pirie, "Bloodtesting preliminary to transfusion: With a note on the distribution among South African natives," *Medical journal of South Africa*, 16(1921), 109–25; and A. H. Tebbult and S. McConnel, "Human isohemagglutinins: Their distribution among some Australian aborigines," *Medical journal of Australia*, 1(1922), 201–208.

42   Georges Popoviciu, "Recherches sérologiques sur les races en Roumanie," *Revue anthropologique*, 35(1925), 152–64.

43   D. J. Buining, "Recherches sur les groupes sanguins aux Indes néerlandaises," *Anthropologie*, 44(1934), 77–91, 315–25; and René Martial, "Les peuples du Caucase: nouvelles orientations dans les études d'anthropologie," *Anthropologie*, 46(1936), 65–89, 303–22. There were, however, several review articles each year on blood group research beginning in 1931. E. Farinaud, "Contribution à l'étude des populations de l'Indochine méridionale française d'aprés repartition des groupes sanguins," *Bulletin de la société d'anthropologie de Paris*, 9e sér, 2(1941), 75–102.

44   *Anthropologie*, 39(1929), 96–97.

45   The prestige of this French journal was such that after the First World War, it became an international publication for research conducted in several countries. Among the formally affiliated societies that published their proceedings in the journal were those of Belgium, Poland, Rumania, and Denmark, as well as the cities of Lisbon, Athens, Buenos Aires, and local societies of the major French provincial cities.

46   For examples of Polish work, see Ludwik Hirszfeld and E. Przesmycki, "Recherches sur l'agglutination normale. De l'isoagglutination des globules rouges chez les chevaux," *Comptes-rendus de la société de biologie* (hereafter cited as *CRSB*), 89(1923), 1360–61; W. Halber and Jan Mydlarski, "Recherches séro-anthropologiques en Pologne," *CRSB*, 89(1923), 1373–75; Hirszfeld and H. Zborowski, "Sur la symbiose sérologique entre la mère et le foetus," *CRSB*, 94(1926), 205–207.

For Michon's work, see Paul Michon, "Sur les variations quantitatives de l'isohémagglutination et les infractions aux schema de Moss," *CRSB*, 92(1925), 37–39; "Nouvelles remarques sur l'isohémagglutination-conservation des stocks-serums. Transfusion possible malgré incompatibilité théorique," *CRSB*, 94(1926), 676–78; "Individualité humorale et groupes sanguins," *CRSB*, 100(1929), 445–47.

Examples of the work of E. Balgaires and Louis Christiaens are, "Le taux des iso-hémagglutinines des sérums O, A et B chez l'adulte," *CRSB*, 126(1937), 29–30; "La distribution des iso-hémagglutinogenes A et B dans le Nord de la France," *CRSB*, 129(1938), 567–68; "Détection des hémo-agglutinogènes M et N dans les quantités minima de sang sec," *CRSB*, 130(1939), 59–61.

The early work of Nicholas Kossovitch included, "Les groupes sanguins chez les tcheques," *CRSB*, 93(1923), 1343–44; and "Recherches sur la race arménienne par l'isohémagglutination," *CRSB*, 97(1927), 69–71.

47 In fact, two researchers at the Pasteur Institute came very close to an independent discovery of human blood groups in 1901. They found that the blood from different human subjects, when mixed, sometimes clumped together; but because of the small number of subjects tested and the fact that they were hospital patients, the conclusion of the researchers was that the agglutination was caused by disease. See Jean Camus and Pagniez, "D'un pouvoir agglutinant de certains sérums humains pour les globules rouges de l'homme," *CRSB*, 58(1901), 242–44. For more on the question of priority in the blood group discovery, see Jan Hirschfeld, "The birth of serology and the discovery of the human ABO system," *Nordisk medicinhistorisk arsbok* (1977), 163–80. For background on French medical training at the turn of the century, see George Weisz, "Reform and conflict in French medical education, 1870–1914," in *The organization of science and technology in France, 1808–1914*, ed. George Fox and George Weisz (Cambridge, England: Cambridge University Press, 1980), 61–94.

48 P. Lepine, "Nécrologie: Nicholas Kossovitch, 1864–1948," *Annales de l'institut Pasteur*, 75(1948), 62; Ludwig Hirszfeld, "The story of one life," unpublished translation by F. R. Camp and F. R. Ellis of *Historia jednego zyeia*, 2nd ed. (Warsaw: Institut Wydawniczny, 1967), 56, 58.

49 Kossovitch, "Les groupes sanguins chez les français," *Revue anthropologique*, 39(1929), 244–59, 374–79; 41(1931), 131–55; Kossovitch and Ferdinand Benoit, "Contribution à l'étude anthropologique et sérologique (groupes sanguins) des juifs modernes," *Revue anthropologique*, 42(1932), 99–125; Kossovitch and Benoit, "Une tribu inconnu du Maroc: les bahloula," *Revue anthropologique*, 45(1935), 347–63.

50 Kossovitch, "Les groupes sanguins chez les français et les regles de l'hérédité," *CRSB*, 102(1929), 494–97.

51 V. Liodt and N. Pojarski, "L'application de l'isohémoagglutination à l'étude des races indigènes de l'Afrique Equatoriale Française," *CRSB*, 101(1929), 889–90; P. Rodé, "Les groupes sanguins chez les races indigènes de l'Afrique Occidentale," *CRSB*, 122(1936), 206–208; and Rodé, "Le phenomène d'agglutination dans les recherches de groupes sanguins chez les lepreux," *CRSB*, 122(1936), 300–302.

52 For Balgaires and Christiaens, see note 46. See also M.-E. Farinaud, "La répartition des groupes sanguins chez les Bauhais, les Djarais et les Sedangs, populations primitives de l'Indochine méridionale," *CRSB*, 131(1939), 1236–38; Farinaud, "Nouvelles recherches sur la distribution

des groupes sanguins parmi les populations de l'Indochine mériodinale: Les 'mois' du Darlac et les Chams," *CRSB*, 131(1939), 1238–40.

53 Leland C. Wyman, and William C. Boyd, "Human blood groups and anthropology," *American anthropologist*, 37(1935), 192–93.

54 William C. Boyd and Lyle G. Boyd, "New data on blood groups and other inherited factors in Europe and Egypt," *American journal of physical anthropology*, 23(1937), 49–70; Julian S. Huxley and Alfred C. Haddon, *We Europeans* (New York: Harpers, 1936), 98–106. Of course, reactions to the extreme claims of Nazi and other racist ideologues, such as those described in Chapter 7 and those that follow, also had much to do with the abandonment of the concept of race. See Montagu, *Man's most dangerous myth*, 435–44; or his "On the phrase 'ethnic group' in anthropology," *Psychiatry*, 8(1945), 27–33; and "Some anthropological terms: A study in the systematics of confusion," *American anthropologist*, 47(1945), 119–33. Nancy Stepan, *The idea of race in science* (London: Macmillan, 1982), raises some questions about the supposed sharp break after the Second World War.

55 Marrus, 17–27. See also Raphael Patai and Jennifer Patai Wing, *The myth of the Jewish race* (New York: Scribner's, 1975).

56 Kossovitch and Benoit, "Contribution à l'étude anthropologique et sérologique (groupes sanguins) des juifs modernes," 99–125; Félix Regnault, "Il n'y a pas une race juive," *Revue anthropologique*, 42(1932), 390–93; Rina Younovitch, "Les caractères sérologiques des juifs asiatiques," *CRSB*, 113(1933), 1101–1103. Patai and Wing use similar categories in describing views on Jews as a race, 21–40.

57 Hirszfeld, *Groupes sanguins*, 152; "The story of one life," 264–67.

58 A contemporary assessment for the general reader is Jean Bernard, *Le sang et l'histoire* (Paris: Buchet/Chastel, 1983).

CHAPTER 9

1 Eugène Apert, "L'eugénique en France," *Pédiatrie*, 19(1940), 17–22; reprinted in *Revue anthropologique*, 50(1940), 205–16, with an obituary notice by Georges Schreiber.

2 Mark H. Haller, *Eugenics: Hereditarian attitudes in American thought* (New Brunswick: Rutgers University Press, 1963), 152–57; Kenneth M. Ludmerer, *Genetics and American society* (Baltimore: Johns Hopkins University Press, 1972), 95–113.

3 There is no biography of Martial, but for a list of his work through 1935, see *Titres et travaux de René Martial* (Paris: Jouve, 1935).

4 René Martial, "Organisation scientifique des usines ou méthode de F. W. Taylor," *Revue d'hygiène et de police sanitaire*, 35(1913), 146–68. See also *L'ouvrier: Son hygiène, son atelier, son habitation* (Paris: Doin, 1909). Martial also wrote a three-part series of articles on "Le progrès de l'hygiène ouvrier" in Germany, Austria, and England that appeared in the *Revue d'hygiène* in 1908 and 1909.

5 Ann-Louise Shapiro, "Private rights, public interest and professional jurisdiction: The French public health law of 1902," *Bulletin of the history of medicine*, 54(1980), 4–22; Martha Lee Hildreth, *Doctors, bureaucrats and public health in France, 1888–1902* (New York: Garland Press, 1986). Martial also showed an early interest in foreign travel, participating in a study trip to Germany and Denmark in 1907.

6 Martial, *Travaux du bureaux d'hygiène de la ville de Douai pendant l'année 1911* (Douai: Lefebvre, 1912).

7 Several times a year during this period, the minutes of the Academy of Medicine reported on correspondence from Martial. See, for example, meetings of July 22, 1913 or January 20, 1914 in the *Bulletin de l'academie de médecine*.

8 Martial and André Cavaillon, "Conditions imposées par la guerre et la prophylaxie," *Montpellier médical*, 36(1917), 729–38. Among the papers sent to the Academy of Medicine was "Sur une épidémie de fièvre typhoïde survenue chez les annamites employés à l'usine de dynamite de Paulilles (Pyrenées Orientales)," *Bulletin de l'académie de médecine* (December 29, 1917). See also, Martial, "Prophylaxie de l'immigration pendant et depuis la guerre," *Annales d'hygiène*, 48(1926), 399–407.

9 René Martial, "Voyage avec des émigrants, du Havre à Buenos Aires," *Bulletin de l'academie de médecine*, 101(1929), 687–93; "Les services d'immigration en Argentine, leur législation et leurs statistiques," ibid., 102(1929), 57–64.

10 *Revue médicale française*, 11(1930), 57.

11 In addition to titles mentioned in Chapter 8, see Georges Dupeux, "L'immigration en France de la fin du XVIIIe siècle à nos jours," in Commission internationale d'histoire des mouvements sociaux et des structures sociales, *Les migrations internationales de la fin du XVIIIe siècle à nos jours* (Paris: CNRS, 1980), 161–74; Gary S. Cross, "The politics of immigration in France during the era of World War I," *French historical studies*, 11(1980), 610–32; Timothy P. Maga, "Closing the door: The French government and refugee policy, 1933–39," *French historical studies* 12(1982), 424–42; and a special issue of *Vingtième siècle*, 7(1985) devoted to immigration in France, with such articles as Charles-Robert Ageron, "L'immigration maghrébine en France: Un survol historique," 59–70; Pierre Guillaume, "Du bon usage des immigrés en temps de crise et de guerre, 1932–40," 117–24; and Olivier Milza, "La gauche, la crise et l'immigration (années 1930–1980)," 127–40.

12 Raymond Millet, *Trois millions d'étrangers en France* (Paris: Librairie de Medici, 1938), 7–15; Gary Cross, *Immigrant workers in industrial France* (Philadelphia: Temple University Press, 1983).

13 Cross, *Immigrant workers*, 64; 146–47. Growing out of this reaction, a deputy specializing in immigration matters, Charles Lambert, wrote *La France et les étrangers* (Paris: Delagrave, 1928), which Charles Davenport found so conducive to the eugenic view that he wrote an article on it in *Eugenical news*, 13(1928), 20.

14 Martial, "Le problème de l'immigration: Examen sanitaire et logement des immigrants," *Revue politique et parlementaire*, 129(1926), 391. See also his articles, "Immigration de la main d'oeuvre agricole et industrielle," *Annales d'hygiène*, 8(1924), 236–41, and "De l'immigration," *Concours médical*, 48(1926), 980–81.

15 Martial, "Immigration de la main d'oeuvre agricole et industrielle," 243–44.

16 Georges Dequidt and Georges Forestier, "Les aspects sanitaires du problème de l'immigration en France," *Revue d'hygiène*, 48(1926), 1001. For more on Dequidt and Forestier, see Lion Murard and Patrick Zylberman, "De l'hygiène comme introduction à la politique expérimentale (1875–1925), *Revue de synthèse*, 115, 3e sér. (1984), 313–41.

17 Madison Grant, *Le déclin de la grande race* (Paris: Payot, 1926).

18 Dequidt and Forestier, 1001–03, 1009–13. Dequidt continued to use such statistics as late as 1929 in a ministry of interior report, "Assistance aux étrangers," cited in Cross, 263.

19 Roger Picard, "Les étrangers en France," *Cahiers des droits de l'homme* (August 25, 1926), 372.

20 Edmond Goglewski, "Les polonais en France avant la seconde guerre mondiale," *Revue du nord*, 242 (1979), 50–51. On recruitment and the stability of Polish communities in France, see Cross, 81–98.

21 Quoted in Dequidt and Forestier, 1026.

22 An example of Lapouge's lament is, "Comment l'anthropo-sociologie, science française, fut assassinée en France," French translation in Lapouge Archives of an article published in *Die Sonne* (December 1929).

23 Lapouge Archives, Grant letters to Lapouge, October 17, 1917, and February 27, 1919; as well as Lapouge letter to Grant, March 23, 1919.

24 Lapouge Archives, Grant letter to Lapouge, November 26, 1920. On the immigration act, in addition to Haller and Ludmerer cited earlier, see E. P. Hutchinson, *Legislative history of American immigration policy, 1798–1965* (Philadelphia: University of Pennsylvania Press, 1981), 174–213. For Lapouge's influence on American eugenicists, see Barry Mehler, "A history of the American Eugenics Society, 1921–40," (PhD dissertation, University of Illinois, 1988), 51–55.

25 *Eugenical news*, 13(1928), 82–84; 14(1929), 69, 78–80; 16(1931), 10–12; 17(1932), 94–95; 19(1934), 39–40.

26 Lapouge Archives, Grant letter to Lapouge, May 8, 1924; March 19, 1925. Grant had written the introduction to Stoddard's book, which was published in France in 1925 with the title, *Le flôt montant des peuples de couleur contre la supériorité mondiale des blancs* (Paris: Payot, 1925).

27 Lapouge Archives, Grant letter to Lapouge, April 22, 1926; November 17, 1926.

28 Lapouge Archives, Grant letter to Lapouge, September 1, 1927.

29 See, for example, "Le problème de l'immigration,," 391–92; "De l'immigration," 981–82; and "Législation et prophylaxie de l'immigration

aux Etats-Unis et dans d'autres pays," *Annales d'hygiène*, 48(1926), 463–69.

30   "La main d'oeuvre étrangère en France," *Annales d'hygiène*, 48(1926), 285.

31   Mauco, 544–54; Cross, *Immigrant workers*, 173, 178.

32   The French also watched American events very closely because of the repercussions on immigration to France. In addition to Martial, "Législation et prophylaxie de l'immigration aux Etats-Unis," cited here, see R. Duthil, "L'immigration aux Etats-Unis et le déclin de l'intelligence américaine," *La grande revue*, 118(1925), 130–34; Pierre Wurtz, *La question d'immigration aux Etats-Unis* (Paris: L. Dreux et M. Schneider, 1925); and Cross, 173–76.

33   Martial, "De l'immigration. Nouvelles formules à adopter," *Concours médical*, 50(1928), 361–64, was the first mention of the phrase, but Martial's fullest development of the idea was in *Traité de l'immigration et de la greffe inter-raciale* (Paris: Larose, 1931).

34   Martial, *Greffe inter-raciale*, 89–93.

35   *Industrial and labour information*, 34(1930), 114–16; 36(1930), 424–26. For more on the legislative reaction, see Bonnet, 201–35, and Cross, 186–94. Examples of press reaction are summarized in *Revue de l'immigration*, 41(1931), 33; 44(1932), 39; 49(1933), 41; and 50(1933), 39.

36   As cited in Françoise Thébaud, "Le mouvement nataliste dans la France de l'entre-deux-guerres," *Revue d'histoire moderne et contemporaine*, 32(1985), 296–97.

37   Martial, *La race française* (Paris: Mercure de France, 1934), 306–07, repeated in later articles.

38   Ibid., 296–98; Martial, "L'immigration et le pouvoir de resorption de la France," *Revue anthropologique*, 43(1933), 351–69; 449–67. The article carried charts of color traits in successive generations of plants to illustrate Mendelian inheritance, and Martial even mentioned Morgan's drosophila research. On the late arrival of Mendelian genetics, see Camille Limoges, "Natural selection, phagocytosis and preadaptation, Lucien Cuénot, 1886–1901," *Journal of the history of medicine*, 31(1976), 176–78; and Denis Buican, "La génétique classique en France devant le néolamarckisme tardif," *Archives internationales d'histoire des sciences*, 111(1983). For background, see Buican's book, *Histoire de la génétique et de l'évolutionnisme en France* (Paris: Presses Universitaires de France, 1984).

39   Georges Lakhovsky, *La civilisation et la folie raciste* (Paris: Editions SACL, 1939), 13–49; 124. This idea has been outlined before in his *Racisme, l'orchestre universel* (Paris: Alcan, 1934), but the new book was in part a response to Martial's ideas.

40   Paul Rivet, article in *Oeuvre*, September 13, 1938, 6.

41   "Politique de l'immigration," *Mercure de France*, (1935), 275.

42   See Chapter 8 and William H. Schneider, "Chance and social setting in the application of the discovery of blood groups," *Bulletin of the history of medicine*, 57(1983), 545–62.

43 *Race française*, 307. See also "L'immigration et le pouvoir de resorption," 263.

44 *La Pologne jadis et de nos jours* (Paris: Gebethner and Wolff, 1927).

45 *Race française*, 307.

46 Nicholas Kossovitch and F. Benoit, "Contribution à l'étude anthropologique et sérologique des juifs modernes," *Revue anthropologique*, 42(1932), 124–25. See also another article in the same issue of the journal by Félix Regnault, "Il n'y a pas une race juif," 390–93.

47 *Race française*, 241.

48 Ibid. 237–40. Paula Hyman, *From Dreyfus to Vichy* (New York: Columbia University Press, 1979), 63–88, has noted that during this period Jews were highly concentrated in Paris (as high as 70–80 percent of all French Jews), which would have tended to exaggerate their presence to observers in the capital, more so than Polish, Italian, or Spanish immigrants, for example, who resided in mining or frontier districts.

49 Martial, "Le parallelisme céphalo-hématique et ses consequences au point de vue de la definition de la race," *Revue anthropologique*, 45(1935), 227–33.

50 This holds true only for the ABO system. At that time, the existence of the Rh system, which in certain ways follows Martial's description, was not yet known. Between the wars there was a great deal of interest in the comparison of blood type between mothers and newborns by Hirszfeld and many others; yet nothing suggested the conclusion about incompatibility that Martial drew for the ABO system.

51 Martial, *Race française*, 323; and repeated in, for example, "Politique de l'immigration," 288.

52 A February 1933 talk at the Hotel Chambon in Paris was reported in *Concours médical* (1933), 613–14; and a talk in March at a meeting of the International Institute of Anthropology was published in July of that year under the title "L'immigration et le pouvoir de resorption de la France," *Revue anthropologique*, 43(1933), 351–69, 449–67. As late as 1932, Martial made no mention of the blood groups even in a popular medical reference book on the heart, blood, and circulatory system, *Appareil circulatoire: sang et humeurs* (Paris: Albin Michel, 1932).

53 Published as *Vie et constances des races* (Paris: Mercure de France, 1939), which contains an extensive bibliography of Martial's other writings. In applying to the Faculty of Medicine for renewal of his course in the 1939–40 academic year, Martial reported that for the previous year,

> the average audience attending after the opening lecture was forty to forty-five. But as for the inaugural lesson, its success was so great that Thesis Hall No. 2 was literally overflowing and a good number of people had to wait in the corridor until the end.

Martial also indicated that he had an extremely loyal following, with some two dozen of those attending giving him their names and addresses in order to stay in touch. France: Archives Nationales, Series

AJ, carton 6277, Martial letter to Prof. Tiffeneau, dean of Faculty of Medicine, May 15, 1939.

54 "L'immigration et le pouvoir de resportion," 351.

55 Ibid.

56 Martial, "Note sur la correlation entre les indices céphaliques des crânes et des groupements sanguins," *Institut international d'anthropologie. 5e congrès (Bruxelles). Rapport* (Brussels: Imprimerie médicale et scientifique, 1936), 61–65; Martial, "Métissage et immigration," in Raymond Turpin, ed. *Prémier congrès latin d'eugénique (1–3 août 1937). Rapport* (Paris: Masson, 1938), 16–40.

57 Martial, "Un precurseur des groupements sanguins: Vacher de Lapouge," *Mercure de France* (1936), 623.

58 *La terre retrouvée*, 8(December 26, 1935), 22–23; 9(March 25, 1936), 4; 9(May 25, 1936), 15.

59 *La terre retrouvée*, 9(February 1, 1937), 20.

60 Julius Brutzkus, "Les groupes sanguins parmi les populations juives," *Congrès international de la population. VII: Problèmes qualitatives de la population* (Paris: Herman, 1938), 73. This is the original paper from which the *Races et racisme* article was reprinted. For more on Brutzkus, see entry in *Encyclopedia Judaica*.

61 Ibid. Note that Brutzkus did not question the biochemical definition of race, only its application to the Jews. Such was the influence of Hirszfeld's concept.

62 Georges Lakhovsky, *La civilisation et la folie racisme* (Paris: Editions SACL, 1939), 139–40.

63 Jean Rostand, *Herédité et racisme* (Paris: Gallimard, 1939), cited by Georges Schreiber in *Races et racisme*, no. 19(December 1939), 46.

64 Joseph J. Spengler, *France faces depopulation: Postlude edition, 1936–1976* (Durham, NC: Duke University Press, 1979), 215–17.

65 Millet, 128–38. Examples of the paramount interest in foreign immigration by the general press are Robert de Beauplan, "Les étrangers en France," *Illustration*, 201(1938), 234–35; a front-page article, "Les étrangers en France," in *Le temps*, November 2, 1938; a series on immigration in the north of France in *Epoque*, January 18–21, 1939; as well as "Les étrangers dans les hôpitaux," *Avenir*, January 24, 1939; "Le problème juif," *Le matin*, February 2, 1939; and "Le problème des étrangers," in *Le temps*, April 15, 1939.

66 Millet, *Trois millions d'étrangers*, 123–38. For examples of the acceptance of Martial's ideas by the medical community, see the *Concours médical* report of the Hotel Chambon conference, (1933), 613–14; and Octave Beliard, "L'oeuvre de Dr. René Martial," *Hippocrate. Revue d'humanisme médical*, 6(1938), 617–27.

67 Michael R. Marrus and Robert Paxton, *Vichy France and the Jews* (New York: Basic Books, 1981), 49–53. For other examples, see Pierre-Marie Dieudonnant, *Je suis partout, 1930–44* (Paris: Table Ronde, 1973) or William R. Tucker, *The fascist ego: A political biography of Robert Brasillach* (Berkeley: University of California Press, 1975).

68   Jean-Marie Baron, *La grande découverte: Les juifs et le sang B* (Paris: Centre de documentation et de propagande, 1938), 8–9.

69   Fernand Chateau, "Races et groupements sanguins," *Mercure de France* (1938), 275–78.

70   Doriot's diatribe was timed to coincide with the aftermath of Kristallnacht in a daily column in *Liberté* entitled "La grande invasion" beginning in November 3, 1938, and running through December. In it he complained of such things as jobs taken by foreigners, the domination of Jews in cinema and medicine, and the infiltration of France by foreign Marxists.

71   A dossier on Montandon in the French National Archives, AN series 317, AP 170, includes an exchange of correspondence with Louis Marin and articles on his speeches clipped from *Gazette de Bruxelles* (May 4, 1938); *Avant-garde* (May 5, 1938); *La terre retrouveé* (June 17, 1938); and *Libre parole* (July 1938).

CHAPTER 10

1   Louis Marin, "Les études portant sur l'homme et l'école d'anthropologie de 1926 à 1956," *Revue anthropologique*, n.s. 2(1956), 174.

2   *Revue anthropologique*, 51(1941), 8–15.

3   Both talks were reported in *Revue anthropologique* 51(1941), 195–96; and *Ethnie française*, 1(1941), 13–14. For the full text, see Otmar von Verscheurer, "L'image héréditaire de l'homme," and Eugen Fischer, "Problème de la race et la législation raciale en Allemagne," in *Etat et santé*, ed. Karl Epting (Paris: Fernand Sorlot, 1942), 59–79, 81–110. Montandon later translated Verscheurer's most influential eugenics work, *Manuel d'eugénique et hérédité humaine* (Paris: Masson, 1943).

4   Joseph Billig, *Le Commissariat général aux questions juives, 1941–1944*, 3 vols. (Paris: Centre de documentation juive contemporaine, 1955–1960). The commisariat is hereafter cited as CGQJ. For its role in a broader context, see Michael Marrus and Robert Paxton, *Vichy France and the Jews,* (New York: Basic Books, 1981), 128–44.

5   Marrus and Paxton, 81–83, 293.

6   Quoted in Marrus and Paxton, 118.

7   Georges Montandon, *Ethnie française* (Paris: Payot, 1935).

8   Joseph Billig, *L'Institut d'étude des questions juives. Inventaire des archives du centre de documentation juive contemporaine,* 3 vols. (Paris: Centre de documentation juive contemporaine, 1974), 3:204. The Institut is hereafter cited as IEQJ.

9   Archives of the Centre de documentation juive contemporaine, hereafter cited as CDJC archives, XCV-122, 24 July 1940.

10   Henri Briand, "Les vraies familles françaises doivent revivre," 1(1941), 5–9; Georges Mauco, "L'immigration étrangère en France et le problème des refugiés," 6(1942), 6–15; and Mauco, "La situation démographique en France," 7(1943), 15–19.

11 Marrus and Paxton, 211.

12 CDJC XXII-13; Marrus and Paxton, p. 211. On the CGQJ view of the need for such public education, see Asher Cohen, "Le peuple aryen vu par la Commissariat général aux questions juives," *Revue d'histoire de la deuxième guerre mondiale*, 36(1986), 45–58.

13 "Le racisme: Loi biologique fondamentale," 1(1942), 31–44; "Les juifs et le sang B," 3(1942), 45–51. There was also a review of *Les métis* by Martial and summaries of articles by Martial appearing in the press such as "Asie," 4(1942), 105; and "Les mariages mixtes," 7(1942), 76.

14 René Martial, *Francais, Qui es-tu?* (Paris: Mercure de France, 1942), i.

15 CDJC archives, LXCIII-162 (14 December 1942), Billig, *CGQJ*, 2:307.

16 *Question juive* (January–February 1943), as cited in Billig, *CGQJ*, 1:307.

17 Billig, *CGQJ*, 2:322–23.

18 See Marrus and Paxton, 284–85, for more on Darquier.

19 For a summary of the dozens of programs whose transcripts survived the war, see Billig, *IEQJ*, 2:325–27.

20 Cited in Billig, *IEQJ*, 2:319–20.

21 Cited in Billig, *IEQJ*, 2:329.

22 Billig, *IEQJ*, 3:204–205. On Montandon's greed, see Billig, *CGQJ*, 1:140.

23 Marrus and Paxton, 246–52.

24 Alfred Fabre-Luce, *Anthologie de la nouvelle Europe* (Paris: Librairie Plon, 1942), xiv–xv; 63–92.

25 See, for example, M. Lamy, *Les applications de la génétique à la médicine* (Paris: G. Doin, 1943); Georges Jeanneny, "Hérédité, génétique, eugénique," *Revue française de gynécologique et d'obstétrique*, 38(1944), 121–44.

26 His earliest exposure to eugenics was undoubtedly as an intern with Weill-Hallé in the 1920s. Examples of the reports published in a proceedings volume edited by Turpin, *Prémier congrès latin d'eugénique (1–3 août 1937). Rapport* (Paris: Masson, 1938), include: Raymond Turpin, A. Caratzali, and H. Rogier, "Etude étiologique de 104 cas de mongolisme et considérations sur la pathogénie de cette maladie," 154–64; Turpin, Caratzali, and M. Gorny, "Contribution à l'étude de l'influence de l'âge et de l'état de santé des procreateurs, du rang et du nombre des naissances, sur les caractères de la progéniture. (Resultat de l'étude de 1,100 familles)," 240–61; and Turpin, Caratzali, and N. Georgescu-Roagen, "Influence de l'âge maternel, du rang de naissance et de l'ordre des naissances sur la mortinatalité," 271–77. Broader prewar writings of Turpin included "La génétique appliquée à la prophylaxie des maladies humains," *Semaine des hôpitaux de Paris*, 12(1936), 381–94, 413–17, and "Le péril pour l'éspèce des mutations germinales," *Semaine des hôpitaux de Paris* (July 1, 1939), 339–47.

27 Turpin, "Eugénisme et guerre," *Bulletin médical* 42(1941), 472.

28 Ibid., 473; Charles Richet, *Le passé de la guerre et l'avenir de la paix* (Paris: Ollendorff, 1907).

29 Turpin, "Eugénisme et guerre," 475.

30 Turpin, "Applications familiales de l'eugénisme," in *La famille et l'enfant: problèmes d'aujourd'hui et de démain* (Paris: Comité nationale de l'enfance, 1941), 189–90.

31 Robert Paxton, *Vichy France* (New York: Norton, 1972), 166–67; Aline Coutrot, "La politique familiale," in *Le gouvernement de Vichy, 1940–42. Colloque sur le gouvernement de Vichy et la révolution nationale* (Paris: Armand Colin, 1972), 161–63.

32 Verine [sic], "La famille," in *France 1941: La révolution nationale constructive. Un bilan et un programme* (Paris: Editions Alsatia, 1941), 192.

33 Coutrot, 254–55.

34 Raymond Fontaine, "La législation recente sur la famille et l'enfant," in *La famille et l'enfant,* 107.

35 Richard Holt, *Sport and society in modern France* (Hamden, CT: Archon Books, 1981), 57–58. Membership in sports organizations actually declined under Vichy. For the measures passed, see Henri Mavit, "Education physique et sport," *Revue d'histoire de la deuxième guerre mondiale,* 14(1964), 89–104.

36 Verine, 194.

37 Coutrot, 252–54; Fontaine, 13; Olivier Wormser, *Les origines doctrinales de la Révolution Nationale* (Paris: Plon, 1971), 111–12.

38 Verine, 199.

39 Coutrot, 245–47. On alcoholism, see J. O. *Lois et décrets* (July 22, 1940, August 24, 1940, and November 6, 1940). The anti-venereal disease decrees were promulgated on January 14, 1941, and March 24, 1941, and tuberculosis sanatoriums were reorganized by decrees of February 14 and October 3, 1943. For background, see Fontaine, 10; Wormser, 110–12, and Raymond Grasset, *Au service de la médecine. Chronique de la santé publique durant les saisons amères (1942–44)* (Clermont-Ferrand: G. de Bussac, 1956), 78–79.

40 J. O. *Lois et décrets,* (December 16, 1942).

41 Ibid.

42 J. O. *Lois et décrets,* (July 29, 1943).

43 *Siècle médical,* March 1, 1943, as reprinted in *Prophylaxie antivénérienne,* 15(1943), 80.

44 Henri Gougerot, "Enquête aupres du corps médical au sujet du certificat prenuptial," *Prophylaxie antivénérienne,* 15(1943), 82.

45 Just Sicard de Plauzoles and A. Cavaillon, "Le corps médical et le certificat prenuptial," *Prophylaxie antivénérienne,* 16(1944), 154–59.

46 Raoul Blondel, "Le certificat prenuptial obligatoire," *Oeuvre,* (March 29, 1943), as reprinted in *Prophylaxie antivénérienne,* 15(1943), 118–19. (Emphasis in the original.)

47 Alain Drouard, "Les trois âges de la fondation française pour l'étude des problèmes humains," *Population,* 38(1983), 1017–37.

48 There are several biographies, none of which, however, can be described as particularly objective or critical. Among them, Robert Soupault, *Alexis Carrel, 1873–1944* (Paris: Plon, 1952) is still the standard work, although Joseph T. Durkin's *Hope for our time: Alexis Carrel on*

man and society (New York: Harper, 1965) makes use of the Carrel papers at Georgetown University. For a more recent assessment, see the entry by George W. Corner in the *Dictionary of scientific biography*.

49 Alexis Carrel, *Man, The unknown* (New York: Harper, 1935), ii.
50 Charles A. Lindbergh, *Autobiography of values* (New York: Harcourt Brace, 1976), 16–17, 132–33; Walter S. Ross, *The last hero: Charles A. Lindbergh* (New York: Harper and Row, 1964), 229–42.
51 A copy of the press release is in the Carrel Archives of Georgetown University, (hereafter cited as Carrel Papers), Box 42, Section 14-3, Folder 19.
52 Ibid.
53 Carrel and Lindbergh, "The culture of whole organs," *Science*, 81(1935), 621–23; *New York Times*, September 29, 1936, 24. For an interesting review of Carrel's book in France, see Jean Rostand, "L'homme, cet inconnu," *Revue hebdomadaire*, 46(1935), 288–300. According to Drouard, the French publisher estimated that by 1980, over 1 million copies of the book had been sold in France.
54 Carrel, ix.
55 Raymond Pearl, "Dr. Carrel ponders the nature and soul of man," *New York Times*, September 29, 1935, vi:3.
56 Carrel, 47–50, 124–25, 213–14.
57 Carrel, 296–97.
58 *Autobiography of values*, 129. Leonard Moseley, *Lindbergh: A biography* (New York: Doubleday, 1976), 218. For a more balanced assessment of the relationship see Ross, 240–42.
59 Carrel, 300.
60 Carrel, 318–19.
61 Mark Haller, *Eugenics: Hereditarian attitudes in American thought* (New Brunswick, NJ: Rutgers University Press, 1963), 42, notes a peak in the hysteria about eliminating the "hereditary criminal" in the early 1900s, when an author such as W. Duncan McKim wrote, "The surest, the kindest and most human means for preventing reproduction among those whom we deem unworthy of this high privilege is a gentle, painless death." For examples of the pervasive concept of eugenic "burden" in the 1920s and 1930s in the United States, see Paul Popenoe and Roswell Johnson, *Applied eugenics,* (New York: Macmillan, 1920), 158–60, 181–83, and Ellsworth Huntington and Leon Whitney, *Builders of America* (New York: Morrow, 1927), 88–110.
62 Intermittent social correspondence can be found in Carrel Papers, Box 45, Section 15-1, Folder 13; Box 49, Section 15-4, Folder 63.
63 Carrel Papers, Box 59, Section 17-1, Folder 48.
64 Carrel Papers, Box 42, Section 14-3, Folder 15. For more on Kellogg, race betterment, and eugenics, see Richard W. Schwartz, *John Harvey Kellogg, MD* (Nashville: Southern Publications, 1970), 220–29, and Gerald Carson, *Cornflake crusade* (New York: Rinehart, 1957), 244–47.
65 See Soupault, 206–35, 247–61, and Durkin, 134ff. An idealized account by one of the bright young researchers who joined the foundation is

Jean-Jacques Gillon, "La fondation française pour l'étude des problèmes humaines," in *Science et théorie de l'opinion publique*, ed. R. Boudon, F. Bourricaud, and A. Girard (Paris: Retz, 1981), 257–68. For a more objective assessment, see Drouard, 1021–26; and for background on French technocracy, especially the work of Jean Coutrot, see Girard Brun, *Technocrates et technocratie en France, 1918–1945* (Paris: Editions Albatros, 1985).

66 Soupault, 231–35.
67 George W. Corner, *History of the Rockefeller Institute, 1901–1953* (New York: Rockefeller Institute Press, 1964), 39–43, 152–60.
68 Carrel, 290–291.
69 Carrel, 292.
70 Carrel, "The making of civilized man" (October 11, 1937), as quoted in Durkin, 135.
71 *Cahiers de la fondation française pour l'étude des problèmes humaines* [hereafter cited as *Cahiers*], 1(1943), 48–49.
72 *Cahiers*, 1(1943), 50–51.
73 Drouard, 1027–29.
74 *Cahiers*, 2(1944), 12. Carrel noted in one of his last letters to the United States, "There are incredible difficulties to surmount, but the organization which we have created is very resilient, because it is composed uniquely of men from 28 to 35 years of age on average. Only a few are 38 to 42." Letter of July 2, 1942, reproduced in Soupault, 244.
75 Durkin, 134.
76 *Cahiers*, 1(1943), 19. The other two projects reported in the first year were on the physical conditions of workers and "putting to use the mental qualities of the population."
77 *Cahiers*, 1(1943), 20–21.
78 *Cahiers*, 2(1944), 24.

CHAPTER 11

1 *Masing Maria* (Tananarive: Volamahitsy, 1956). Based on the place of publication, this was likely his land of refuge, after such close collaboration with the Germans.
2 On American and British human genetics, see Daniel J. Kevles, *In the name of eugenics* (NY: Knopf, 1985), 193–211, 251–68. A recent collection of studies on continuity in German research is Heidrun Kaupen-Haas, *Der Griff nach der Bevölkerung:Aktualität und Kontinuität nazistischer Bevölkerungspolitik* (Nördlingen: Delphi Politik, 1986).
3 See Lucien Jame's obituary in *Prophylaxie sanitaire et morale*, 41(1969), 5–9. Examples of Sicard's articles are "L'eugénisme français," *Prophylaxie antivénérienne*, 17(1945), 527–33; and "Prophylaxie du crime par l'eugénique et la puericulture," *Prophylaxie sanitaire et morale*, 28(1956), 82–89.
4 J. O. *Lois et décrets* (November 5, 1945), as cited in *Prophylaxie antivénérienne*, 18(1946), 160–62. It should be noted that the advisory com-

mission of the provisional government came close to eliminating the requirement of an examination altogether, because of its possible hindrance to marriage and potential eugenic uses, according to René Savatier, "Etude juridique," *Cahiers Laennec*, 17(1957), 11.

5 J. O. (November 5, 1945).

6 Ibid.

7 For examples, see Georges Schreiber, "La nouvelle réglementation du certificat médical prenuptial," *Presse médicale* (March 23, 1946), 194; Pierre Baude, *Examen médical prenuptial en France* (Paris: Thèse en médecine, 1947); P. Giacardy, "Dans quelle mésure la loi sur le sérologie prenuptiale et prenatale est-elle appliqué?" *Prophylaxie antivénérienne*, 22(1950), 338–39; Yvonne Carniol-Dreyfus, "Le certificat prenuptial," *Progrès médical*, 83(November 24, 1955), 407–408, which was based on a doctoral law thesis at Lyons in 1953; and an entire issue of the *Cahiers Laennec*, 17, no. 4(Nov. 1957) devoted to the examination. For a more sanguine view of the lack of eugenic danger posed by the law, from the perspective of twenty-five years of implementation, see Roger Nerson, "L'influence de la biologie et de la médecine moderne sur le droit civil," *Revue trimestrielle de droit civil*, 68(1970), 677–80.

8 Jean-Jacques Gillon, "Sondage sur la protection maternelle et infantile," *Concours médical*, 75(1953), 2787–96. As mentioned in Chapter 10 (n. 65), Gillon had been head of one of the research teams of Carrel's Fondation française pour l'étude des problèmes humaines.

9 P. Freour, M. Sérise, P. Coudray, and C. Cahuzac, "Le certificat prenuptial et l'opinion," *Hygiène mentale*, 48(1959), 220–21.

10 Lacomme and Grasset, "A propos du certificat d'examen médical avant le mariage," *Revue médical française*, (1943), 187–88.

11 *Cahiers de la fondation française pour l'étude des problèmes humaine*, 3(1945), 28.

12 Alfred Sauvy, *Richesse et population* (Paris: Payot, 1943), 82.

13 Alain Drouard, "Les trois âges de la fondation pour l'étude des problèmes humains," *Population*, 38(1983), 1037, n. 30.

14 *Population*, 1(1946), 187.

15 Alfred Sauvy, *De Paul Reynaud à Charles de Gaulle* (Paris: Casterman, 1972), 178. In cutting back the foundation staff to half its size, Sauvy eliminated the whole biology research team except Sutter.

16 Drouard, 141–43. For an example, see Raymond Mandé, "A propos d'une enquête pour le recensement des enfants anormaux," *Cahiers*, 4(1945), 84–94.

17 See, for example, "Le facteur 'qualité' en démographie," *Population*, 2(1946), 299–315; "Les avortements legaux eugéniques en Suède, en Danemark, en Suisse," *Population*, 3(1947), 575–79; and "Problèmes sanitaires posés par l'immigration," *Documents sur l'immigration* (Paris: Presses Universitaires de France, 1947), 197–223.

18 Jean Sutter, *Eugénique* (Paris: PUF, 1950); "L'évolution de la taille des polytechniciens (1801–1954)," *Population*, 13(1958), 373–406. For a complete bibliography see Albert Jacquard, ed. *Génétique et population:*

Hommage à Jean Sutter (Paris: PUF, 1971). For brief sketches of Sutter's life, see the obituaries by Sauvy and Jean Bourgeois-Pichat in *Population*, 25(1970), 749–52, and Jacquard in *Population*, 26(1971), 717–20.

19 Kevles, 164–75; Gar Allen, "The eugenics record office at Cold Spring Harbor, 1910–1940. An essay in institutional history," *Osiris*, 2nd ser., 2(1986), 250–54.

20 This conclusion is based only on a search of the Carrel papers at Georgetown University.

21 The views on immigration recently stated by French politician Jean-Marie LePen fit well with Martial's earlier ideas.

Selected bibliography

ARCHIVES AND GOVERNMENT

Alliance israelite universelle (Paris). Maurice Moch archives.
American Philosophical Society (Philadelphia). Charles Davenport papers.
Centre de documentation juive contemporaine (Paris). Archives.
France. Archives nationale. Série AJ15. Museum national d'histoire naturelle.
France. Archives nationales. Série AJ16. Ministère de la santé: Faculté de médecine.
France. Archives nationales. Série AN317. Louis Marin papers.
France. Bibliothèque nationale. Ms N.A.Fr. 24523.
France. Faculté de médecine (Paris). Archives.
France. *Journal officiel. Lois et décrets.*
France. *Journal officiel. Documents parlementaires.*
France. Ministère de la santé. *Bulletin du secretariat d'état à la santé. Receuil des textes officiels concernant la protection de la santé publique.* 1942.
France. Museum national d'histoire naturelle. Edmond Perrier papers.
France. Office national d'hygiène sociale. *Rapports annuels.* 1925–33.
Georgetown University. Alexis Carrel papers.
Institut de France. Académie des sciences. Dossiers of Edmond Perrier, Charles Richet.
Jewish Theological Seminary (New York). Documents of French history.
Montpellier. Université Paul Valéry. Georges Vacher de Lapouge archives.
Rockefeller Foundation Archives. Series RG 1.1.
Strasbourg. Archives municipales. Fondation Ungemach.

PERIODICALS (systematically searched)

American journal of physical anthropology. 1919–39.
Annales d'hygiène publique. 1900–25.
Anthropologie. 1919–39.
Cahiers de la fondation française pour l'étude des problèmes humaine. 1943–45.
Cahiers des droits de l'homme. 1900–40.
Cahiers du bolchevisme. 1925–39.
Chronique médicale. 1900–14.
Comptes rendus de la société de biologie. 1919–39.
Etudes. 1920–39.

Eugenics review. 1900–39.
Eugénique. 1912–26.
L'Humanité. 1920–39.
Industrial and labour information. 1923–39.
Mercure de France. 1919–39.
Prophylaxie antivénérienne. 1928–69.
Question juive. 1941–43.
Races et racisme. 1937–39.
Revue anthropologique. 1880–1940 [1880–90 title varies].
Revue de l'alliance nationale contre la dépopulation. 1896–1940 [title varies].
Revue de l'immigration. 1928–33.
Terre retrouvée. 1930–39.

BOOKS AND JOURNAL ARTICLES APPEARING BEFORE 1945

Abeau, Tilly. "Les ravages de l'article 317 contre l'avortement." *Cahiers du bolchevisme*, 6 (1931), 789–92.

Achard, M. "Décès de M. Charles Richet." *Comptes rendus de la société de biologie*, 120 (1935), 927–29.

Alexandresco, Virginie. "Enseignement officiel et particulier de la puericulture et vulgarisation de l'hygiène enfantile en Roumanie," *Annales de médicine et de chirurgerie infantile*, 11 (1907), 474–79.

Anias, Juan. "Contribution à l'étude du certificat prénuptial." Medical dissertation, University of Paris, 1935.

Apert, Eugène. "Afterwar medical problems: The preservation of the race," *Monde médical*, 27 (1917), 1–10.

——. ed. *Examen médicale en vue de mariage*. Paris: Flammarion, 1927.

——. "Eugénique en France," *Pédiatrie*, 9 (1940), 17–22.

——. "Eugénique en France." *Revue anthropologique*, 50 (1940), 205–16.

——. "Applications familiales de l'eugénique: Le certificat prénuptial," *Revue de l'Alliance nationale contre la dépopulation*, 43 (1942), 183–89.

Apert, Eugène, et al. *Eugénique et sélection*. Paris: Félix Alcan, 1922.

"Eugène Apert: Nécrologie," *Revue anthropologique*, 50 (1940), 205–16.

Arostegul, G. "Puericultura," *Gaceta medica catalana*, 28 (1905), 275–300.

Aubrun, H. "Le certificat prénuptial obligatoire," *Paris médical*, 68 (1928), 284–86.

Bachimont, Charles. "Documents pour servir à l'histoire de la puericulture interuterine." Medical dissertation, University of Paris, 1898.

Balgaires, E., and Louis Christiaens. "Le taux des iso-hémagglutinines des serums O, A et B chez l'adulte," *Comptes rendus de la société de biologie*, 126 (1937), 29–30.

——. "La distribution des iso-hémagglutinogènes A et B dans le Nord de la France," *Comptes rendus de la société de biologie*, 129 (1938), 567–68.

——. "Détection des hémo-agglutinogènes M et N dans les quantités minima de sang sec," *Comptes rendus de la société de biologie*, 130 (1939), 59–61.

Bar Paul. "Adolphe Pinard," *Gynécologié et obstétrique*, 29 (1934), 497–512.

Baron, Jean-Marie. *La grande découverte: Les juifs et le sang B*. Paris: Centre de documentation de propagande, 1938.

Beauplan, Robert de. "Les étrangers en France," *Illustration*, 201 (1938), 234–35.

Beliard, Octave. "L'oeuvre du Dr. René Martial," *Hippocrate. Revue d'humanisme médical*, 6 (1938), 617–27.

Bertillon, Jacques. *La dépopulation de la France*. Paris: Félix Alcan, 1911.

——. "La taille en France," *Revue scientifique*, 23 (1885), 481–88.

——. "Sur la natalité en France," *Bulletin de la société d'anthropologie*, 4e sér. 2 (1891), 366–85.

——. "Puericulture à bon marché," *Revue d'hygiène*, 19 (1897), 311–20.

Bertillon, Suzanne. *La vie d'Alphonse Bertillon*. Paris: Gallimard, 1941.

Biardeau, Laure. "Le certificat prénuptial." Medical dissertation, University of Paris, 1930.

Biauté. "Folie degénérescence et dépopulation," *Gazette médical de Nantes*, 26 (1908), 613–17.

Bied-Charreton, René. "Le problème national No. 1: Dénatalité et dépopulation," *Etudes*, 239 (1939), 471–89.

Binet, Alfred. "Recherche sur la technique de la mensuration de la tête vivante," *L'année psychologique*, 7 (1900), 314–429.

Bloch, Adolphe. "De la transformation d'une race dolichocéphalique en une race brachycéphalique, et vice versa," *Bulletin de la société d'anthropologie*, 5e, sér. 2 (1901), 73–83.

——. "Sur un prétendue découverte anthropologique aux Etats-Unis," *Bulletin de la société d'anthropologie*, 6e, sér. 2 (1911), 206–207.

Blondel, Raoul. "Le certificat prénuptial obligatoire," *Prophylaxie antivénérienne*, 15 (1943), 118–19.

Boas, Franz. *Report on changes in bodily form of descendants of immigrants*. Washington: Government Printing Office, 1911.

Boudin, J. "De l'acroissement de la taille et des conditions d'aptitude militaire en France," *Mémoires de la société d'anthropologie de Paris*, 1e, sér. 2 (1865), 221–59.

Boulanger, L. "Au sujet du certificat d'aptitude matrimoniale," *Vie médicale*, 6 (1925), 297–302.

Bounak, V. V. "Le mouvement eugénique en Russie." In *Institut international d'anthropologie, 2e session de Prague, 14–21 septembre 1924*, 536–39. Paris: Librairie Noury, 1926.

Bourgeois, Léon. "Lettres sur le mouvement social," *Nouvelle revue*, 93 (1895), 390–98, 642–48.

Bouthoul, Gaston. *La population dans le monde*. Paris: Payot, 1935.

Boverat, Fernand, "Qualité et quantité," *Revue de l'Alliance nationale contre la dépopulation*, 32 (1931), 399–403.

——. "Eugénisme. Dangers des mésures preconisées pour éviter la naissance des enfants anormaux," *Revue de l'alliance nationale contre la dépopulation*, 34 (1933), 69–73.

——. *La race blanche en danger de mort*. Paris: Editions de l'alliance nationale pour l'accroisement de la population française, 1933.

——. "Les communistes français et la natalité," *Revue de l'alliance nationale contre la dépopulation*, 37 (1936), 35–42.

——. *La résurrection par la natalité*. Lyons: Hachette, 1942.

Boyd, William C., and Lyle G. Boyd. "New data on blood groups and other inherited factors in Europe and Egypt," *American journal of physical anthropology*, 23 (1937), 49–70.

Brandenburg, G. "Du certificat d'aptitude du mariage." Medical dissertation, University of Paris, 1926.

Briand, Henri. "Quelques réflexions sur le certificat et l'examen prénuptial," *Revue anthropologique*, 41 (1931), 63–69.

——. "Une conference du Professeur Eugen Fischer à Paris," *Revue anthropologique*, 51 (1941), 195–96.

——. "Les vraies familles françaises doivent revivre," *L'Ethnie française*, 1 (1941), 5–9.

——. "Education physique et sauvegarde de la race," *Revue anthropologique*, 51 (1941), 8–15.

Brieux, Eugène. "Damaged goods." In *Three plays by Brieux*. New York: Brentanos, 1911.

Broca, Paul. "Sur la prétendue dégénérescence de la population française," *Revue des cours scientifiques de la France et à l'étranger*, 4 (1866–67), 307–309.

——. "Les sélections," *Mémoires d'anthropologie*, 3 (1877), 244–45.

Brouillard, René. "L'eugénique et morale catholique," *Interdiocesaine*, (April 1930), 113–19.

——. "Causerie de morale," *Etudes*, 207 (1931), 441–54, 578–600.

Bruno, Alexandre. *Contre la tuberculose. La mission Rockefeller en France et l'effort français*. Paris: Villages sanatoriums de hautes altitudes, 1925.

Brutzkus, Julius. "Les groupes sanguins parmi les populations juives," *Congrès international de la population. VII: Problèmes qualititatives de la population*, 72–82. Paris: Hermann, 1938.

Budin, Paul. "Note sur l'allaitement des nouveaux-nés," *Bulletin de l'académie de médicine*, 3e sér, 28 (1892), 99–114.

Buining, D. J. "Recherches sur les groupes sanguins aux Indes néerlandaises," *Anthropologie*, 44 (1934), 77–91, 315–25.

Cabanès, Henri. "Le mariage, doit-il être réglementé?" *Chronique médicale*, 10 (1903), 449–95.

Camus, Jean, and Pagniez(?), "D'un pouvoir agglutinant de certains sérums humains pour les globules rouge," *Comptes rendus de la société de biologie*, 58 (1901), 242–44.

Capdepont, Charles. "La doctrine de la dégénérescence et ses contradictions," *Revue de stomatologie*, 15 (1908), 26–30, 129–33.

Caron, Alfred. *L'hygiène des nouveau-nés dans ses rapports avec le développement physique et moral des individus au point de vue de l'amélioration de l'éspèce*. Paris: Plon, 1858.

——. *Puericulture ou la science d'élever hygièniquement et physiologiquement les enfants*. 2nd ed. Rouen: E. Orville, 1866.

Carrel, Alex. *Man, The unknown*. New York: Harper, 1935.

Carrel, Alexis, and Charles Lindbergh. "The culture of whole organs," *Science*, 81 (1935), 621–23.

Cattier, Fernand. "Enseignement de la puericulture," *Revue pédagogique*, 85 (1924), 132–38.

Cazalis, Henri. *Des risques pathologiques du mariage. Des hérédités morbides et l'examen médicale avant le mariage.* Brussels: Charles van de Weghe, 1902.

Chachuat, Maurice. *Le mouvement du "birth control" dans les pays Anglo-Saxons.* Paris: Marcel Giard, 1934.

Chambers, Theodore. "Eugenics and the war," *Eugenics review,* 6 (1914–15), 272–90.

Champouillon, M. "Etude sur le developpement de la taille et de la constitution de la population civile dans l'armée," *Receuil des mémoires de médicine chirurgicale et pharmacie militaire,* 3e sér., 22 (1869).

Chateau, Fernand. "Races et groupements sanguins," *Mercure de France,* (1938), 275–78.

Chesterton, G. K. *Eugenics and other evils.* London: Cassell and Co., 1922.

Chipau, André. "La lutte contre les taudis," *Cahiers du bolchevisme,* 13 (1936), 1250–57.

Coca, Arthur F., and O. Diebert. "A study of the occurrence of the blood groups among the American Indians," *Journal of immunology,* 8 (1923), 487–93.

Commission catholique du congrès de la natalité. *Eugénisme, stérilisation: Leur valeur morale.* Paris: Editions Spes, 1930.

——. *Où en-sommes nous? La doctrine familiale de l'église catholique.* Paris: Editions mariage et famille, 1932.

Comité national d'études sociales et politiques. *Les problèmes relatifs à l'immigration.* Paris: Comité national d'études sociales et politiques, 1925.

——. *Mariage et certificat prénuptial.* Paris: Comité national d'études sociales et politiques, 1928.

Conray, Jacques. "L'examen prénuptial." Medical dissertation, University of Lyons, 1938.

Couvelaire, Alexandre. "Quelques mots sur l'eugénique et les consultations prénuptiales," *Bulletin médical,* 44 (1930), 693–94.

Crane, R. Newton. "Marriage laws and statutory experiments in the United States," *Eugenics review,* 2 (1910), 61–73.

Cuénot, Lucien. "L'hérédité des caractères acquises," *Revue générale des sciences,* 32 (1921), 544–50.

——. "Génétique et adaptation." In *Eugenics, genetics and the family,* scientific papers at the Second International Congress of Eugenics. New York, September 22–28, 1921, 1:29–58. Baltimore: Williams and Wilkins, 1923.

——. "Eugénique," *Revue lorraine d'anthropologie,* 8 (1935–36), 5–24.

——. *Invention et finalité en biologie.* Paris: Flammarion, 1941.

D'Heucqueville, Georges. "Points de vue sur la stérilisation chirurgicale," *Annales de médicine legale,* 15 (1935), 208–14.

Darwin, Leonard. "Eugenics during and after the war," *Eugenics review,* 7 (1915–16), 91–106.

Dassonville, J., and L. DeGeuser. *Les laureats des Prix Cognacq-Jay.* Paris: Eds. Spes, 1926.

Davenport, Charles, "Marriage laws and customs," in *Problems in eugenics,* 151–55. London: Eugenics Education Society, 1912.

De Beauplan, Robert. "Les étrangers en France," *Illustration,* 201 (1938), 234–35.

De Bivort de la Sandée, J. "Le communisme et la famille," *Etudes*, 233 (1937), 52–62.

De Quatrefages, Armand. *Les émules de Darwin*. Paris: Félix Alcan, 1894.

Dennery, Etienne. *Foules d'Asie: Surpopulation japonaise, expansion chinoise, émigration indienne*. Paris: A. Colin, 1930.

Dequidt, Georges, and Georges Forestier. "Les aspects sanitaires du problème de l'immigration en France," *Revue d'hygiène*, 48 (1926), 999–1049.

Descamp, Desiré. "Le problème de la population," *Revue socialiste*, 23 (1896), 257–85.

Xe congrès international d'hygiène et de démographie à Paris en 1900: Compte rendu. Paris: Masson, 1901.

Drieu La Rochelle, Pierre. "Discours aux français sur les étrangers," *Revue hebdomadaire*, 7 (1926), 141–61.

Du Bruy, Bouessel. "De la necessité du certificat prénuptial." Medical dissertation, University of Paris, 1927.

Duclaux, Emile. *Hygiène sociale*. Paris: Félix Alcan, 1902.

Dujarric de la Rivière, Raymond, and Nicholas Kossovitch. *Les groupes sanguins*. Paris: J.-B. Ballière, 1936.

Duthil, R. "L'immigration aux Etats-Unis et le déclin de l'intelligence américaine," *La grande revue*, 118 (1925), 130–34.

"Encyclical Letter . . . on Christian marriage." *Sixteen encyclicals of Pope Pius XI*. Washington: National Catholic Welfare Conference.

Epting, Karl, ed. *État et santé*. Paris: Fernand Sorlot, 1942.

Espinas, Alfred. *Les sociétés animales*. Paris: Félix Alcan, 1877.

Etienne, Jacques. "Du certificat prénuptial." Medical dissertation, University of Paris, 1931.

Fabre-Luce, Alfred. *Anthologie de la nouvelle Europe*. Paris: Librairie Plon, 1942.

Faguet, Emile. "Le diplôme conjugal," *Revue politique et littéraire*, 18 (1902), 231–34.

Farinaud, M.-E. "La répartition des groupes sanguins chez les Bauhais, les Djarais et les sedangs, populations primitives de l'Indochine méridionale," *Comptes rendus de la société de biologie*, 131 (1939), 1236–38.

——. "Nouvelles recherches sur la distribution des groupes sanguins parmi les populations de l'Indochine méridionale: Les 'moïs' du Darlac et les Chams," *Comptes rendus de la société de biologie*, 131 (1939), 1238–40.

——. "Contribution à l'étude des populations de l'Indochine méridionale française d'après la répartition des groupes sanguins," *Bulletin de la société d'anthropologie de Paris*, 9e sér, 2 (1941), 75–102.

Fessard, G. *La main tendue: Le dialogue catholique-communiste, est-il possible?* Paris: Bernard Grasset, 1937.

Fetscher, Rainer. *Grundzüge der Rassenhygiene*. Dresden: Deutsche Verlag für Volkswohlfahrt, 1924.

Fischer, Eugen. "Le problème de la race et la législation raciale allemande." In *Etat et santé*, 81–110. Ed. Karl Epting. Paris: Fernand Sorlot, 1942.

Fitère, Armand. *Répopulation et eugénique*. Toulouse: Occitana, 1924.

Flloko, Pauli. "Protection de la race et le certificat prénuptial." Medical dissertation, University of Paris, 1934.

Fontaine, Raymond. "La législation récente sur la famille et l'enfant." In *La famille et l'enfant: problèmes d'aujourd'hui et de demain*, 9–15. Paris: Comité nationale de l'enfance, 1941.

Forest, Louis. "L'utilité de l'examen médical en vue de mariage." In *L'examen médical en vue de mariage* 31–35. Ed. Eugène Apert. Paris: Flammarion, 1926.

Fouillée, Alfred. *Science sociale contemporaine*. Paris: 1880.

Frachon, B. "Contre la xénophobie," *Cahiers du bolchevisme*, 7 (1932), 734–41.

Fruhinsholz, Albert. "L'enseignement de la puericulture aux maitresses et aux élèves." In IIIe congrès international d'hygiène scolaire (Paris 2–7 août 1910), 399–405. Paris: A. Maloine, 1910.

Galton. Francis. *English men of science: Their nature and nurture*. London: Macmillan, 1873.

——. *Inquiry into human faculty and its development*. New York: Macmillan, 1883.

——. *Life, letters and labours of Francis Galton*. 2 vols. Ed. Karl Pearson. Cambridge, England: Cambridge University Press, 1924.

"Garanties sanitaires du mariage," *Bulletin de la société de prophylaxie sanitaire et morale*, 3 (1903), 271–324, 339–85, 392–420, 470–88, 531–54.

Gebuhrer, Max. "Contribution à la question du certificat prénuptial." Medical dissertation, University of Strasbourg, 1935.

Gide, Charles. "Solidarité économique." In *Essai d'une philosophie de solidarité*. Ed. Alfred Croiset. Paris: Félix Alcan, 1902.

Glass, D. V. *Population policies and movements in Europe*. Oxford: Oxford University Press, 1940.

Godart, Justin, "A l'association d'études sexologiques," *Siècle médicale*, 7 (1933), 10.

Gontier, René. *Vers un racisme français*. Paris: Editions Denoël, 1939.

Gougerot, Henri. "Conférence par T.S.F.: Creons le certificat médical de mariage," *Prophylaxie antivénérienne*, 1 (1929), 380–83.

——. Enquête auprès du corps médical au sujet du certificat prénuptial, *"Prophylaxie antivénérienne*, 15(1943), 80–82.

Grant, Madison. *Le déclin de la grande race*. Paris: Payot, 1926.

Gravier, Charles. "Un souvenir de M. Edmond Perrier," *Bulletin du museum national d'histoire naturelle*, 27 (1921), 498–504.

Grellety, Lucien. "Psychologie du mariage–l'examen des jeunes mariés," *Revue de psychiatrie, neurologie et hypnologie*, 1 (1890), 202–204.

Grimbert, Charles. "Les psychopathies ou anomalies mentales et l'eugénisme," *Revue de philosophie*, 25 (1930), 129–40.

Halber, W., and Jan Mydlarski. "Recherches séro-anthropologiques en Pologne," *Comptes rendus de la société de biologie*, 89 (1923), 1373–75.

Haldane, C. B. S. "Report of the meeting of the International Federation of Eugenics Organizations," *Eugenical news*, 11 (1926), 137–39.

Hamburger, Maurice, *Léon Bourgeois, 1851–1925*. Paris: M. Rivière, 1932.

Hardy, G. [pseudonym of Gabriel Giroud]. "The situation in France." In *Sixth international neo-Malthusian and birth control conference*, 33–40. Ed. Margaret Sanger. New York: American Birth Control League, 1925.

——. *Paul Robin, sa vie, ses idées, son action*. Paris: Mignolet et Storz, 1937.

Haskovec, Ladislaus. "Le certificat médical prematrimonial," *Institut international d'anthropologie. 2e session de Prague, 14–21 septembre 1924*, 455–59. Paris: Noury, 1926.

Haury, Paul. "Une natalité suffisante, est-ce la guerre?" *Revue de l'alliance nationale contre la dépopulation*, 35 (1934), 33–40.

———. "Le destin des races blanches," *Revue de l'alliance nationale contre la dépopulation*, 36 (1935), 267–72.

Heger-Gilbert, Félix. "La stérillisation des fonctions genitales," *Bulletin de la société française sanitaire et morale*, 28 (1928), 65–74.

Henry, Louis. "La puericulture au congrès de l'alliance d'hygiène sociale d'Arras," *Revue philanthropique*, 16 (1904), 146–58, 271–91.

Hervieu, Louise. *Le malade vous parle*. Paris: Editions Noël, 1943.

Heuyer, Louis. "Conditions de santé à envisager au point de vue du mariage dans les maladies." In *L'examen médicale en vue du mariage*, 123–36. Ed. Eugène Apert. Paris: Flammarion, 1926.

Hirszfeld, Ludwig. *Konstitutionsserologie und Blutgruppenforschung*. Berlin: Springer, 1928.

Hirszfeld, Ludwig, and Hanna Hirszfeld. "Essai d'application des méthodes sérologiques au problème des races," *Anthropologie*, 29 (1919), 505–37.

Hirszfeld, Ludwig, and E. Przesmycki. "Recherches sur l'agglutination normale. De l'isoagglutination des globules rouges chez les chevaux," *Comptes rendus de la société de biologie*, 89 (1923), 1360–61.

Hirszfeld, Ludwig, and H. Zborowski. "Sur la symbiose sérologique entre la mére et le foetus," *Comptes rendus de la société de biologie*, 94 (1926), 205–207.

Houssay, Frédéric. "Eugénique, sélection et determinisme des tares." In *Problems in eugenics*, 155–61. London: Eugenics Education Society, 1912.

Huber, Michel. *La population de la France pendant la guerre*. Paris: PUF, 1931.

———. "Lucien March, 1859–1933," *Journal de la société de statistique de Paris*, 32 (1933), 269–80.

———. "Quarante années de la statistique générale de la France, 1896–1936," *Journal de la société de statistique de Paris*, 36 (1937), 179–89.

Huntington, Ellsworth, and Leon Whitney. *Builders of America*. New York: Morrow, 1927.

Huxley, Julian S., and Alfred C. Haddon. *We Europeans*. New York: Harpers, 1936.

Ichok, G. "L'hygiène à l'étranger. La stérilisation des indésirables aux Etats-Unis d'Amérique," *Revue d'hygiène*, 52 (1930), 271–76.

Jarach, M. "Cours de puericulture," *Revue pédagogique*, 42 (1903), 67–68; 43 (1904), 270–72.

Jeanneny, Georges. "Hérédité, génétique, eugénique," *Revue française de gynécologique et d'obstétrique*, 39 (1944), 121–44.

Jordan, Edouard. "Limites, dangers et contradictions de l'eugénique," *Nourisson*, 17 (1939), 20–27.

———. "Eugénisme et morale," *Cahiers de la nouvelle journée*, 19 (1931), 1–176.

———. "Natalité dirigée," *Etudes*, 231 (1937), 762–74.

———. ed. *L'église et l'eugénisme*. Paris: Editions mariage et famille, 1930.

Kahn, Gustave. "Fecondité," *Revue blanche*, 20 (1899), 285–93.

Klotz-Forest. "La prophylaxie anticonceptionnelle est-elle légitime?" *Chronique médicale*, 11 (1904), 689–99.

Kossovitch, Nicholas. "Les groupes sanguins chez les tcheques," *Comptes rendus de la société de biologie*, 93 (1923), 1343–44.

———. "Recherches sur la race arménienne par l'isohémagglutination," *Comptes rendus de la société de biologie*, 97 (1927), 69–71.

———. "Les groupes sanguins chez les français et les règles de l'hérédité," *Comptes rendus de la société de biologie*, 102 (1929), 494–97.

———. "Les groupes sanguins chez les français," *Revue anthropologique*, 39 (1929), 244–59, 374–79; 41 (1931), 131–55.

Kossovitch, Nicholas, and Ferdinand Benoit. "Contribution à l'étude anthropologique et sérologique des juifs modernes," *Revue anthropologique*, 42 (1932), 99–125.

———. "Une tribu inconnu du Maroc: Les bahloula," *Revue anthropologique*, 45 (1935), 347–63.

Kroeber, Alfred. "Blood group classification," *American journal of physical anthropology*, 18 (1934), 377–94.

Lacomme, M., and Raymond Grasset. "A propos du certificat d'examen médical avant le mariage institué par la loi du 16 décembre 1942," *Revue médicale française*, 12 (1943), 185–88.

Laffont, A., and J. Audit, "Eugénique." In *Encyclopédie médico-chirurgicale*, vol. 6-2, 1–24. Paris: Masson, 1934.

Lakhovsky, Georges. "Que doit-on penser du racisme?" *Illustration*, 201 (1933) 107–108.

———. *Racisme, l'orchestre universel*. Paris: Félix Alcan, 1934.

———. *La civilisation et la folie raciste*. Paris: Editions SACL, 1939.

Lambert, Charles. *La France et les étrangers*. Paris: Delagrave, 1928.

Lamy, M. *Les applications de la génétique à la médicine*. Paris: G. Doin, 1943.

Landouzy, Louis. "A propos de l'hérédité et de sa signification clinique," *Revue pratique d'obstétrique et de gynécologie*, 21 (1906), 94–96.

———. "Aperçus de médicine sociale," *Revue de médicine* 25 (1905), 955–77.

Landry, Adolphe. "L'eugénique," *Revue bleue*, (1913), 779–83.

Laumonnier, J. "Eugénique," *Larousse mensuel*, no. 65 (July, 1912), 454–55.

———. "Le prémier congrès d'eugénique," *Gazette des hôpitaux*, 85 (1912), 1475–77.

Le Dantec, Félix. "Les théories néo-lamarckiennes," *Revue philosophique*, 44 (1897), 449–75, 561–90.

Légrain, Paul-Maurice. *Dégénérescence sociale et l'alcoolisme*. Paris: Masson, 1895.

———. *L'hérédité et l'alcoolisme*. Paris: O. Doin, 1889.

Legueu, Félix. "Le certificat prénuptial," *Progrès médical*, 44 (1929), 2273–78.

Leroy, Edgar. "Le certificat prénuptial à la campagne," *Mouvement sanitaire*, 6 (1930), 75–83.

Letulle, Maurice. "L'oeuvre de Landouzy," *Presse médicale* 26 (1917), 265–67.

Levrat, Etienne. "Stérilisation et eugénique," *Toulouse médical*, 31 (1930), 1–11.

Levy, Georges. "Le problème de la santé publique en France," *Cahiers du bolchevisme*, 14 (1937), 48–61.

——. "Pour une politique de protection de la famille et de l'enfance," *Cahiers du bolchevisme*, 16 (1939), 362–73.

Lindsay, J. A. "The eugenic and social influence of the war," *Eugenics review*, 10 (1918–19), 133–44.

Liodt, V., and N. Pojarski, "L'application de l'isohémoagglutination à l'études des races indigènes de l'Afrique equatoriale française," *Comptes rendus de la société de biologie*, 101 (1929), 889–90.

Lombroso-Ferrero, Gina. *Criminal man according to the classifications of Cesare Lombroso*. NY: G. P. Putnam's Sons, 1911.

Louis, J. H., and D. L. Henderson. "The racial distribution of isohaemagglutination groups," *Journal of the American medical association*, 79 (1922), 1422–24.

[Lowenthal]. "La lutte contre la dégénérescence: stérilisation et castration," *Paris médical*, 95 (1935), 250–54.

Magnan, Valentin, and Alfred Filassier. "Alcoolisme et dégénérescence." In *Problems in eugenics*, 354–67. London: Eugenics Education Society, 1912.

Magnan, Valentin and Paul-Marie Légrain. *Les dégénérés*. Paris: Rueff, 1895.

Manouvrier, Léonce. "L'indice céphalique et la pseudo-sociologie," *Revue anthropologique*, 9 (1899), 233–59, 280–96.

Manuila, Sabin and Georges Popoviciu. "Recherches sur les races roumanes et hongrois en Roumanie par l'isohémagglutination," *Comptes-rendus de la société de biologie*, 90 (1924), 542–43, 1069–73.

March, Lucien. *Commission de la dépopulation. Sous-commission de la natalité. Rapport sur les causes professionnelles de la dépopulation*. Melun: Imprimerie administrative, 1905.

——. "Pour la race. Infertilité et puériculture," *Revue du mois*, 10 (1910), 551–82.

——. "Deux congrès interessants d'hygiène sociale," *Revue politique et parlementaire*, 74 (1912), 531–51.

——. "Some attempts toward race hygiene in France during the war," *Eugenics review*, 10 (1918–19), 195–212.

——. "The consequences of war and the birthrate in France." In *Eugenics, genetics and the family. Scientific papers at the Second International Congress of Eugenics, New York, September 22–28, 1921*, 243–65. Baltimore: Williams and Wilkins, 1923.

Marchand, Henri-Jean. "L'évolution de l'idée eugénique." Medical dissertation, University of Bordeaux, 1933.

Margueritte, Victor. *Prostituée*. Paris: E. Pasquelle, 1907.

Martial, René. *L'ouvrier: Son hygiène, son atelier, son habitation*. Paris: O. Doin, 1909.

——. *Travaux du bureaux d'hygiène de la ville de Douai pendant l'année 1911*. Douai: Lefebvre, 1912.

——. "Organisation scientifique des usines ou méthode de F. W. Taylor," *Revue d'hygiène et de police sanitaire*, 35 (1913), 146–68.

——. "Immigration de la main d'oeuvre agricole et industrielle," *Annales d'hygiène*, 8 (1924), 236–41.

——. "Prophylaxie de l'immigration pendant et depuis la guerre," *Annales d'hygiène*, 48 (1926), 399–407.

——. "Le problème de l'immigration: Examen sanitaire et logement des immi-grants," *Revue politique et parlementaire*, 129 (1926), 391–402.

——. "Législation et prophylaxie de l'immigration aux Etats-Unis et dans d'autres pays," *Annales d'hygiène*, 48 (1926), 463–69.

——. "La main d'oeuvre étrangère en France," *Annales d'hygiène*, 48 (1926), 282–301.

——. *La Pologne jadis et de nos jours*. Paris: Gebethner and Wolff, 1927.

——. "De l'immigration. Nouvelles formules à adopter," *Concours médical*, 50 (1928), 361–64.

——. "Voyage avec des émigrants, du Havre à Buenos Aires," *Bulletin de l'aca-démie de médicine*, 101 (1929), 687–93.

——. "Les services d'immigration en Argentine, leur législation et leurs statis-tiques," *Bulletin de l'academie de médicine*, 102 (1929), 57–64.

——. *Traité de l'immigration et de la greffe inter-raciale*. Paris: Larose, 1931.

——. *Appareil circulatoire: Sang et humeurs*. Paris: Albin Michel, 1932.

——. "L'immigration et le pouvoir de résorption de la France," *Revue anthropo-logique*, 43 (1933), 351–69, 449–67.

——. *La race française*. Paris: Mercure de France, 1934.

——. *Titres et travaux de René Martial*. Paris: Jouve, 1935.

——. "Politique de l'immigration," *Mercure de France*, 259 (1935), 267–94.

——. "Le parallelisme céphalo-hématique et ses consequences au point de vue de la definition de la race," *Revue anthropologique*, 45 (1935), 227–33.

——. "Les peuples du Caucase: Nouvelles orientations dans les études d'anthro-pologie," *Anthropologie*, 46 (1936), 65–89, 303–22.

——. "Note sur la correlation entre les indices céphaliques des crânes et des groupements sanguins." In *Institut international d'anthropologie. 5e congrès (Brux-elles), Rapport*, 61–65. Brussels: Imprimerie médicale et scientifique, 1936.

——. "Un precurseur des groupements sanguins: Vacher de Lapouge," *Mercure de France*, 272 (1936), 620–25.

——. "Metissage et immigration." In *Premier congrès latin d'eugénique (1–3 août 1937), Rapport*, 16–40. Ed. Raymond Turpin. Paris: Masson, 1938.

——. *Vie et constances des races*. Paris: Mercure de France, 1939.

——. *Français, qui es-tu?* Paris: Mercure de France, 1942.

——. "Le racisme: Loi biologique fondamentale," *L'ethnie française*, 1 (1942), 31–44.

——. "Les juifs et le sang B," *L'ethnie française*, 3 (1942), 45–51.

Martial, René, and André Cavaillon. "Conditions imposé par la guerre et la pro-phylaxie," *Montpellier médical*, 36 (1917), 729–38.

Martin, Henri. "Le certificat prénuptial," *Bulletin de la société medicale de S. Luc. S. Côme et S. Damen*, 35 (1929), 33–45.

Martineau, Henri. *Le roman scientifique d'Emile Zola*. Paris: Baillière, 1907.

Martinetti, Maria. "Sulla puericultura intrauterina," *Rivista di igiene e sanita pub-blica*, 12 (1901), 940–53.

Massis, Henri. *Comment Emile Zola composait ses romans*. Paris: Fasquelles, 1906.

Mauco, Georges. *Les étrangers en France*. Paris: Armand Colin, 1932.

——. "L'immigration étrangère en France et le probléme des refugiés," *L'ethnie française*, 6 (1942), 6–15.

——. "La situation démographique en France," *L'ethnie francaise*, 7 (1943), 15–19.

Maurel, E. "Contribution à l'étude de l'eugénique," *Province médicale*, 24 (1913), 113–15.

Merrill, Theodore. "Centralized French endeavor in the field of social hygiene," *Journal of social hygiene*, 9 (1923), 257–66.

Meyer, André. "Notice nécrologique sur M. Charles Richet (1850–1935)," *Bulletin de l'académie de médecine*, 115 (1936), 51–64.

Michon, Paul. "Sur les variations quantitatives de l'isohemagglutination et les infractions aux schema de Moss," *Comptes rendus de la société de biologie*, 92 (1925), 37–39.

——. "Nouvelles remarques sur l'isohemagglutination-conservation des stock-serums," *Comptes rendus de la société de biologie*, 94 (1926), 676–78.

——. "Individualité humorale et groupes sanguins," *Comptes rendus de la société de biologie*, 100 (1929), 445–47.

Millet, Raymond. *Trois millions d'étrangers en France*. Paris: Librairie de Medicis, 1938.

Milne-Edwards, Henri. *Leçons sur la physiologie et l'anatomie comparée*. 14 vols. Paris: Masson, 1857–1881.

Montandon, Georges. *Ethnie française*. Paris: Payot, 1935.

Montet, Eugène. "Pour l'hygiène sociale," *Annales d'hygiène publique*, n.s., 4 (1923), 3–4.

Muller, H. J. *Hors de la nuit*. Paris: Gallimard, 1938.

Nisot, Marie-Thérèse. *La question eugénique dans les divers pays*. 2 vols. Brussels: G. van Campenhout, 1927–29.

——. "La stérilisation des anormaux," *Mercure de France*, 209 (1929), 595–608.

Nordau, Max. *Degeneration*. New York: Howard Fertig, 1968.

Nordmann, Charles. "Les grand fleaux humains," *Revue des deux mondes*, 6e sér., 20 (1914), 205–16.

——. "La croisade des américains contre la tuberculose en France," *Revue scientifique*, 47 (1918), 457–68.

Oualid, William. "Control of foreign workers in France," *Industrial and labour information*, 7 (1923), 2–10.

Pairault, André. "Immigration et race," *Revue de l'immigration*, 25 (1930), 1–3.

Papillaut, Georges. "Le VIe congrès d'anthropologie criminelle," *Revue de l'école d'anthropologie* [*Revue anthropologique*], 19, (1909), 28–40.

——. "Galton et la biosociologie," *Revue anthropologique*, 21 (1911), 56–65.

Pearson, Karl. *La grammaire de la science*. Trans. Lucien March. Paris: Félix Alcan, 1912.

Pelletier, Madelaine. "Qu'est'ce que la dégénérescence?" *Médecine moderne*, 16 (1905), 281–82.

——. "La prétendue dégénérescence des hommes de génie," *Médecine moderne*, 17 (1906), 25–26.

——. "Les dégénérés dans l'armée," *Médecine moderne* 18 (1907), 36–37.

Penel, J. "La stérilisation eugénique en Amérique," *Hygiène mentale*, 25 (1930), 173–88.

Perrier, Edmond. "Role de l'association dans le regne animal," *Revue scientifique*, 17 (1879), 556.

———. *Colonies animales et la formation des organismes*. Paris: Masson, 1881.

———. *A travers le monde vivant*. Paris: Flammarion, 1916.

———. *La vie en action*. Paris: Flammarion, 1918.

———. *Les origines de la vie et de l'homme*. Paris: Flammarion, 1920.

———. *La terre avant l'histoire*. Paris: Flammarion, 1920.

Picard, Roger. "Les étrangers en France," *Cahiers des droits de l'homme*, 26 (1926), 372.

Pichou, Alfred. "L'élite," *Revue internationale de sociologie* 4 (1896), 583–84.

———. "La religion de l'élite," *Revue internationale de sociologie*, 15 (1907), 597–618.

Piechaud, Ferdinand, and Henri Marchaud. "La loi allemande de stérilisation," *Journal de médecine de Bordeaux*, 11 (1934), 103–104.

Pinard, Adolphe. "De l'assistance des femmes enceintes, des femmes en couches et des femmes accouchées," *Revue d'hygiène et police sanitaire*, 12 (1890), 1098–1112.

———. "Note pour servir à l'histoire de la puericulture intra-uterine," *Bulletin de l'academie de médecine*, 34 (1895), 593–97.

———. "A propos du développement de l'enfant," *Revue scientifique*, 34 (1896), 109–11.

———. "De la puericulture pendant la grossesse," *Revue d'hygiène*, 20 (1898), 1072–79.

———. "De la conservation et l'amélioration de l'éspèce," *Bulletin médical*, 13 (1899), 141–46.

———. "Cours de puericulture," *Revue pédagogique*, 42 (1903), 67–68; 43 (1904), 270–72.

———. "Rapport sur un arrêté municipal pris par M. Morel de Villiers, médecin et maire de la commune de Villiers-le-Duc (Côte d'Or)" *Bulletin de l'academie de médecine*, 3e sér., 51 (1904), 222–36.

———. "Prophylaxie de l'hérédo-syphilis," *Annales de gynécologie et d'obstétrique*, 62 (1905), 201–205.

———. "Note sur les causes de la faible mortalité infantile dans la ville du Creusot," *Annales de gynécologie et d'obstétrique*, 62 (1905), 523–30.

———. "Des aptitudes du mariage envisagées au point de vue physique, moral et social," *Revue pratique d'obstétrique et de paediatrique*, 19 (1906), 7–16.

———. "De l'eugénnetique," *Bulletin médical*, 26 (1912), 1123–27.

———. *La puericulture du premier âge*. 6th ed. Paris: Armand Colin, 1913.

Pinard, Adolphe, and Charles Richet. "Rapport sur les causes physiologiques de la diminution de la natalité en France," *Annales de gynécologie et d'obstétrique*, 59 (1903), 15–24, 93–121.

Pirie, James Hunter Harvey. "Bloodtesting preliminary to transfusion: With a note on the distribution among South African natives," *Medical journal of South Africa*, 16 (1921), 109–25.

Popenoe, Paul, and Roswell Johnson. *Applied eugenics*. New York: Macmillan, 1920.

Popoviciu, Georges. "Recherches sérologiques sur les races en Roumanie," *Revue anthropologique*, 35 (1925), 152–64.

Popovsky, Nicholas. "Contribution à l'étude des législations français qui pourra intervenir à l'occasion d'un examen pré-nuptial." Medical dissertation, University of Paris, 1932.

Poulton, E. B. "The disabled sailor and soldier and the future of our race," *Eugenics review*, 9 (1917–18), 218–22.

Problems in eugenics: First international eugenics congress, 1912. London: Eugenics Education Society, 1912.

Quillent, E. "A la santé du proletariat. L'action antialcoolique," *Revue socialiste*, 30, (1914), 519–26.

Rabaud, Etienne. "Origine et transformation de la notion de dégénéré," *Revue de l'école d'anthropologie [Revue anthropologique]*, 17 (1907), 37–46.

Raymond, D. "La dépopulation et la misère de l'enfance" *Cahiers du bolchevisme*, 13 (1936), 101–109.

Raynaud, André. "Contribution à l'étude du certificat prénuptial." Medical dissertation, University of Marseilles, 1933.

Regnault, Félix. "Il n'y a pas une race juif," *Revue anthropologique*, 42 (1932), 390–93.

Reichler, Max. *Jewish eugenics*. New York: Bloch Publishing, 1916.

Richet, Charles. "Accroissement de la population française," *Revue des deux mondes*, 3e sér. 50 (1882), 900–32; 51 (1882), 587–616.

———. "Faut-il laisser la France périr?," *Revue bleue* (1896), 620–22.

———. *Le passé de la guerre et l'avenir de la paix*. Paris: Ollendorff, 1907.

———. *Sélection humaine*. Paris: Félix Alcan, 1919.

———. "Memoires sur moi et les autres." Unpublished manuscript, 1920.

———. "Charles Richet, autobiographie." In *Les biographies médicales*, 5: 157–88. Ed. P. Busquet and Maurice Genty. Paris: J.-B. Ballière, 1932.

———. *Souvenirs d'un physiologiste*. Yonne: J. Peyronnet, 1933.

———. *Au secours*. Paris: Peyronnet, 1935.

Rivet, Paul. "Les données de l'anthropologie." In *Nouveau traité de psychologie*, 1:55–101. Ed. Georges Dumas. Paris: Félix Alcan, 1930.

Rodé, P. "Les groupes sanguins chez les races indigènes de l'Afrique occidentale," *Comptes rendus de la société de biologie*, 122 (1936), 206–208.

Rodé, P. "Le phenomène d'agglutination dans les recherches de groupes sanguins chez les lepreux," *Comptes rendus de la société de biologie*, 122 (1936), 300–302.

Roger, Henri. "Charles Richet," *Presse médicale*, 43 (1935), 2043–45.

Rostand, Jean. "L'homme, cet inconnu," *Revue hebdomadaire*, 46 (1935), 288–300.

———. *Hérédité et racisme*. Paris: Gallimard, 1939.

Roubakine, Alexandre. "Sur la prétendue 'dépopulation' de la France," *Bulletin de l'académie de médecine*, 113 (1935), 143–47, 219–27, 492–504, 516–19.

Ruyer, Raymond. "Une législation eugéniste," *Revue de metaphysique et de morale*, 3 (1937), 659–78.

Sanger, Margaret. *Margaret Sanger: An autobiography*. New York: Norton, 1938.

Sauvy, Alfred. *Richesse et population*. Paris: Payot, 1943.

Scheifley, William H. *Brieux and contemporary French society.* New York: G. P. Putnam's Sons, 1917.

Schiff, Paul, and Pierre Mareschal. "Hérédité psychopathique et stérilisation eugénique," *Annales médico-legales,* 89 (1931), 71–78.

Schreiber, Georges. "A la fédération internationale d'eugénique," *Revue anthropologique,* 45 (1935), 78–92.

——. "Examen médical prénuptial devant la société française d'eugénique," *Vie médicale,* 7 (1926), 2411–14.

——. "L'examen médical prénuptial dans les differents pays," *Bulletin médical,* 41 (1927), 170–74.

——. "La stérilisation humain aux Etats-Unis," *Revue anthropologique,* 39 (1929), 260–81.

——. "Le certificat médical prénuptial: Comment l'instituer en France?" *Prophylaxie antivénérienne,* 11 (1939), 594–601.

——. "L'eugénique en France," *Nourisson,* 30 (1940), 89–102.

See, Henri. *Histoire de la ligue des droits de l'homme, 1898–1926.* Paris: Ligue des droits de l'homme, 1927.

Sicard de Plauzoles, Just. *Principles d'hygiène sociale.* Paris: Editions médicales, 1927.

——. "Le droit à la vie saine," *Cahiers des droits de l'homme,* 27 (1927), 103.

——. "Le certificat prénuptial," *Prophylaxie antivénérienne,* 1 (1929), 347–52.

——. "L'avenir de l'éspèce humain. La surpopulation, c'est la guerre," *Prophylaxie antivénérienne,* 7 (1935), 69–99.

Sicard de Plauzoles, Just, and A. Cavaillon. "Le corps médical et le certificat prénuptial," *Prophylaxie antivénérienne,* 16 (1944), 154–59.

Sinclair, Upton. *Sylvia's marriage.* Chicago: John C. Winston, 1914.

Snyder, Louis H. "Human blood groups: Their inheritance and racial significance," *American journal of physical anthropology,* 9 (1926), 233–63.

Spillmann, L. "De l'utilité du certificat pré-nuptial," *Revue d'hygiène sociale,* 12 (1933), 65–85.

Steffan, Paul, and Siegmund Wellisch. "Die geographische Verteliung der Blutgruppen," *Zeitschrift für Rassenphysiologie,* 2 (1930), 114–45; 3 (1931), 184–7; 5 (1932), 180–85; 6 (1933), 28–35.

Stoddard, Lothrop. *Le flôt montant des peuples de couleur contre la superiorité mondiale des blancs.* Paris: Payot, 1925.

Strauss, Paul. "La puericulture," *Revue des revues,* 32 (1900), 125–40, 229–37.

Swarc, G. "La stérilisation sexuelle et l'eugénique," *Hygiène mentale,* 29 (1934), 228–34.

Tarboureich, Ernest. *La cité future.* Paris: Stock, 1902.

Tebbult, A. H., and S. McConnel. "Human isohemagglutinins: Their distribution among some Australian aborigines," *Medical journal of Australia,* 1 (1922), 201–208.

Thomas, Paul. "Le certificat d'aptitude matrimonial," *Vie médicale,* 5 (1924), 1621–22.

Tisserand, M. "A propos des mesures appliqués depuis quatres ans en Allemagne pour veiller à la protection de la race," *Concours médical,* 61 (1939), 1087–89; 1161–62.

Toledano, André. "La question eugénique," *Revue de l'alliance nationale pour l'accroisement de la population française*, 29 (1928), 50–53.

Toulemon, André. "Le suffrage dit 'universel' et la natalité," *Etudes*, 231 (1937), 588–60.

Toulouse, Edouard. "Le problème humaine," *Le journal* (November 2, 1931).

Toulouse, Edouard, and A. Courtois. "La stérilisation chirurgicale du point de vue médico-legale," *Bulletin de la société de sexologie*, 2 (1935), 316–24.

Turpin, Raymond. "La génétique appliquée à la prophylaxie des maladies humains," *Semaine des hôpitaux de Paris*, 15 (1936), 386–94; 413–17.

——, ed. *Prémier congrès latin d'eugénique (1–3 août 1937)*. Rapport. Paris: Masson, 1938.

——. "Le péril pour l'espèce de mutations germinales," *Semaine des hôpitaux de Paris*, 15 (1939), 339–47.

——. "Eugénisme et guerre," *Bulletin médical*, 42 (1941), 471–75.

——. "Applications familiales de l'eugénisme." In *La famille et l'enfant: Problèmes d'aujourd'hui et de demain*, 177–90. Paris: Comité nationale de l'enfance, 1941.

Turpin, Raymond, A. Caratzali, and H. Rogier. "Etude étiologique de 104 cas de mongolisme et considérations sur la pathogénie de cette maladie." In *Prémier congrès latin d'eugénique (1–3 août 1937)*. Rapport, 154–64. Ed. Turpin. Paris: Masson, 1938.

Turpin, Raymond, A. Caratzali, and M. Gorny. "Contribution à l'étude de l'influence de l'âge et de l'état de santé des procreateurs, du rang et du nombre des naissances, sur les caractères de la progéniture." In *Prémier congrès latin d'eugénique (1–3 août 1937)*. Rapport, 240–61. Ed. Turpin. Paris: Masson, 1938.

Turpin, Raymond, A. Caratzali, and N. Georgescu-Roagen. "Influence de l'âge maternel, du rang de naissance et de l'ordre des naissances, sur la mortinatalité." In *Prémier congrès latin d'eugénique (1–3 août 1937)*. Rapport, 271–77. Ed. Turpin. Paris: Masson, 1938.

Vacher de Lapouge, Georges. "L'anthropologie et la science politique; Leçon d'ouverture du cours libre d'anthropologie de 1886–87," *Revue d'anthropologie* (1887), 136–57.

——. "La dépopulation de la France," *Revue d'anthropologie* (1887), 69–80.

——. *Sélections sociales*. Paris: A. Fontemoing, 1896.

——. *L'aryen et son rôle social*. Paris: A. Fontemoing, 1899.

——. *Resumé des travaux scientifiques*. Poitiers: Société d'imprimerie et de librairie, 1909.

——. "La race chez les populations melangées." In *Eugenics, genetics and the family: Scientific papers of the second international congress of eugenics*, 1–6. Baltimore: Williams and Wilkins, 1923.

——. "A eugenic birthrate for France." In *Sixth international neo-Malthusian and birth control conference*, 227–31. Ed. Margaret Sanger. New York: American Birth Control League, 1925.

Vallin, E., and A.-J. Mastin. "De la déclaration obligatoire des maladies transmissibles, ses conséquences nécessaires." In *Xe congrè international d'hygiène et de démographie à Paris en 1900. Compte rendu*, 733–57. Paris: Masson, 1901.

[Verine]. "La famille." In *France 1941: La révolution nationale constructive. Un bilan et un programme*, 191–214. Paris: Editions Alsatia, 1941.

Verwaeck, Louis, and Jules LeClercq. "Le certificat prénuptial," *Annales de médecine legale,* 9 (1929), 297–337.

Verzar, Frigyes, and Oskar Weszecky. "Rassenbiologische Untersuchungen mittels isohaemagglutinen," *Biochemische Zeitung,* 126 (1921), 33–39.

Vignes, Henri. "Certificat du mariage ou vulgarisation des notions d'eugéniques." In *Institut international d'anthropologie, 2e session de Prague, 14–21 septembre 1924,* 459–96. Paris: Noury, 1926.

——. "Stérilisation des inadaptés sociaux," *Revue anthropologique,* 42 (1932), 228–44.

——. "Les indications de la loi allemande de stérilisation eugénique," *Presse médicale,* 42 (1934), 825–27, 971–73.

——. "Intoxication alcoolique et ses effets sur la race," *Revue anthropologique,* 51 (1941), 33–42.

Virebeau, Georges. *Les juifs et leurs crimes.* Paris: Office de propagande nationale, 1938.

Vishnevski, Boris. "Anthropology in the U.S.S.R. in the course of 17 Years (1917–1934)," *American journal of physical anthropology,* 21 (1936), 1–17.

Von Verscheurer, Otmar. "L'image héréditaire de l'homme." In *Etat et santé,* 59–79. Ed. Karl Epting. Paris: Sorlot, 1942.

——. *Manuel d'eugénique et hérédité humaine.* Paris: Masson, 1943.

Wallich, Victor. "A propos de l'histoire de la puericulture," *Annales de gynécologie et d'obstétrique,* 2e sér. (1906), 19–23.

Weill-Hallé, Benjamin. "La puericulture et son évolution," *Presse médicale,* 37 (1929), 217–20.

——. "L'Ecole de puericulture," *Revue française de puericulture,* 1 (1933), 21–41.

Williams, Linsly R. "La fondation Rockefeller dans la lutte contre la tuberculose en France," *Revue du musée social* (1922), 33–64.

Wolf, Ch. "Stérilisation eugénique," *Presse médicale,* 44 (1936), 1228–32.

Wurtz, Pierre. *La question d'immigration aux Etats-Unis.* Paris: L. Dreux et M. Schneider, 1925.

Wyman, Leland C., and William C. Boyd. "Human blood groups and anthropology," *American anthropologist,* 37 (1935), 192–93.

Younovitch, Rina. "Les caractères sérologiques des juifs asiatiques," *Comptes rendus de la société de biologie,* 113 (1933), 1101–1103.

BOOKS AND JOURNAL ARTICLES APPEARING AFTER 1945

Ackerknecht, Erwin H. "Hygiene in France, 1815–1848," *Bulletin of the history of medicine,* 22 (1948), 117–55.

Adams, Mark B., ed. *The wellborn science.* New York: Oxford University Press, 1990.

——. "The eugenics record office at Cold Spring Harbor, 1910–1940. An essay in institutional history," *Osiris,* 2nd ser., 2(1986), 225–64.

Ageron, Charles-Robert. "L'immigration maghrébienne en France, un survol historique," *XXe siècle,* 7 (1985), 59–70.

Allen, Garland. "From eugenics to population control," *Science for the people,* 13 (1980), 22–28.

Ariés, Philippe. *Centuries of childhood*. London: Jonathan Cape, 1962.

Armengaud, André. "Mouvement ouvrier et néo-malthusien au debut du XXe siècle," *Annales de démographie historique*, 3 (1966), 7–21.

——. *La population française aux XIXe siècle*. Paris: PUF, 1971.

——. "L'attitude de la société à l'égard de l'enfant au XIXe siècle," *Annales de démographie* (1973), 303–12.

Aron, J.-P. "Taille, maladie et société: Essai d'histoire anthropologique." In *Anthropologie du conscrit français d'apres les comptes numériques et sommaires du recruitment (1819–1820)*. Ed. J.-P. Aron, P. Dumont, E. Leroy-Ladurie. Paris: Mouton, 1972.

Audit, Jean. *L'eugénique et l'euthénique*. Paris: J.-B. Ballière, 1953.

Baader, Gerhard. "Das 'Gesetz zur Verhütung erbkranken Nachwuchses' – Versuch einer kritische Deutung." In *Zusammenhang Festschrift für Marielene Putscher*, 865–75. Ed. Otto Baue and Otto Glanden. Cologne: Wienland, 1984.

——. "Sozialhygienische Theorie und Praxis in der Gewerbehygiene in Berlin der weimarer Zeit," *Koroth*, 8 (1985), 24–37.

Baguley, David. *Fecondité d'Emile Zola*. Toronto: University of Toronto Press, 1973.

Barrows, Susanna. "After the Commune: Alcoholism, temperance and literature in the early Third Republic." In *Consciousness and class experience in nineteenth-century Europe*, 205–18. Ed. John Merriman. New York: Holmes and Meier, 1979.

——. *Distorting mirrors: Visions of the crowd in late nineteenth-century France*. New Haven: Yale University Press, 1981.

Barzun, Jacques. *Race: A study in superstition*. 2nd ed. New York: Harper and Row, 1965.

Bejin, André. "Le sang, le sens, et le travail," *Cahiers internationaux de sociologie*, 72 (1982), 325–45.

——. "Toward the semantic history of social Darwinsim: Georges Vacher de Lapouge's theory of 'social selections,' " *Graduate faculty philosophy journal*, 9 (1983), 129–50.

Bernard, Philippe, and Henri Dubief. *The decline of the Third Republic, 1914–1938*. Cambridge, England: Cambridge University Press, 1985.

Bernard, Jean. *Le sang et l'histoire*. Paris: Buchet/Chastel, 1983.

Betts, Raymond F. *Assimilation and association in French colonial theory, 1890–1914*. New York: Columbia University Press, 1961.

Bezucha, Robert J. "The moralization of society: The enemies of popular culture in the 19th Century." In *The wolf and the lamb: Popular culture in France*, 175–87. Ed. Jacques Beauroy. Saratoga: Anima Libri, 1976.

Billig, Joseph. *L'institut d'étude des questions juives. Inventaire des archives du centre de documentation juive contemporaine*. 3 vols. Paris: Centre de documentation juive contemporaine, 1974.

——. *Le commissariat général aux questions juives, 1941–1944*. 3 vols. Paris: Centre de documentation juive contemporaine, 1955–1960.

Blacker, C. P. *Eugenics: Galton and after*. London: Duckworth, 1952.

Blanckaert, Claude. "Edmond Perrier et l'étiologie du 'polyzoisme' organique," *Revue de synthèse*, 95–96 (1979), 353–76.

——. "L'anthropologie au féminin: Clémence Royer (1830–1902)," *Revue de snythèse,* 105 (1982), 23–39.

Boesiger, Ernest. "Evolutionary biology in France at the time of the evolutionary synthesis." In *The evolutionary synthesis,* 309–20. Ed. Ernst Mayr and William Provine. Cambridge: Harvard University Press, 1982.

Boissel, Jean. "Autour du gobinisme," *Annales du CESERE,* 4 (1981), 91–120.

——. "Georges Vacher de Lapouge: Un socialiste revolutionnaire darwinien," *Nouvelle école,* 38 (1982), 59–84.

——. "A propos de l'indice céphalique," *Revue d'histoire des sciences,* 35 (1982), 289–317.

Boltanski, Luc. *Prime education et morale de classe.* Paris: Mouton, 1969.

Bonnet, Jean-Charles. *Les pouvoirs publiques français et l'immigration dans l'entre-deux-guerres.* Lyons: Centre d'histoire économique et sociale de la région lyonnaise, 1976.

Borel, Jacques. *Du concept de dégénérescence à la notion d'alcoolisme dans la médecine contemporaine.* Montpellier: Causes et Cie., 1968.

Bowler, Peter J. *The eclipse of Darwinism.* Baltimore: Johns Hopkins University Press, 1983.

——. "E. W. MacBride's Lamarckian eugenics and its implications for the social construction of scientific knowledge," *Annals of science,* 41 (1984), 245–60.

Brédin, Jean-Denis. *The affair.* New York: Geroge Braziller, 1986.

Brun, Girard. *Technocrates et technocratie en France, 1918–1945.* Paris: Editions Albatros, 1985.

Brunschwig, Henri. *French colonialism, 1871–1914, myths and realities.* London: Pall Mall Press, 1966.

Brush, Stephen G. *The temperature of history.* New York: Burt Franklin, 1978.

Buican, Denis. "La génétique classique en France devant le néo-lamarckisme tardif," *Archives internationales d'histoire des sciences,* 111 (1983), 300–24.

——. *L'Histoire de la génétique et de l'évolutionnisme en France.* Paris: PUF, 1984.

Byrnes, Robert F. "The French publishing industry and its crisis in the 1890s," *Journal of modern history,* 23 (1951), 232–44.

Caen, Marcel. "La naissance d'un mot: Puericulture," *L'hôpital et l'aide sociale,* 22 (1963), 551–52.

Cameron, Rondo. "Economic growth and stagnation in France, 1815–1914," *Journal of modern history,* 30 (1958), 1–13.

Carniol-Dreyfus, Yvonne. "Le certificat d'examen médical prénuptial," *Prophylaxie sanitaire et morale,* 26 (1954), 124–29.

Caron, François. *An economic history of modern France.* New York: Columbia University Press, 1979.

Carson, Gerald. *Cornflake crusade.* New York: Rinehart, 1957.

Carter, A. E. *The idea of decadence in French literature, 1830–1900.* Toronto: University of Toronto Press, 1958.

Chamla, M. C. "L'accroisement de la stature en France, 1880–1960," *Bulletin de la société d'anthropologie,* 11e sér. (1964), 201–78.

Chase, Allen. *The legacy of Malthus.* New York: Alfred Knopf, 1977.

Chevalier, Louis. *Labouring classes and dangerous classes.* Princeton: Princeton University Press, 1981.

Christophe, Paul. *1936: Les catholiques et le front populaire*. Paris: Desdée, 1979.

Clark, Linda L. *Social Darwinism in France*. Montgomery: University of Alabama Press, 1984.

——. *Schooling the daughters of Marianne*. Albany: SUNY Press, 1984.

Cobo, Modesto Sanemeterio. "L'Ecole d'anthropologie de Paris." Dissertation: Ecole d'anthropologie, 1975.

Cohen, William B. *The French encounter with Africans*. Bloomington: Indiana University Press, 1980.

Coleman, William. *Death is a social disease: Public health and political economy in early industrial France*. Madison: University of Wisconsin Press, 1982.

Colombat, Jean. *La fin du monde civilisé: Les prophéties de Vacher de Lapouge*. Paris: Vrin, 1946.

Conry, Yvette. *L'introduction du darwinisme en France au XIXe siècle*. Paris: Vrin, 1974.

Corbin, Alain. *Les filles de noce*. Paris: Aubier, 1978.

Corner, George W. *History of the Rockefeller Institute, 1901–1953*. New York: Rockefeller Institute Press, 1964.

Coutrot, Aline. "La politique familiale." in *Le gouvernement de Vichy, 1940–42. Colloque sur le gouvernement de Vichy et la révolution nationale*, 245–63. Paris: Armand Colin, 1972.

Couvelaire, Roger. "Epigrammes familiales et violons imaginaires." Paris: privately printed, n.d.

Crosby, Alfred W. *The Columbian exchange*. Westport, CT: Greenwood Press, 1972.

Cross, Gary S. "The politics of immigration in France during the era of World War I," *French historical studies*, 11 (1980), 610–32.

——. *Immigrant workers in industrial France*. Philadelphia: Temple University Press, 1983.

De la Haye Jousselin, Henri. *Georges Vacher de Lapouge (1854–1936). ·Essai de bibliographie*. Paris: privately printed, 1986.

A decade of progress in eugenics: Third international congress of eugenics. New York: Garland Press, 1984.

Desrosières, Alain. "Histoires de formes: Statistiques et sciences sociales avant 1940," *Revue française de sociologie*, 26 (1985), 294–97.

Dieudonnant, Pierre-Marie. *Je suis partout, 1930–44*. Paris: Table Ronde, 1973.

Digeon, Claude. *La crise allemande de la pensée française, 1870–1914*. Paris: PUF, 1959.

Donzelot, Jacques. *Policing of families*. New York: Pantheon, 1980.

Drouard, Alain. "Les trois âges de la fondation française pour l'étude des problèmes humains" *Population* 38 (1983), 1017–37.

Dumont, Martial, and Pierre Morel. *Histoire de l'obstétrique et de la gynécologie*. Lyons: SIMEP Editions, 1968.

Dupeux, Georges. "L'immigration en France de la fin du XVIIIe siècle à nos jours." In *Les migrations internationales de la fin du XVIIIe siècle à nos jours*, 161–74. Paris: Editions du CNRS, 1980.

Durkin, Joseph T. *Hope for our time: Alexis Carrel on man and society*. New York: Harper, 1965.

Dyer, Colin. *Population and society in twentieth century France.* New York: Holmes and Meier, 1978.

Elwitt, Sanford. "Social reform and social order in late nineteenth century France: The musée social and its friends," *French historical studies* 11 (1980), 431–51.

Eugenics, genetics and the family: Second international eugenics congress. 2 vols. New York: Garland Press, 1985.

Eugenics in race and state: Second international eugenics congress, 1921. New York: Garland Press, 1985.

Evans, Richard J. "Prostitution, state and society in imperial Germany," *Past and present* 7 (1976), 106–29.

Fancher, Raymond E. "Alphonse de Candolle, Francis Galton, and the early history of the nature–nurture controversy," *Journal of the history of the behavioural sciences* 19 (1983), 341–52.

Farrall, Lyndsay A. "The origins and growth of the English eugenics movement, 1862–1925," PhD dissertation, Indiana University, 1970.

———. "The history of eugenics: a bibliographic review," *Annals of science,* 36 (1979), 111–23.

Foucault, Michel. *The history of sexuality.* New York: Pantheon, 1978.

Fredenson, Patrick. "Un tournant, Taylorien de la Société française, 1900–1914," *Annales ECS,* 42(1987), 1031–60.

Freeden, Michael. "Eugenics and progressive thought: A study in ideological affinity," *Historical journal,* 22 (1979), 645–71.

———. "Eugenics and ideology," *Historical journal,* 26 (1983), 959–62.

Freeman, Gary P. *Immigrant labor and racial conflict in industrial societies: The French and British experience, 1945–1975.* Princeton: Princeton University Press, 1979.

Friedlander, Ruth. "Benedict-Augustin Morel and the development of the theory of degeneresence." PhD dissertation, University of California, 1973.

Froggatt, P. and N. C. Nevin. "Galton's law of ancestral heredity – its influence on the early history of genetics" *History of science,* 4 (1971), 1–27.

Fruhinsholz, Albert. "Adolphe Pinard, puericulteur français," *Médecine de France,* 21 (1951), 3–9.

Gani, Léon. "Jules Guesde, Paul Lafargue et les problèmes de population," *Population,* 34 (1979), 1023–43.

Ganier, Raymond. *Une certaine France; L'antisemitisme 40–44.* Paris: Ballard, 1978.

Gardner, James F. "Microbes and morality: The social hygiene crusade in New York City, 1892–1917." PhD dissertation, Indiana University, 1974.

Gillon, Jean-Jacques. "La fondation française pour l'étude des problèmes humaines." In *Science et théorie de l'opinion publique,* 257–68. Ed. R. Boudon, F. Bourricaud, and A. Giard. Paris: Retz, 1981.

Goglewski, Edmond. "Les polonais en France avant la seconde guerre mondiale," *Revue du nord,* 242 (1979), 649–62.

Goldstein, M. S. "Franz Boas, 1858–1942," *American journal of physical anthropology,* 56 (1981), 491–93.

Gordon, Linda. "The politics of population: Birth control and the eugenics movement," *Radical America,* 8 (1974), 61–97.

Gould, Stephen Jay. *The mismeasure of man.* New York: W. W. Norton, 1981.

Graham, Loren R. "Science and values: The eugenics movement in Germany and Russia in the 1920s," *American historical review,* 82 (1977), 1133–64.

———. *Between science and values*. New York: Columbia University Press, 1981.

Grasset, Raymond. *Au service de la médecine. Chronique de la santé publique durant les saisons amères (1942–1944)*. Clermont-Ferrand: G. de Bussac, 1956.

Grether, Judith K. "Sterilization and eugenics: An examination of early twentieth century population control," PhD dissertation, University of Oregon, 1980.

Guillaume, Pierre. "Du bon usage des immigrés en temps de crise et de güerre, 1932–1940," *XXe siècle*, 7 (1985), 117–25.

Haley, Bruce. *The healthy body and Victorian culture*. Cambridge: Harvard University Press, 1978.

Haller, Mark H. *Eugenics: Hereditarian attitudes in American thought*. New Brunswick: Rutgers University Press, 1963.

Hansen, Eric C. *Disaffection and decadence: A crisis in French intellectual thought, 1848–1898*. Washington, DC: University Press of America, 1982.

Harvey, Joy. "Evolution transformed: Positivists and materialists in the société d'anthropologie de Paris from the Second Empire to Third Republic." In *The wider domain of evolutionary thought*, 289–310. Ed. D. Oldroyd and I. Langham. D. Reidel, 1982.

———. "Races specified, evolution transformed." PhD dissertation, Harvard University, 1983.

Hayward, J. E. S. "Solidarity: The social history of an idea in nineteenth century France," *International review of social history*, 4 (1959), 261–84.

———. "The official social philosophy of the French Third Republic: Léon Bourgeois," *International review of social history*, 6 (1961), 19–48.

Herzog, William. *From Dreyfus to Petain*. New York: Octagon Books, 1976.

Hildreth, Martha Lee. *Doctors, bureaucrats and public health in France, 1888–1902*. New York: Garland Press, 1986.

Hirschfeld, Jan. "The birth of serology and the discovery of the human ABO system," *Nordisk medicinhistorisk arsbok* (1977), 163–80.

Hirszfeld, Ludwig. "The story of one life." Unpublished translation by F. R. Camp and F. R. Ellis of *Historia jednego zygia*, 2nd ed. Warsaw: Institut Wydawnicszny, 1967.

Holt, Richard. *Sport and society in modern France*. Hamden, CT: Archon Books, 1981.

Humbert, Jeanne. "Deux grandes figures du mouvement pacifiste et néo-malthusien: Eugène Humbert, Sebastian Faure," *La voix de la paix* (1970), 3–11.

———. "Gabriel Giroud," *Grande reforme* (1946).

Huss, Marie-Monique. "Pro-natalism in the interwar period in France: An elite or a popular preoccupation?" London: unpublished manuscript, 1984.

Hutchinson, E. P. *Legislative history of American immigration policy, 1798–1965*. Philadelphia: University of Pennsylvania Press, 1981.

Hyman, Paula. *From Dreyfus to Vichy: The remaking of French Jewry, 1906–1939*. New York: Columbia University Press, 1979.

Jackson, Julian. *The politics of depression in France, 1932–1936*. Cambridge, England: Cambridge University Press, 1985.

Jacob, François. *The logic of life*. New York: Random House, 1982.

Jacquard, Albert, ed. *Génétique et population: Hommage à Jean Sutter*. Paris: PUF, 1971.

Jacquemet, Gerard. "Médecine et 'maladies populaires' dans le Paris de la fin du

XIXe siècle." In *L'haleine des faubourgs*, 349–64. Ed. Lion Murard and Patrick Zylberman. Fontenay-sur-bois: Recherche, 1978.

Jones, Gareth Stedman. *Outcast London*. Oxford: Clarendon Press, 1971.

Jones, Greta. "Eugenics and social policy between the wars," *Historical journal*, 25 (1982), 717–28.

Joseph, Laurence A. *Henri Cazalis: Sa vie, son oeuvre, son amitié avec Mallarmé*. Paris: A.-G. Nizet, 1972.

Juri, Marilisa. *Charles Richet, physiologiste, 1850–1935*. Zurich: Juris Drück, 1965.

Kevles, Daniel J. *In the name of Eugenics*. New York: Knopf, 1985.

Kienreich, Werner. "Die Wiener Gesellschaft für Rassenpflege im Lichte ihrer 'Nachrichten,' " *Psychologie und Gesellschaftskritik*, 3 (1979), 61–73.

Kindleberger, Charles. *Economic growth in France and Britain, 1851–1950*. Cambridge: Harvard University Press, 1964.

Kriskis, Martine. "L'antisemitisme de droite en France à l'époque de la nuit de cristal à travers les journaux politico-littéraires et la littérature antisemite." Master's thesis, University of Paris, 1972–73.

La Berge, Ann F. "Public health in France and the French public health movement, 1815–48." PhD dissertation, University of Tennessee, 1974.

Lalouette, Jacqueline. "Le discours bourgeois sur les 'debits de boissons' aux alentours de 1900." In *L'haleine des faubourgs*, 315–48. Ed. Lion Murard and Patrick Zylberman. Fontenay-sur-bois: Recherche, 1978.

Landes, David. "French entrepreneurship and industrial growth in the nineteenth century," *Journal of economic history*, 9 (1949), 45–61.

Latour, Bruno. *Les microbes. Guerre et paix*. Paris: A. M. Metailié, 1984.

Ledbetter, Roseanne. *A history of the Malthusian league*. Columbus: Ohio University Press, 1976.

Ledermann, Sully. *Alcool, alcoolisme, alcoolisation*. 2 vols. Paris: PUF, 1956–64.

Léonard, Jacques. *La vie quotidienne du médecin de province au 19e siècle*. Paris: Hachette, 1977.

——. *France médicale: Médecins et malades au XIXe siècle*. Paris: Gallimard, 1978.

——. *La médecine entre les savoirs et les pouvoirs: Histoire intellectuelle et politique de la médecine française au XIXe siècle*. Paris: Aubier Montaigne, 1981.

——. "Eugénisme et darwinisme." In *De Darwin au darwinisme: Science et idéologie*, 187–207. Ed. Yvette Conry. Paris: J. Vrin, 1983.

——. "Le premier congrès international d'eugénique et ses consequences françaises," *Histoire des sciences médicales*, 17 (1983), 141–46.

Lepine, P. "Nécrologie: Nicholas Kossovitch, 1864–1948," *Annales de l'institut Pasteur*, 75 (1948), 62.

Lewis, Martin Deming. "One hundred million Frenchmen: The 'assimilation' theory in French colonial policy," *Comparative studies in society and history*, 4 (1962), 129–53.

Lilienthal, Georg. "Rassenhygiene im Dritten Reich: Krise und Wende," *Medizinhistorische Journal*, 14 (1979), 114–34.

——. *Der Lebensborn*. Stuttgart: G. Fischer, 1985.

Limoges, Camille. "Natural selection, phagocytosis and preadaptation, Lucien Cuénot, 1886–1901," *Journal of the history of medicine*, 31 (1976), 176–214.

——. "A second glance at evolutionary biology in France." In *The evolutionary synthesis*, 309–21. Ed. Ernst Mayr and William Provine. Cambridge: Harvard University Press, 1982.

Lindbergh, Charles A. *Autobiography of values*. New York: Harcourt Brace, 1976.

Ludmerer, Kenneth M. *Genetics and American society*. Baltimore: Johns Hopkins University Press, 1972.

MacAloon, John J. *The great symbol: Pierre de Coubertin and the origin of the modern Olympic games*. Chicago: University of Chicago Press, 1981.

MacFadyen, Dugald. *Sir Ebenezer Howard and the town planning movement*. Manchester: Manchester University Press, 1970.

Maga, Timothy P. "Closing the door: The French government and refugee policy, 1933–39," *French historical studies* 12 (1982), 424–42.

Malinas, Yves. "Zola, precurseur de la pensée scientifique du XXe siècle," *Cahiers naturaliste*, 16 (1970), 108–20.

——. "Zola et les hérédités imaginaires," *Ouest médicale*, 24 (1971), 549–59, 1105–09, 1323–37, 1403–10, 1477–83, 1615–21, 1785–90, 1937–46, 2106–16.

——. *Zola et les hérédités imaginaires*. Paris: Expansion scientifique française, 1985.

Mande, Raymond. "A propos d'une enquête pour le recensement des enfants anormaux." *Cahiers de la fondation française pour l'étude des problèmes humaines*, 4 (1945), 84–94.

Mandell, Richard D. *Paris 1900*. Toronto: University of Toronto Press, 1967.

Marin, Louis. "Les études portant sur l'homme et l'ecole d'anthropologie de 1926 à 1956," *Revue anthropologique*, n.s. 2 (1956), 169–79.

Marrus, Michael R. *The politics of assimilation*. New York: Oxford University Press, 1971.

——. "Social drinking in the belle epoque," *Journal of social history*, 7 (1974), 115–41.

Marrus, Michael R., and Robert Paxton. *Vichy France and the Jews*. New York: Basic Books, 1981.

Martindale, Colin. "Degeneration, disinhibition, and genius," *Journal of the history of the behavioral sciences*, 8 (1972), 177–82.

Martino, P. *Le naturalisme français*. Paris: Armand Colin, 1965.

Mavit, Henri. "Education physique et sport," *Revue d'histoire de la deuxième guerre mondiale*, 14 (1964), 89–104.

Mayr, Ernst. "The arrival of neo-Darwinism in France." In *The evolutionary synthesis*, 321–28. Ed. Mayr and William B. Provine. Cambridge: Harvard University Press, 1980.

——. *The growth of biological thought*. Cambridge, MA: Belknap Press, 1982.

McDougall, Mary Lynn. "Protecting infants: The French campaign for maternity leaves, 1890–1913," *French historical studies*, 13 (1983), 79–105.

McLaren, Angus. "Revolution and education in the late nineteenth century: The early career of Paul Robin," *History of education quarterly*, 21 (1981), 317–35.

——. *Sexuality and social order*. New York: Holmes and Meier, 1983.

Medvedev, Zhores A. *The rise and fall of T. D. Lysenko*. New York: Praeger, 1969.

Mehler, Barry. "A history of the American Eugenics Society, 1921–1940." PhD dissertation, University of Illinois, 1988.

Milza, Olivier. "La gauche, la crise et l'immigration (années 1930–années 1980)," *XXe siècle*, 7 (1985), 127–40.

Mitchell, Allan. *German influences in France after 1870.* Chapel Hill: University of North Carolina Press, 1979.

———. *Victors and vanquished.* Chapel Hill: University of North Carolina Press, 1984.

Montagu, Ashley. "Some anthropological terms: A study in the systematics of confusion," *American anthropologist*, 47 (1945) 119–33.

———. "On the phrase 'ethnic group' in anthropology," *Psychiatry*, 8 (1945), 27–33.

———. *Man's most dangerous myth*, 5th ed. New York: Oxford University Press, 1974.

———, ed. *Frontiers of anthropology.* New York: G. P. Putnam's Sons, 1974.

Mortimer, Edward. *The rise of the French Communist Party, 1920–1947.* London: Faber and Faber, 1984.

Moseley, Leonard. *Lindbergh: A biography.* New York: Doubleday, 1976.

Mourant, A. E., Ada C. Kopec, and Kazamiera Domaniewska-Sobczak. *The distribution of human blood groups and other polymorphisms*, 2nd ed. New York: Oxford University Press, 1976.

Murard, Lion, and Patrick Zylberman. *Petit travailleur indefatigable.* Paris: Recherches, 1976.

———. "La cité eugénique," in *L'haleine des faubourgs*, 423–53. Ed. Murard and Zylberman Fontenay-sur-bois: Recherches, 1977.

———. "De l'hygiène comme introduction à la politique expérimentale (1875–1925)", *Revue de synthèse*, 3e sér., 115 (1984), 313–41.

———. "La raison de l'expert ou l'hygiène comme science sociale appliquée," *Archives européenes de sociologie*, 26 (1985), 58–59.

———. "L'autre guerre (1914–18): France sous l'oeil d'Amérique," *Revue d'histoire*, 276 (1986), 367–98.

———. "La mission Rockefeller en France et la création du comité national de defense contre la tuberculose (1917–23)," *Revue d'histoire moderne et contemporaine*, 34 (1987), 257–81.

Nagel, Gunter. *Georges Vacher de Lapouge: Ein Beitrag zur Geschichte des Sozialdarwinismus in Frankreich.* Freiburg: H. F. Verlag, 1975.

Nerson, Roger. "Les progrès scientifiques et l'evolution du droit familial." In *Le droit privé au milieu du XXe siècle*, 1:403–31. Paris: Librairie générale de droit, 1950.

———. "L'influence de la biologie et de la médecine sur le droit civil," *Revue trimistrielle de droit civil*, 68 (1970), 661–83.

Noakes, Jeremy. "Nazism and eugenics: The background to the Nazi sterilization law of 14 July 1933." In *Ideas into politics*, 75–94. Ed. Roger J. Bullen et al. London: Croom Helm, 1984.

Nogueres, Henri. *Histoire de la résistance en France*, 5 vols. Paris: Robert Laffont, 1976.

Noonan, John T. *Contraception.* Cambridge: Harvard University Press, 1965.

Nowak, Kurt. *"Euthanasie" und Sterilisierung im Dritten Reich.* Göttingen: Vandenhoeck Ruprecht, 1984.

Nye, Robert A. "Heredity or milieu: The foundation of modern European criminological theory," *Isis*, 67 (1976), 335–55.

———. "Degeneration, neurasthenia and the culture of sport in belle epoque France," *Journal of contemporary history*, 17 (1982), 51–68.
———. *Crime, madness, and society in modern France*. Princeton: Princeton University Press, 1984.
Offen, Karen. "Depopulation, natalism and feminism," *American historical review*, 89 (1984), 653–71.
Ogden, P. E., and Marie-Monique Huss. "Demography and pronatalism in France in the 19th and 20th centuries," *Journal of historical geography*, 8 (1982), 283–98.
Ory, Pascal. *Les collaborateurs, 1940–45*. Paris: Editions du Seuil, 1976.
Patai, Raphael, and Jennifer Patai Wing. *The myth of the Jewish race*. New York: Scribner's, 1975.
Paul, Harry. *The sorcerer's apprentice: The French scientists' image of German science, 1840–1919*. Gainesville: University of Florida Press, 1972.
Paxton, Robert. *Vichy France*. New York: Norton, 1972.
Perrot, Michelle. *Les grèves en France, 1870–1890*, 2 vols. Paris: Mouton, 1974.
Poliakov, Leon. *The Aryan myth*. New York: New American Library, 1977.
Prestwich, P. E. "French workers and the temperance movement," *International review of social history*, 25 (1980), 35–52.
Rabinbach, Anson. "The body without fatigue: A nineteenth-century utopia." In *Political symbolism in modern Europe*, 46–62. Ed. Seymour Drescher et al. New Brunswick: Transaction, 1982.
Reed, James. *From private vice to public virtue: The American birth control movement and American society since 1830*. New York: Basic Books, 1978.
Reid, Donald. *The miners of Decazeville*. Cambridge: Harvard University Press, 1983.
Reynolds, Sian. "Who wanted the crèches? Working mothers and the birth rate in France, 1900–1950." Unpublished manuscript: Oxford, n.d.
Roger, Jacques, ed. "Les néo-lamarckiens français," *Revue de synthèse*, 95–96 (1979), 279–468.
Roll-Hansen, Niels. "Eugenics before World War II. The case of Norway," *History and philosophy of the life sciences*, 2 (1981), 269–98.
Romerein, Jan Marius. *The watershed of two eras: Europe in 1900*. Middletown, CT: Wesleyan University Press, 1978.
Ronsin, Frances. "Liberté – natalité. Reaction et répression anti-malthusiennes avant 1920." In *Haleine des faubourgs*, 365–93. Ed. Lion Murard and Patrick Zylberman. Fontenay-sur-bois: Recherche, 1978.
———. *La grève des ventres*. Paris: Aubier, 1980.
Rosenberg, Charles. "Charles Benedict Davenport and the beginning of human genetics," *Bulletin of the history of medicine*, 35 (1961), 266–76.
———. *Trial of the assasin Guiteau*. Chicago: University of Chicago Press, 1968.
———. "The bitter fruit: Heredity, disease and social thought in nineteenth century America," *Perspectives in American history*, 8 (1974), 189–235.
Ross, Walter S. *The last hero: Charles A. Lindbergh*. New York: Harper and Row, 1964.
Rostand, Jean. "Zola: homme de verité," *Cahiers des naturalistes*, 3 (1957), 361–66.
———. *Biologie et humanisme*. Paris: Gallimard, 1964.

Roussy, Gustave. "Charles Richet (1850–1935)," *Bulletin de l'académie de médecine*, 129 (1945), 725–31.

Sauvy, Alfred. *De Paul Reynaud à Charles de Gaulle*. Paris: Casterman, 1972.

Savatier, René. *Les métamorphoses économiques et sociales du droit privé d'aujourd'hui*. Paris: Dalloz, 1952.

———. "Etude juridique [d'examen prénuptial]," *Cahiers laennec*, 17 (1957), 10–20.

Schaffer, Daniel. *Garden cities for America*. Philadelphia: Temple University Press, 1982.

Schiller, Francis. *Paul Broca: Founder of French anthropology, Explorer of the brain*. Berkeley: University of California Press, 1979.

Schneider, William H. "Colonies at the 1900 world's fair," *History today*, 31 (1981), 31–36.

———. *An empire for the masses: The French popular image of Africa, 1870–1900*. Westport, CT: Greenwood Press, 1982.

———. "Towards the improvement of the human race: The history of eugenics in France," *Journal of modern history*, 54 (1982), 268–91.

———. "Chance and social setting in the application of the discovery of blood groups," *Bulletin of the history of medicine*, 57 (1983), 545–62.

———. "Henri Laugier, The science of work and the workings of science in France, 1920–1940," *Cahiers pour l'histoire du CNRS*, 5(1989), 7–34.

Schreiber, Georges. "La nouvelle réglementation du certificat médical prénuptial," *Presse médicale*, 54 (1946), 194.

Schwartz, Richard W. *John Harvey Kellogg, MD*. Nashville: Southern Publications, 1970.

Scott, John A. *Republican ideas and the liberal tradition in France, 1870–1914*. New York: Columbia University Press, 1951.

Searle, Geoffrey R. *Eugenics and politics in Britain, 1900–1914*. Noordhoff: International Publishing, 1976.

———. "Eugenics and politics in Britain in the 1930s," *Annals of science*, 36 (1979), 159–69.

Seeman, Bernard. *The river of life*. New York: Norton, 1961.

Shapiro, Ann-Louise. "Private rights, public interest and professional jurisdiction: The French public health law of 1902," *Bulletin of the history of medicine*, 54 (1980), 4–22.

Shorter, Edward, and Charles Tilly. *Strikes in France 1830–1968*. New York: Cambridge University Press, 1974.

Sicard de Plauzoles, Just. "L'eugénisme français," *Prophylaxie antivénérienne*, 17 (1945), 527–33.

———. "Prophylaxie du crime par l'eugénique et la puericulture," *Prophylaxie sanitaire et morale*, 28 (1956), 82–89.

Soloway Richard A. "Neo-Malthusians, eugenists, and the declining birthrate in England, 1900–1918," *Albion*, 10 (1978), 264–86.

———. "Counting the degenerates: The statistics of race degeneration in Edwardian England," *Journal of contemporary history*, 17 (1982), 137–64.

———. *Birth control and the population question in England, 1877–1930*. Chapel Hill: University of North Carolina Press, 1982.

Sorlin, Pierre. *'La croix' et les juifs*. Paris: Grasset, 1967.

Soucy, Robert. *Fascist intellectual, Drieu LaRochelle*. Berkeley: University of California Press, 1977.

Soupault, Robert. *Alexis Carrel, 1873–1944*. Paris: Plon, 1951.

Spengler, John Joseph. *France faces depopulation: Postlude edition, 1936–1976*. Durham, NC: Duke University Press, 1979.

Stebbin, Robert E. "France." In *The comparative reception of Darwin*, 139–44. Ed. Thomas Glick. Austin: University of Texas Press, 1974.

Stengers, Jean. "Les pratiques anti-conceptionnelles dans le mariage aux XIXe et au XXe siècle," *Revue belge de philologie et d'histoire*, 49 (1971), 1119–74.

Stepan, Nancy. *The idea of race in science*. London: Macmillan, 1982.

Sternhell, Zev. *La droite revolutionnaire, 1885–1941: Les origines françaises du fascisme*. Paris: Editions du Séuil, 1978.

Sulleron, Claude. "La littérature au XIXe siècle et la famille." In *Renouveau des idées sur la famille*, 60–80. Ed. Robert Prigent. Paris: PUF, 1954.

Sussman, George. *Selling mother's milk*. Champaign-Urbana: University of Illinois Press, 1982.

Sutcliffe, Anthony. *Towards the planned city: Germany, Britain, the United States and France, 1780–1914*. New York: St. Martins, 1981.

Sutter, Jean. "Le facteur 'qualité' en démographie," *Population*, 2 (1946), 299–315.

———. "Problèmes sanitaires posés par l'immigration." In *Documents sur l'immigration*, 197–222. Paris: PUF, 1947.

———. "Les avortements legaux eugéniques en Suède, en Danemark, en Suisse," *Population*, 3 (1947) 575–79.

———. *Eugénique*. Paris: PUF, 1950.

———. "L'evolution de la taille des polytechniciens (1801–1954)," *Population*, 13 (1958), 373–406.

Suzuki, Zenji. "Genetics and the eugenics movement in Japan," *Japanese studies in the history of science*, 14 (1975), 157–64.

Swart, Koenraad W. *The sense of decadence in nineteenth century France*. The Hague: Martinus Nijhoff, 1964.

Swinburne, R. G. "Galton's law – formulation and development," *Annals of science*, 21 (1965), 15–31.

Taguieff, Pierre-André, ed. *G. Vacher de Lapouge et l'anthroposociologie en France*. Paris: Editions du CNRS, in press.

Talmy, Robert. *Histoire du mouvement familiale en France, 1896–1939*, 2 vols. Paris: Union nationale des caisses des allocutions familiales, 1962.

Thébaud, Françoise. "Le mouvement nataliste dans la France de l'entre-deux-guerres: L'alliance nationale pour l'accroisement de la population française," *Revue d'histoire moderne et contemporaine*, 32 (1985), 276–301.

Thomann, K. D. "Otmar von Verscheurer – ein Hauptvertreter der faschistischen Rassenhygiene." In *Medizin im Faschismus*, 36–52. Ed. A. Thom and H. Spaar. Berlin: VEB Verlag Volk und Gesundheit, 1983.

Thompson, Larry V. " 'Lebensborn' and the eugenic policy of the 'Reichsführer-SS'," *Central European history*, 4 (1971), 54–77.

Thorez, Maurice. *Oeuvres*, 16 vols. Paris: Editions sociales, 1952.

Thullier, Guy. "Un anarchiste positiviste: Georges Vacher de Lapouge." In *L'idée de race dans la pensée politique française contemporaine,* 48–65. Ed. Pierre Guiral and Emile Temine. Paris: Editions du CNRS, 1977.

Tucker, William R. *The fascist ego: A political biography of Robert Brasillach.* Berkeley: University of California Press, 1975.

Tutzke, Dieter. *Alfred Grotjahn.* Leipzig: G. Teubner, 1979.

Valabregue, Catherine. *Contrôle des naissances et planning familial.* Paris: Table Ronde, 1960.

Walter, Richard D. "What became of the degenerate? A brief history of a concept," *Journal of the history of medicine,* 11 (1956), 422–29.

Weber, Eugen. *The nationalistic revival in France, 1905–1914.* Berkeley: University of California, 1959.

——. "Gymnastics and sport in *fin-de-siècle* France: Opium of the classes?" *American historical review,* 76 (1971), 70–98.

——. *France fin-de-siècle.* Cambridge: Harvard University Press, 1986.

Weindling, Paul. "Theories of the cell state in imperial Germany." In *Biology, medicine and society, 1840–1940,* 99–155. Ed. Charles Webster. Cambridge, England: Cambridge University Press, 1981.

——. "Die preussische Medizinalverwaltung und die 'Rassenhygiene,'" *Zeitschrift für Sozialreform,* 29 (1984), 675–87.

——. "Weimar eugenics: The Kaiser Wilhelm Institute for Anthropology, Human heredity and eugenics in social context," *Annals of science,* 42 (1985), 303–18.

——. *Health, race and German politics between national unification and Nazism, 1870–1945.* Cambridge, England: Cambridge University Press, 1989.

Weingart, Peter. "The rationalization of human behavior: The institutionalization of eugenic thought in Germany," *Journal of the history of biology,* 20 (1987), 159–93.

Weisz, George. "Reform and conflict in French medical education, 1870–1914." In *The organization of science and technology in France, 1808–1914,* 61–94. Ed. George Fox and George Weisz. Cambridge, England: Cambridge University Press, 1980.

Williams, Roger L. *The mortal Napoleon III.* Princeton: Princeton University Press, 1971.

Williams, Elizabeth. "The science of man: Anthropological thought and institutions in nineteenth-century France." PhD dissertation, Indiana University, 1983.

Winter, J. M. "The fear of population decline in western Europe, 1870–1940," in *Demographic patterns in developed societies,* 173–97. Ed. P. W. Hiorns. London: Taylor and Francis, 1980.

Wormser, Olivier. *Les origines doctrinales de la révolution nationale.* Paris: Plon, 1971.

Zeldin, Theodore. *France 1848–1945.* 2 vols. New York: Oxford University Press, 1973–1977.

Index

Third Republic, The, 14, 23, 29, 61,
207
and neo-Lamarckism, 73
Thorez, Maurice, 201–2, 204–6. *See
also* French Communist Party
Toulouse, Edouard, 45, 182–84
Traits, blending of inherited, 5. *See
also* Heredity
Tuberculosis, 132, 133
and blood type, 225
campaigns against, 49–50, 120–21,
135–36
as cause of degeneration, 22–23
Turpin, Raymond, 265–66, 286

Ungemach Gardens, 124–28
Ungemach, Leon, 124
Union française pour la defense de la
race (UFDR), 262

Vaillant-Couturier, Paul, 202–4. *See
also* French Communist Party
Valery, Paul, 264
Vallat, Xavier, 258
Vallois, Henri, 224
Venereal disease
action against, 50–53, 120
as cause of degeneration, 22
and premarital examination law,
270–71
and syphilis, 52, 132, 133, 164, 205
and war, 265
Verscheurer, Otmar von, 1, 257
Verzar, Frigyes, 223

Vichy regime, 10
family and health policies, 28, 207,
266–71
and premarital examination law,
147, 154, 172
and racism, 238
Vienne, Marie Bequet de, 67
Vignes, Henri, 153, 188, 257
Villermé, Louis, 18
Vincent, George, 141
Vincent, Paul, 289–90

Wallich, Victor, 64, 69
War
First World, 27, 102–3, 114–22,
222, 284
Second World, 256
Weil, Pierre-Emile, 224
Weil-Hallé, Benjamin, 122, 321n26
Weismann, August, 73, 323n52
Weszeczky, Oskar, 223
Wilhelm II (Kaiser), 209
Williams, Linsly R., 140
Worms, René, 59, 62, 86

Ybarnegaray, Jean, 268

Zola, Emile, 182, 299n24, 305n99
depiction of heredity, 71–72
ideas of degeneration of, 17
and regeneration, 28, 41
Au Bonheur des Dames, 17
Four Gospels, 28, 41
Germinal, 17
J'Accuse, 184
L'Assomoir, 17

Printed in the United States
By Bookmasters